Dissolving wedlock

The divorce rate has been rising throughout the twentieth century, with a significant increase since 1971, so that now some 45 per cent of marriages will end in divorce. How and why has this happened? How has the law and the state changed to accommodate and facilitate this and what changes in society's attitudes have affected family breakdowns? To answer these important questions Colin Gibson takes an interdisciplinary approach to examine the history, demography, sociology, politics and policy of divorce.

The first half of *Dissolving Wedlock* traces the interaction between social change, marriage patterns, family law and parliamentary legislation from the eighteenth century to the present. The second half looks at family patterns and policy choices and examines such matters as the welfare and financial support of children and their carers in the light of the new Child Support Act, and the two-tier court system for handling the casualties of broken marriages.

Dissolving Wedlock will be invaluable reading to all lecturers and students of social policy, sociology and social work as well as to professionals and lawyers working in the field of divorce.

Colin Gibson is Lecturer in Sociology at Royal Holloway College, University of London.

D1381953

Dissolving wedlock

Colin S. Gibson

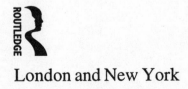

London and New York

First published in 1994
by Routledge
11 New Fetter Lane, London EC4P 4EE

Simultaneously published in the USA and Canada
by Routledge
29 West 35th Street, New York, NY 10001

© 1994 Colin S. Gibson

Typeset in Times by
LaserScript Limited, Mitcham, Surrey
Printed and bound in Great Britain by
Mackays of Chatham PLC, Chatham, Kent

British Library Cataloguing in Publication Data

A catalogue record for this book is available from the British Library.

Library of Congress Cataloging in Publication Data

Gibson, Colin, 1937–
    Dissolving wedlock/Colin Gibson.
    p.   cm.
    Includes bibliographical references and index.
    1. Divorce–England–History. 2. Divorce–Wales–History.
    3. Marriage–England–History. 4. Marriage–Wales–History.
    5. Marriage law–England. 6. Marriage law–Wales.
    I. Title.
    HQ876.G6 1994
    306.89'0942–dc20
                                                    93–7386
                                                       CIP
ISBN 0–415–03225–3
       0–415–03226–1 (pbk)

To Yvonne

Contents

Tables

Preface

This book is essentially a socio-legal study of marriage breakdown in England and Wales over the last three centuries. The contents affirm the interdisciplinary method of investigation. With such an analytical approach the sociologist risks vacating the protective academic boundary of a recognized discipline. None the less, a persuasive tapestry illuminating how and why the various socio-legal facets of marriage breakdown have come to be necessitates interweaving the historical, demographic, sociological, legal, political and policy threads of continuity and change.

Use has been made of my doctorate submission in 1972 to London University. The thesis was supervised by Professor (now Lord) McGregor, and I gratefully acknowledge his influence. Earlier academic years were happily spent in the stimulating company of Lord McGregor of Durris within the Legal Research Unit, London University; and the Centre for Socio-Legal Studies, Oxford University. Apprenticeship brought awareness of the importance of understanding the past in explaining the present, and I hope some element of this conviction emerges in the book.

Thanks are due to those who undertook the typing. Mrs Judy Gerling efficiently typed the first six chapters. Mrs Joyce Acher remains a loyal friend who transformed the residue of the remaining script into publishable form. Both generously requested remuneration should be made to their favoured charities. Ms Belinda Davis, Mrs Lynda Hussey, Mrs Elizabeth Pinn and Mrs Sheila Sweet have all helped towards the final text.

The work has taken too much commitment and time for the well-being of my marriage. The understanding and cheerful encouragement of Yvonne has helped the book along, as have her suggestions on earlier drafts. Warning messages began to appear: Carol Clewlow's novel *A Woman's Guide to Adultery* on my pillow, a Christmas present voucher for a hot air balloon trip. The restorative is completion.

Introduction

This century has seen all citizens obtain the right to elect their government. A democratic state should be aware of the impact of its laws and legal structure, and be sensitive to their improvement. Legislative perception relies upon awareness of both the nation's social condition and the links between law and structure.

The book's interactive central themes are first, the factors that have led to the current law and procedure governing marriage breakdown, and second, the social consequences of the law in action. Within this pattern our legal institutions and lawmakers have generally provided a series of *ad hoc* responses to impelling human wants and pressures rather than internally initiate reform. The last two centuries have witnessed the social and occupational structure of England and Wales (henceforth England for brevity) metamorphose from a rural society to a sixfold populated urban industrial state. This transformation has remoulded family patterns and individual expectations. These changing personal attitudes, values and habits have been the catalyst motivating matrimonial law reform.

The constituent major concepts continuously emerging within the evolving social fabric of this study are the family (nuclear, reconstituted, extra-marital and lone-parent), morality, secularization, gender, social class and family breakdown. There are many forms of family but this work largely focuses on the nuclear – or conjugal – family. Such a modern household generally consists of a married couple and their children. Yet this uniform picture is increasingly being refuted by the growing prevalence of lone-parent families and extra-marital cohabitation. Lone-parent families are commonly the product of marital breakdown; in earlier times – as Chapters 4 and 8 record – death more readily shattered the family.

The second half of the book examines some of the realities and choices for a society where divorce is experienced by one in three spouses. Divorce has become progressively easier; it is now the privately accepted and publicly approved remedy for irretrievably broken marriages. The final chapter argues that the decline of the national corporate identity together with the joint advance of consumer freedom of choice and individualism are the underlying structural facets behind the rising divorce rate. These changes have become associated with heightened personal expectation and demand for marital happiness. A glance into likely future trends suggests lifelong marriage will no longer be the central institutional underpin of the twenty-first-century family as it had been in 1950.

Unhappy spouses have divorce by consent through a procedure which is cheap, accessible, quick and offering minimal judicial interference. Judges have digested and approved the Law Commission's 1966 (par. 15) philosophy that an objective of a good divorce law was 'to enable the empty legal shell (of an irretrievably broken marriage) to be destroyed with the maximum fairness, and the minimum bitterness, distress and humiliation'. Chapter 11 reports the legal evidence of twenty-five years on. Three-quarters of the 153,000 decrees granted in 1990 were still obtained on the accusatorial 'facts' of fault. All this occurs against a background in which only a minute number of spouses attempt to deny or defend in court the alleged breakdown. Dissolution has become the petitioner's assured outcome.

A fundamental change in the official approach is reflected in the trans-formation of the divorce process from a High Court judicial trial in 1967 to become by 1977 an administrative process known as special procedure. Annually filed petitioners had surged fourfold in seventeen years: from 32,000 in 1961 to 170,000 in 1977, the year when special procedure finally became the general procedure. The weight of demand overwhelmed the ritualistic courtroom adjudicative framework. The legal processing of private matrimonial troubles was radically, rapidly and silently recast into a low-cost paper exercise no longer requiring the court attendance of either the spouses or their lawyers. A measure of the radical shift in public attitude is obtained by comparing current practice with the belief of the last Royal Commission on Marriage and Divorce. They reported in 1956 that the proper buttressing of marriage and family life required that petitioners should come before the authority and presence of a High Court judge. Now we have postal divorce. The standard procedure as it operated in Court Three of Somerset House on the morning of 23 April 1992 was documented by the national newspapers. Judge Angel took four minutes to pronounce thirty decree nisis – the first of which formally ended the marriage of Princess Anne and Captain Phillips. The clerk gave proper dignity to the proceedings, reading the Princess's full name, title and honours; meanwhile the petitioner was carrying out royal engagements in Hampshire. All citizens, be they patricians or plebeians, are swept quickly and invisibly through the common process of dissolution. The state's direct and visual regulatory capacity has all but disappeared.

Divorce is causing an increasing number of mothers and children to encounter the financially insecure world of lone-parent families. The English experience has been that over the decade 1980–9 a million and a half children under the age of sixteen witnessed the dissolution of their parents' marriage. A third are below (for 1989) the age of five. How effectively the law protects the future welfare and economic condition of lone parents and children is the concern of Chapter 12. Though divorce removes the direct legal bonds of the marriage it does not dissolve the discord that often continues on through maintenance and child-contact disputes. The issue of maintenance remains at the centre of the parental obligation debate, though it has long ceased to be a major source of financial support for lone-parent families. Today, maintenance payments form less than 10 per cent of a lone parent's income. In essence it is the presence of social security which actually underwrites the financial subsistence the courts have pledged. The existence of income support blankets the fiction that maintains the average male wage earner can support two households. As a result a father's legal obligation to maintain his dependants, and the moral duty of the community to provide welfare and social security benefits for needy and disadvantaged citizens are covered by three overlapping systems of law: dissolution in the divorce courts, the matrimonial jurisdiction offered by magistrates, and social security law under the Department of Social Security. Into this tripartite frame has recently been added a fourth figure. The escalating outflow of public expenditure upon lone-parent families galvanized Parliament into placing trust in the regulatory powers of the newly formed Child Support Agency. From April 1993 the Agency began to enforce paternal support obligations. Many divorced men utilize their freedom to marry again and thereby take on further obligations and responsibilities. The question of who should support lone mothers and dependent children highlights the general conflict between individual freedom and responsibility in an open society and state interference and control. This interaction between private troubles and public issues is a recurring theme of the book. Chapter 13 analyses some of the related problems.

Such discussions need to be set against our knowledge of family life and habit, and this evidence forms the consideration of marriage patterns in the twentieth century which constitutes Part III. Only a combination of statistical ignorance, historical incomprehension and legal disregard could set the 600 divorce petitions of 1900 against some 192,000 petitions of 1990 as evidence of Victorian family permanency. Chapter 8 presents the major demographic and social patterns, and examines changes within the modern family. For instance, increasing extra-marital cohabitation over the last two decades refutes Parliament's legislative expectation of greater marriage conformity following the divorce reforms of 1969. The propensity of lower-income marriage to record above average levels of breakdown creates an important element within the social form of divorce recorded in Chapter 9. The pattern of high divorce rates and low income has direct relevance to the legal and social policy issues concerning maintenance and family support. The majority of divorcing men and women form further relationships with new partners. Why such reconstituted families present special characteristics becomes the contents of Chapter 10.

The first half of the work traces from the Reformation to the present day the link between family law, marriage patterns and Parliamentary legislation. It sets out the main markers in the interaction between social change and the law which have led to the present legal structure for resolving marital breakdown in England and Wales.

Legal regulation of marriage breakdown since the eighteenth century features the inequality of access to divorce between both rich and poor and husband and wife. This work gives discriminative treatment to the changing legal status, social position and attitudes of women. As Mrs Hartley (1913: 356) recorded eighty years ago:'Whenever divorce is difficult, there woman's lot is hard and her position is low.' Wives were only offered formally equal terms of divorce in 1923, the opportunity to utilize the proffered remedy via the introduction of legal aid in 1951, and the financial means to survive as a lone-parent family through the right to state support without stigma in 1948.

Part II (Divorce or separation) maps out why both the law and procedure for divorce were transformed from a restrictive, difficult and humiliating civil process requiring the vigilance of High Court judges and the attendance of barristers into the directly accessible administrative process of modern times. Until the 1960s the majority of matrimonial hearings continued to be adjudicated by lay magistrates. The consequences of a socially divisive legal framework which sanctioned separation but harshly restricted divorce and the chance of a fresh marriage becomes a recurring theme of this section.

The Victorian population multiplied in the new industrial towns and conurbations. Effective government required the counting of heads. Poverty and low physical standards visible within the expanding labouring population aided the development of large-scale private inquiries and official censuses, surveys and commissions of inquiry. Legislators and civil servants were presented with factual evidence of the family's demographic reality and public condition. Ignorance of the social and moral consequences of legal and procedural barriers to divorce could no longer be a sustainable apology for legislative non-involvement. Parliament was eventually pressurized to entice within official regulations those whose extra-marital behaviour transgressed established norms. Nevertheless, substantive and meaningful reform only occurred in the second half of this century.

How the present divorce law came to be introduced as a moral corrective allowing legal internment of long dead marriages forms the focus of Chapter 7. The principal institution which converted to a more liberal divorce stance during the 1960s was the Church of England. Chapters 5 and 6 examine the impact of the two-tier court system for dealing with the matrimonial casualties of different social classes between 1857 and 1945. Why at the beginning of this century were there forty times as many wives seeking matrimonial relief from the recently formed summary court jurisdiction than the Divorce Court? Poverty and a restrictive divorce law limited the access of most potential petitioners. Women faced the additional barrier of the continuing double standard. Evidence of consequent extra-marital unions caused Establishment concern for the breakdown of family morality. The ongoing legal and social restrictions to dissolution between the First and Second World Wars meant official divorce statistics continued to hide the true extent of marital breakdown. Chapter 6 argues that unsuccessful applications for assistance to the Poor Person's Procedure indicate a wide level of spousal unhappiness.

The year 1858 witnessed the introduction of a civil judicial divorce procedure within the newly formed Divorce Court in London. Part I (Before civil divorce) traces the 1857 statute's pedigree from its medieval roots in the canon law doctrine of marital indissolubility administered in the Roman Church's ecclesiastical courts. The formally divorceless state of post-Restoration England was not sustainable for those with titles and property to protect, and there developed the curious provision of Parliamentary divorce. Chapter 3 examines the various restraining facets of a long and costly process initially intended for wealthy cuckold husbands within a patriachial society. In 1792 Westminster granted three divorces as Paris shook to the cries of liberty, equality and fraternity.

Chapter 4 discusses how customary practice arose to ameliorate the state's *de facto* denial of divorce and the consequent right to marry again. It also examines why Parliament intervened in the Church's province by insisting on formal regulation to govern the formation of marriage; and the reason this logically led on to the introduction of civilly contracted marriage in 1836, followed by civil divorce in 1857. The law of divorce still remained as established in Parliamentary private Act procedure. But the anachronistic post-Reformation survival of the Courts Christian matrimonial jurisdiction did come to an end in 1857. The causes of this termination concerns Chapter 2. Ecclesiastical influence was not to be readily removed, though adulterous wives were no longer formally recorded as being seduced by the Devil! For seven centuries the ecclesiastical courts' regulations and practices had been the matrimonial law of the land. The opening chapter presents the earthly realities of the courts' spiritual foundation and temporal authority. Canon law's principle of marital indissolubility was to remain a dominant influence upon official public attitudes until the 1970s.

Part I
Before civil divorce

1 Ecclesiastical influence and jurisdiction in matrimonial matters

In pre-Reformation Europe the regulation of family matters was recognized to be the province of the Roman Church. Clerics taught the rules of spiritual survival in a sinful world; their prescriptions were to channel the newly baptized from the cradle to the grave and beyond. In this world, marriage allowed the human sexual needs and habits of ordinary people to be regulated behind the protection of a sacramental shield. The Church directed that marriage was monogamous and for life, within which the proper consequence of sexual intercourse was the bearing of children. Rome's authority and teaching on such matters was generally acknowledged and upheld by the sovereigns and governors of Europe. It is against this broad canvas that a brief examination of the regulation of marriage and divorce in pre-Reformation England has to be set.

In Anglo-Saxon Britain both the Church and the state accepted full divorce with the right of remarriage (divorce *a vinculo matrimonii*) (Young 1876: 179). This recognition remained until the coming of the Normans. Very little is known about how family law was regulated, though probably it was administered by bishops and abbots sitting alongside magistrates in the civil courts. As a result of Norman settlement, the rule of canon law over local law in matters of marriage began to be established. The canon law of marriage became English law around the beginning of the twelfth century, from which time the ecclesiastical courts alone had the right to give judgment on matrimonial matters (Pollock and Maitland 1968: 367–8). The historical journey from a pre-Reformation structure until modern times will observe the fetter of papal dogma on English matrimonial law. Understanding of this bond between canon law and the regulation of marriage is essential to any study of the development of divorce law and practice in this country.

ECCLESIASTICAL COURTS AND CANON LAW

The early medieval Church based its earthly blueprint for Christian society upon Roman civil law, which in time was modified by ecclesiastical needs to form canon law. By the Middle Ages ecclesiastical law had become labyrinthine, intertwining the elements of civil law, canon law, common law and statute into an esoteric conglomerate of laws and dogma. It was no wonder that Lord Bryce

(1901: 416) found that 'to pass from the civil law of Rome to the ecclesiastical law of the Dark and Middle Ages is like quitting an open country, intersected by good roads, for a tract of mountain and forest where rough and tortuous paths furnish the only means of transit.' Nevertheless, canon law was to regulate some of the most important affairs of citizens' lives. Administration and enforcement of canon law was by means of the ecclesiastical courts. The courts derived their authority from the pope rather than the sovereign: as Lord Justice James observed in *Niboyet v. Niboyet* (1878, 4 P.D 1), 'the jurisdiction of the Court Christian was a jurisdiction over Christians who, in theory, by virtue of their baptism, became members of the one Catholic and Apostolic Church.'

Obedience to the Church's teaching and authority was a normal factor in the government of everyday life, as well as being an essential element for spiritual salvation. One of the main principles of canon law was the doctrine that marriage was a sacrament that represented the everlasting union of Christ with his Church. Because this spiritual bond was indestructible, so equally permanent were the bonds of matrimony. No earthly power had the right to put asunder a properly formed and consummated marriage; only death could terminate wedlock. This was the doctrine which led to the principle of marital indissolubility and gave the Church exclusive authority to deal with matrimonial causes.

THEORY AND PRACTICE OF ANNULMENT

The Roman Church's rule of matrimonial indissolubility applied to all unions that had been consummated into holy matrimony. But dogmatic inflexibility was softened by the presence of a legitimate escape route from the bonds of unhappy wedlock. This was through the doctrine of nullity whereby a marriage could be declared void. Each spouse was made once more single as though the union and its progeny had been conjured away through the mist of matrimony that was held never to have occurred. Nullity could be due to either a flaw in the marriage ceremony or an impediment to the union of the husband and wife. In the former case it was sufficient to prove that the marriage ceremony was deficient in formalities or that there had been duress. The second way was to show that there existed a relationship, either by blood (consanguinity) or by affinity through marriage, between the spouses. A marriage was invalid if, through the prohibited degrees of consanguinity, a person unwittingly married anyone descended from their great-great-grandparents; or by affinity as a result of one spouse's sexual union – before or after marriage – with a third party who was related within the four degrees of descent to one's spouse. For such latter reason the marriage of Roger Donnington was declared invalid because before its celebration he had had sexual intercourse with a third cousin of his future wife. The awesome complexity of the laws regarding consanguinity and affinity have been described by Joseph Jackson (1969: 286) as 'a mixture of mathematics and mysticism, based on the view that sexual intercourse made man and woman one flesh, and so related to one another regardless of marriage'. A marriage could also be annulled if there was proof of a previous binding contract to marry another.

Within the closely bound rural society that formed medieval England it was not too difficult to show that the marriage offended the Church's prohibition on either consanguinity or affinity. The medieval world of convoluted canonical casuistry allowed a dispensable impediment to be revealed in almost every unhappy marriage in consideration of a supporting benefaction. The compelling consideration preventing the marriage of Henry VIII being annulled by the Pope – by reason of quasi-affinity created by Katherine's prior betrothal to Arthur, Henry's dead brother – was that Katherine's nephew, the Emperor Charles V, was the most powerful man in Europe.

After the Reformation the Protestant countries of Europe, other than England, accepted that marriage was a civil contract to be regulated by the state. On the Continent and in Scotland the Protestant reformers rejected marriage as a sacrament, holding that its significance was secular. Church courts disappeared from the Protestant states of Switzerland and Germany and the countries of Denmark and Norway. Of the countries that repudiated Catholicism at this time, it was only England which retained the canon law as her law of marriage. In Scotland, John Knox argued that adultery was so heinous a crime that the victim was entitled to divorce and the guilty spouse deserved death (a provision which would make divorce seem redundant).

The matrimonial law of England and Wales was almost changed to reflect a more liberal attitude. In the reign of Henry VIII, Parliament had authorized a review of the existing pre-Reformation canon law in light of Protestant teaching. The ecclesiastical law Commissioners produced a reformed code of canons, known as the *Reformatio Lequm Ecclesiasticarum*. Acceptance of the section entitled *De Adulteriis et Divortiis* would have brought the theological thinking of the Anglican Church and the divorce laws of England into line with that of other Protestant countries. The code recommended that complete divorce should be allowed on the grounds of adultery, desertion, cruelty, long absence and deadly hatred between the spouses. In addition, it would have permitted the innocent spouse to remarry. These proposals were never implemented, proving unacceptable to the majority of both Parliamentary and Anglican opinion, and so the existing canon law remained unaltered. The revised Anglican Canons of 1604 expressly prohibited divorce *a vinculo*, only providing for annulments and separations: the latter being divorce *a mensa et thoro*. Paradoxically, 'a principal effect of the Reformation on marriage in England was the abolition of the very evasions, fictions and loopholes which had made the medieval system tolerable in practice' (McGregor *et al.* 1970: 1).

The purpose of Henry VIII's break with Rome was not to free the people from religious direction; nor did the Church of England claim to be a new Church. Its defenders saw the Established Church as embodying in itself the powers and traditions of the early, untarnished, Catholic Church. This background helps to explain why the same ecclesiastical courts that existed in pre-Reformation England continued unaltered. Lord Hardwicke could declare of the ecclesiastical courts' jurisdiction that the 'authority they exercise in matrimonial cases is the general law of the land . . .' (*Hill v. Turner* [1737], 1 Atk. 515). English matrimonial law remained that as laid down within the ecclesiastical courts until 1857. With this in mind, it is necessary to understand the powers and procedures of the ecclesiastical courts.

ECCLESIASTICAL COURTS' AUTHORITY

The origins of ecclesiastical courts are found in the Norman reform of English church administration. Wishing to increase his own power, William I ordered in 1076 that canon law and common law should not thereafter be dispensed in the same court and that all ecclesiastical transactions should be transferred to a separate ecclesiastical court in each diocese (Johnstone 1851). In carrying out William's orders, the first Norman Archbishop of Canterbury, Lanfranc, took as his guide the existing Continental canon law. Canon law laid emphasis on the authority of the bishop over the people of his diocese in both spiritual and secular matters that concerned Christian teaching. This resulted in ecclesiastical courts being administered by the bishops, who had sole jurisdiction over spiritual matters. This authority included pleas affecting episcopal jurisdiction, as well as causes concerning the government of souls. Realizing that the law in the twelfth century was developing into a complexity beyond their own handling, the bishops began to transfer their judicial duties to men appointed for their knowledge and training in law. This transfer provided the foundation for a new body of lawyers proficient in the practice of both civil (the law of Continental Europe, with its roots in ancient Roman state law) and ecclesiastical law (Cohen 1915: 73). It was the civilian lawyers who provided the legal expertise in the church courts.

By the late thirteenth century, the common law courts dealt with matters arising from family relationships which came under the headings of real property or breach of the peace. The church courts' civil jurisdiction covered the administration of estates of deceased persons and construction of wills of personality, and matrimonial matters: these were issues that came within the spheres of religion and morality.

The church courts' now established right and authority to deal exclusively with matrimonial matters allowed them to make the following decrees: divorce *a mensa et thoro*, restitution of conjugal rights, nullity and jactitation of marriage. They could also deal with issues involving contracts of marriage and espousals. But they did not have the right to dissolve a validly contracted marriage. Canon law would not countenance divorce *a vinculo matrimonii*. This was a divorce dissolving the marriage bond and giving one or both of the spouses the right to marry again during the lifetime of the former partner. The only legally approved course within the Courts Christian by which a valid marriage consortium could be set aside – but not extinguished – was by the making of a divorce *a mensa et thoro*. The sentence of separation – literally from bed and board – enabled the complaining spouse to live apart from the defendant spouse. This order allowed the marriage to remain in name, if not in form; it was similar to what we know today as judicial separation. The decree was available to either husband or wife upon proof of the other's committal of one or more matrimonial offences; these being adultery, cruelty, unnatural offences or heresy and apostacy but, surprisingly, not desertion.

COURT ADMINISTRATION AND PROCEDURE

For ecclesiastical purposes England and Wales were divided into the provinces of Canterbury and York, each under its own archbishop. Each province operated a complex demarcation of court authority, with provinces divided into dioceses, dioceses into archdeaconeries, archdeaconeries into rural deaneries. By the early nineteenth century there were altogether about four hundred ecclesiastical courts, of which twenty-six were consistory courts; twenty-two in the province of Canterbury and four in the province of York (Reports 1832: 567). It was only the consistory courts, together with the two Archbishops courts, that had the jurisdiction to deal with matrimonial suits. Matrimonial appeals were heard by the two metropolitan courts, these being the Court of Arches at London (province of Canterbury) and the Chancery court at York.

By 1800, the work passing through the ecclesiastical courts had fallen dramatically, and consequently demand for advocates and proctors, who undertook a similar role to that now taken by solicitors, was severely reduced. In 1833, the advocates numbered only between twenty and thirty, their membership forming a minute 1 per cent of the common law barristers practising at the Bar.

At the commencement of Victoria's reign, the ecclesiastical courts' jurisdiction and procedure was a residual from medieval times. The process was inquisitorial in form. Only written evidence was accepted by the ecclesiastical courts. This canonical procedure depended on the collection and collation of depositions (the sworn statements of witnesses) by the judge. Three main stages followed the making of a matrimonial complaint. In the first stage the defendant received the 'libel', this being similar in design to a divorce petition of today. The libel contained the allegations being made, together with the related facts and the supporting evidence. It might be that a wife charging her husband with adultery would produce letters written by him as evidence of the allegation that he had fathered illegitimate children since the marriage.

The second stage allowed witnesses from both parties to be examined in private by a court official called an examiner, upon questions previously set by the judge. Their replies were sent to the other side, and yet further delay was caused by the necessity of giving each party the right to comment on these depositions. As the taking of evidence and cross-examination were by deposition, a protracted case would result in many pages of hand-written evidence and a costly court fee for the complainant. A typical court record of a divorce *a mensa et thoro* hearing examined by the writer consisted of some 120 pages, three-quarters of which were depositions or exhibits coming from twelve witnesses providing evidence in support of the complainant's allegations. When the judge was satisfied that all the necessary evidence to the 'libel' and later 'rejoinders' and 'answers' had been obtained, he closed this stage of the proceedings.

The third stage consisted of the judge studying the gathered documents, pleas, exhibits, depositions and interrogatories before hearing the argument of the advocates of both sides. There was no jury, the judge giving both verdict and sentence.

The standard sentence for divorce *a mensa et thoro*, in this case awarded to a husband upon his wife's adultery, was as follows:

> That the said M.A.K., after the solemnization and consummation of the said Marriage being altogether unmindful of her conjugal vows not having the fear of God before her eyes and being instigated and seduced by the Devil did at the times libellate or some or one of them commit the foul crime of adultery and thereby violated her conjugal vow – Wherefore and by reason of the Premises we do pronounce decree and declare that the said N.K. Esquire ought by Laws to be divorced from bed and board and mutual cohabitation with the said M.A.K. his wife until they shall be reconciled to each other.

The slow and expensive hearing effectively debarred complaints from those with low incomes. Those able to meet the legal and court fees, endure the delay and convince the judge of their accusation, were rewarded with a decree that provided little real benefit to the successful spouse. Divorce *a mensa et thoro* allowed neither spouse the right to enter a second marriage during the other's lifetime. Rather, the somewhat unworldly court's expectation was that the parties would become reconciled and reunited. Additionally, a successfully complaining wife might obtain an order for maintenance, but she was denied a practical means of enforcing payment. It was not surprising that the spiritual courts' matrimonial jurisdiction was seldom resorted to.

COST OF MATRIMONIAL PROCEEDINGS

Witnesses to the Ecclesiastical Courts' Commission of 1832 gave details of the high costs and delays in matrimonial proceedings (Report 1832: 69). Similar evidence came before the Campbell Commission of 1853; for instance, John Shephard, Deputy Registrar of the London consistory court, provides information about fifty-four cases heard in his court over six years from 1845 to 1850. Analysis of these hearings shows that the majority (57 per cent) took more than six months from commencement to conclusion (Report 1853: 30). When it came to a formal opposition of the allegations, only a minority (20 per cent) of the defendant spouses offered a defence, though the husband was more likely to defend the charge formally (33 per cent of wife suits) compared with wife defendants (12 per cent of husband suits). The husband was liable to meet his wife's legal expenses either in bringing or defending a case. But this was of little help to the impoverished wife of an ordinary wage-earning husband lacking property or capital. Even if the husband could pay his wife's legal costs, she still had to have his address to which both court papers and legal bills could be served.

The hearing of the suit would normally take place in the diocesan consistory court in which the defendant spouse lived, for under the Statute of Citations Act of 1531, residence was the condition precedent of the ecclesiastical courts' jurisdiction. Poor people could seek legal help by suing *in forma pauperis* if they were worth less than £5, but this pauper procedure had remained unchanged for three centuries and had now become of little practical benefit.

All the available evidence indicates that resort to the ecclesiastical courts was an expensive matter in the first half of the nineteenth century. Randel Lewis, writing as a lawyer in 1805, observed that few suits were judicially determined for under £300. A defended case could drag on for up to two or three years and cost anything from £300 to thousands of pounds. How enormous the legal bill might be is indicated in the two-year drawn-out contested suit between the Countess and Earl of Portsmouth. The Countess's taxed costs of 1828 amounted to £3,820, the itemized expenses unfolding to form a bill of 104 feet in length (Slatter 1953: 144).

Even in an unopposed suit the minimum costs in the consistory court of London were likely to vary from £120 to £140 (Report 1853: 21). There seems little chance that ecclesiastical courts were used by working-class folk when the average wage paid to the manufacturing labourer in the 1830s was only the equivalent of 70p a week (Bowley 1900: 70).

MAINTENANCE AND ITS ENFORCEMENT

The wife's right to maintenance lay within the authority of the ecclesiastical courts until 1857. The decision of a majority of English common law judges hearing the case of *Manby v. Scott* (*Smith's Leading Cases*, 13th edn, vol. 2: 418) in 1663 held that the wife had no remedy or independent right to maintenance via the common law courts, but only to the relief offered by the ecclesiastical jurisdiction.

Yet the foundation of the wife's right to maintenance was set in common law, through status acquired by marriage. The parties to a marriage, as a consequence of entering into that status, were (and are) under an obligation to cohabit. By marrying, a man voluntarily contracted a new status from which followed an obligation to support his wife and children according to his estate and condition. Though the common law recognized the husband's obligation to maintain his wife, it nevertheless refused the means of enforcement against recalcitrant husbands. If any doubts remained by the mid-seventeenth century as to what the civil courts' attitude to marriage and its consequences were, they were removed by the *Manby v. Scott* decision. The authority of the ecclesiastical courts to be the established jurisdiction to handle matrimonial matters was now certain.

Manby v. Scott remained a precedent for the proposition that a wife's right to alimony was enforceable exclusively in the ecclesiastical courts until Parliament intervened two centuries later in 1857. None the less, alimony could not be ordered by the ecclesiastical courts until separation had occurred upon the fault of the husband. Church courts were concerned only with incidents of the matrimonial relationship, and an order for alimony was ancillary to the decree of separation.

Upon marriage, the wife's personal property passed to her husband unless it was held for her by settlement, as would be the case for heiresses from wealthy families. But the great mass of wives did not have this protection and could not be financially independent of their husbands. For this reason ecclesiastical courts recognized that, unless the wife was to be a pauper, it was essential to provide the means to live separate from her husband in accordance with the decree divorce *a mensa et thoro*. The requirements of 'guilt' and 'innocence' were basic to the courts' resolution of maintenance. A wife who established the moral wayward-ness of her husband could expect maintenance to be 'dealt out with as much liberality as precedent will warrant' (Poynter 1824: 251). The court would not order alimony if the wife was living in an adulterous relationship, this being so flagrant a disregard of matrimonial conduct as to forfeit all claims of support upon the husband. The only exception to this latter policy was if the wife had wealth in her own right before marriage, in which case, Poynter explains, 'the allotment of alimony would be no more than, with some regard to her former situation, and the fortune she brought, would be absolutely necessary for maintenance'. This justice reflected the Courts Christian pedigree of canon law morality infused with the patriarchal tenets of the common law.

If the parties could not agree voluntarily on the amount to be paid, then the wife would be required to file an affidavit setting out details of her husband's financial position together with her own dowry and current monetary circumstances. From this information the judge would utilize his broad discretion when deciding the amount of maintenance to be ordered. The normal practice of the judge was to order an amount that was around one-third of the husband's income, though the amount could fall below or exceed this proportion according to the spouses' conduct. A jeweller with an income of £300 was ordered to pay his wife £80 per annum permanent alimony in 1791, while the Countess of Pomfret in 1796 obtained one-third of her husband's yearly £12,000 income. In this latter case the Countess might well have felt aggrieved, for the Earl's income was largely due to her wealth. But it was held that she had obtained rank through marriage while the husband had the dignity of the peerage to support.

Judges were unwilling to be too severe on 'guilty' husbands whose wealth came from the matrimonial embracement of their wives' financial assets. In 1813, Mrs Smith obtained a decree of separation on the grounds of her husband's adultery and cruelty. A great part of Mr Smith's yearly income of £1,500 was due to his wife's wealth, while Mrs Smith had a separate income of £300 per year. Sir John Nicolls, sitting on appeal in the Court of Arches, observed:

> It is a rule of equity that no man shall take advantage of his own wrong. Perhaps it would be but just that when the husband violates the matrimonial engagement, and the fortune was originally belonging to the wife, that he should give up the whole of it. Courts, however, have not gone that length; yet

in such a case as the present the Court would give as large an allotment as in any.

(Smith v. Smith [1813] 2 Phillim. 235)

The wife received from the court a further £550 a year in addition to the original £450 alimony. Such cases of gross injustice reflected the attitude of the common law that the husband's sovereignty over his wife legitimated the annexation of her legal identity and the impounding of her possessions.

Alimony was seen as a personal allowance paid by the husband for the maintenance and support of his wife and, as such, it was 'allotted from year to year' (Coote, 1847: 349). It was neither the property of the wife nor a debt due from the husband and consequently could not be enforced through proceedings in the common law courts. The reason why alimony was not a debt at law was a consequence of the common law's wish to avoid involvement and possible confrontation with the spiritual jurisdiction of the ecclesiastical courts. Alimony was intended to provide for no more than the wife's day-to-day needs; for the courts held that the mutual obligations of marriage had only been suspended and that the parties were expected to resume cohabitation. The former belief and the latter hope justified the courts' practice not to enforce arrears of many years standing.

The ecclesiastical courts could not enforce their financial orders effectively, as alimony could not be made an assignable or chargeable asset, for the courts had no authority over the husband's property. Non-payment could only be punished by ecclesiastical censure of excommunication. If this action failed, and the excommunicated person remained unyielding, the judge might obtain the recalcitrant's imprisonment by notifying the contempt to the Court of Chancery. But, as the next section shows, it was rare for threats of heavenly censure or earthly punishment to be the means of extracting alimony from defiant husbands.

The ineffective enforcement procedure of the ecclesiastical courts debilitated their authority. The only sanction the courts had directly at their disposal was excommunication. This was a threat of spiritual ostracism which caused little fear to most men. The earthly consequences were that an excommunicant could not be buried in a churchyard; nor could he within common law serve upon juries, be a witness in court, or bring action to recover land or money due to him (Blackstone 1783: 102). Marchant (1969: 221), writing of the sixteenth and seventeenth centuries, records: 'The average contumacious person lived and died excommunicate. If he was poor, the legal disabilities would weigh lightly on him.' The result was that 'church discipline by itself had little compulsive effect on the poorer classes. Excommunication hardly touched them.'

As far back as Tudor times the ecclesiastical courts had found it hard to secure attendance of cited offenders; if successful, the authorities faced further difficulty in exacting obedience to its orders (Price 1942: 106–8). These courts simply did not have the administrative means of enforcing their command. Why disrespect was shown to ecclesiastical censure is explained by Archdeacon Hale (1847: 1): penance, suspension and even excommunication, being 'punishments which affect only the mind and conscience; they have little influence upon persons who have no respect for religion.'

Refusal to obey the order of the court might lead to the issue of a writ of excommunication for contumacy. If an excommunicated person refused to submit to the church court within forty days, the judge could then signify the contempt by issuing a *significavit* against him. Notification of contempt, by the ecclesiastical court to the Court of Chancery, resulted in the latter issuing a writ *de excommunicato* (or *de contumace* after 1813) *capiendo*. The sheriff could now imprison the offender until such time as he, or she, submitted. In one case a woman had been confined eleven years at Nottingham because she refused to admit she was not a married woman (*Hansard* 1813, vol. 26, col. 707).

This was the enforcement procedure laid down but in practice the required time, money and resolution restricted the process. The courts' defective enforcement machinery was underlined by the Lord Chancellor's belief in 1831 that excommunication had become a *brutum fulmen* (an empty threat). It was not the ultimate deterrent of imprisonment but the threat of excommunication that was the *de facto* means of enforcement of an ecclesiastical court order.

The weakness of the ecclesiastical courts' overall jurisdiction was apparent to the 1832 Ecclesiastical Courts Commission: 'It does appear wholly inconsistent with any sound principles of Jurisprudence, that exclusive right of adjudication on certain subjects should be vested in any Court, and yet that Court be left without the means of carrying its decrees and orders into effect' (Report 1832: 67). The tone of the Report suggests that imprisonment was seldom used in matrimonial matters and, indeed, confirmation is provided by a return of all ecclesiastical court imprisonments in the three years 1827–9. Only two out of the sixty-nine committals were matrimonial, one case being of a barrister imprisoned for three days for not paying costs of £64 in a separation case brought by his wife; the second was that of a labourer who spent one week in prison for 'not answering in a cause of Divorce and Separation'. The question as to how effective was the process for enforcing the matrimonial decrees and orders of the courts is answered by the Commission: 'As the law now stands in these Courts, justice is liable to be defeated in various ways, especially in Matrimonial Suits.' The Courts Christian, in short, had no effective practical means of enforcing an order for maintenance.

The basic position of the common law remained unchanged until 1857; the temporal courts would not recognize any separation which had not been decreed by the spiritual courts (Prater 1834: 42). Nor would the former courts interfere with the latters' refusal to grant divorce *a vinculo*. The one institution that had authority to disregard ecclesiastical law was Parliament. After the Restoration the practice developed of petitioning the House of Lords by private Bill for an absolute divorce. The detailed requirements of this curious procedure are discussed in Chapter 3; sufficient to say the route was slow and costly. The few who proceeded from the ecclesiastical courts to the House of Lords and a private Act of divorce highlighted the social injustice of the matrimonial laws of

England and Wales to all but a few citizens, and underlined the iniquitous position of women.

The structure and working of the church courts had been formulated for the needs and conditions of medieval times. But over the centuries their initial purpose of saving souls had been muddied. By the beginning of the nineteenth century the courts had become an anachronism, unable to provide the worldly legal needs of a rapidly expanding industrial society.

2 Decline of the ecclesiastical courts

The question arises as to whether the ecclesiastical courts' matrimonial jurisdiction was in anyway adequate to deal with the generality of unhappy marriages. Who would wish to use a procedure that was both costly and slow, and offered no practical benefit to the successful complainant? Nor did a divorce *a mensa et thoro* – referred to by Lewis in 1805 as the 'suit for alimony' – offer any realistic advantage to separated middle-class wives left without financial means of support. For if the husband would not voluntarily support his wife it was unlikely that the court order would be respected through threat of spiritual censure. A more likely explanation was that a middle-class wife who was cruelly treated, or found her husband's adultery intolerable, sought the Church's seal to live apart from him in a time when violation of spiritual standards of matrimonial accord might result in ostracism within her social strata. The ecclesiastical decree would show the wife to be morally blameless. Similar argument explains the husband's resort to the ecclesiastical court. But all this is conjecture. Unfortunately, many of the post-Reformation ecclesiastical records that have survived destruction at the hands of librarians seeking space in overcrowded archives remain uncatalogued and intractable. However, study of available sources suggests the ecclesiastical courts' matrimonial jurisdiction was seldom used.

THE BUSINESS OF THE COURTS

Even before the Reformation there seems to have been little resort to the ecclesiastical courts' matrimonial jurisdiction, this being due mainly to the already very high cost of proceedings (Woodcock 1952: 85; Morris 1963: 157). The records at York show that by the time of the Stuarts, matrimonial hearings had almost completely disappeared (1 per cent) at York, while there were no such cases coming before the courts at Norwich and Nottingham (Marchant 1969: 20, 62, 194).

Suits for defamation and tithe formed the main part of the seventeenth-century consistory courts' work. Cases of defamation were brought by victims – mostly women – of slanderous gossip usually concerning alleged immorality, blasphemy or cursing. The ecclesiastical courts were the self-appointed guardians of the people's morals. Their powers were such that they could punish fornication and adultery, as the registers of Sutton Valance church in Kent record: 'November 15th, 1717. On which day Eliz. Stace did public penance for ye foul sin of adultery committed with Tho. Hutchins junr. in Sutton Valance Church, as did Anne Hynds for ye foul sin of fornication committed with Theo. Daws' (Tate 1969: 146).

By the end of the eighteenth century the records of the consistory court of Exeter show that the court's work consisted almost exclusively of tithe (50 per cent) and faculties (49 per cent) hearings (Warne 1969: 84). Testamentary hearings, which had formed over half of the cases heard by the Exeter court in 1759, were no longer heard by 1792; this being due to the necessity of such work being transferred to London's Prerogative Court with its advantage of professional advocates at nearby Doctors' Commons. There is no mention in either year of hearings for divorce *a mensa et thoro* having taken place at Exeter, such hearings being extremely rare. The cases heard and the changes experienced at Exeter were similar to those of other ecclesiastical courts throughout the country. Whereas cases involving allegations of fornication and bastardy had formed 39 per cent of Exeter's hearings in 1759, they had disappeared by 1792. That this was indeed the position for all the courts was confirmed by the Ecclesiastical Courts' *Report* of 1832. The ecclesiastical courts' original purpose of spiritual guidance and discipline had disappeared.

The majority of consistory courts, most of whom lacked the legal expertise provided by Doctors' Commons (the Inn of Court for Doctor's of Laws – known as Civilians – established near St Paul's, London), were, in practice, no more than staging posts when it came to deciding matrimonial suits; passing the hearing of the suit on to either London's consistory court or Court of Arches by means of letters of request. Research by T.E. James (1961: 64–5) on the eighteenth century records of the Court of Arches indicates that matrimonial hearings at this court averaged three a year, of which only one was a divorce *a mensa et thoro*. These figures are too small to base any firm conclusion apart from the rarity of such proceedings in everyday life.

Professor James's researches also led him to observe: 'Indeed it is difficult to understand how the practice and procedure in matrimonial causes was preserved in the outlying Courts' (James 1961: 59). The answer to this poser is that resort to the matrimonial jurisdiction possessed by the consistory courts outside London had, by the early nineteenth century, almost completely vanished.

Official returns from ecclesiastical courts show their paucity of matrimonial work. In the four years 1840 to 1843 an average of forty matrimonial suits were annually commenced in England and Wales – with at least seven not proceeded with; three-quarters of all cases were heard in London (Report 1844). This was typical of the work passing through the ecclesiastical courts in this period, similar results having been obtained by the Ecclesiastical Commission for the three years 1827, 1828 and 1829. Out of the 1,903 causes commenced in these three years, only 101 (5 per cent) were classified as matrimonial causes. The Commissioner's Report (1832: 567) does not indicate what proportion of the 101 cases were for divorce *a mensa et thoro* only, but even the improbable assumption that they all were only produces a yearly average of thirty-three. Much of this work came to the London consistory court or the Court of Arches (acting as a provincial court), for together they heard 57 per cent of all matrimonial hearings. The result was that the remaining twenty-five consistory courts outside London did not average even one matrimonial hearing per year. This meant that the great majority of district courts lacked experience of administering and judging such matters. Nearly half (46 per cent) of all matrimonial and professionally lucrative testamentary causes, but only 3 per cent of unremunerative 'other' causes, were commenced in London. The result was that only the London advocates at Doctors' Commons were able to support a skilled Bar and Bench. Within Doctors' Commons, the judges and advocates were usually competent to fulfil their duties; at the outlying courts the position was seldom satisfactory. Outside Doctors' Commons, the great majority of diocesan court judges were legally untrained clerks in holy orders assisted by proctors.

POLITICAL CHANGE

By 1800 the church courts had long lost their original purpose of enforcing moral and spiritual obligation. In medieval times sacred and temporal values had entwined in a society submissive to one Catholic faith. The new creed of Protestantism encouraged examination of the individual conscience and the limits of personal obligation towards state authority. Three centuries later there were many who repudiated the doctrines of the Church of England and its establishment both as the religion and as a constitutional pillar of the state. The stimulation of religious vigilance and the re-examination of Established faith were the consequences of dissent. Such troubled consciences loosened the bonds providing conformity and cohesion and hastened the process of secularization.

The base and form of political power was also being challenged. Industrial changes of the late eighteenth century had brought prosperity to merchants and manufacturers of the middle class. Although the landed interests were represented in Parliament, those of the newly formed wealthy, but landless, middle class were not. Support for middle-class discontent over their lack of enfranchisement was provided by the classical economists and Utilitarian philosophers. David Ricardo expounded his theory of rent in *The Principles of Political Economy and Taxation* (1817), arguing that the landlord was no more than a parasite who gave nothing in return for his unearned rent. When James Mill wrote in 1821 that it was in 'the Representative System alone the securities of good government are to be found', what he was really advocating was the replacement of aristocratic by middle-class political leadership.

The actual source of conflict was not between classes with differing interests and divergent forms of wealth but between opponents and defenders of property. Lord Francis Jeffrey appreciated the reality when he observed: 'The real battle is not between Whigs and Tories, Liberals and Illiberals and such gentlemen-like denominations, but between property and no-property–Swing and the law' (Cockburn 1852: 223). The middle class objected to the discrepancy between the privileges and power of the aristocratic landowners compared with the owners of industrial property. Thus the middle class had to attack the aristocracy without wishing, or appearing to wish, to attack the principle of private property itself. The middle class knew that behind them were those who wished to abolish the private ownership of all land and property. Among the great landowners, the one most open to attack and least capable of defence was the Established Church. Within the Georgian Church a fifth of all incumbents were related to the gentry by either birth or marriage (Virgin 1989: 139). The Church as a landowner acted as other members of the territorial aristocracy, though the latter were in a less anomalous position over the collection of tithes than a cleric who, in the words of the *Quarterly Review* in 1830, was 'at once the plaintiff and the priest, the prosecutor and the pastor, the guardian of the flock and the sharer in the fleece' (Mathieson 1923: 19). Farmers had reason to dislike this dominion. The enclosure movement and agrarian improvements had created greater profit for the farmer who promptly had it clawed away by tithe payment to the Church.

CHURCH REFORM

Many of the middle class saw the distortion of matrimonial laws as only one element in their belief that the Church of England received wealth, and wielded power, out of all proportion to its true historical role. Whether the charges were true or false, this is what the critics of the Established Church felt. Their attacks concentrated on the Church's property and function, holding that Establishment was an instrument of the governing classes. The weakness of the Church had been noted in 1826 by Bentham when, in *Mother Church Relieved by Bleeding; or, Vices and Remedies*, he declared: 'The life then of this Excellent person being in her gold, taking away her gold you take away her life' (cited in Brose 1959: 23). The Church of England became the scapegoat upon which the middle class projected much of their discontent and apprehension. Tories fearing disestablishment, farmers rendering tithes, evangelicals seeking a spiritual renewal, Utilitarians proclaiming proficiency, dissenters incensed by political exclusion: all had reasons to seek change in the power and structure of the Church of the nation.

The Church Establishment at this time, as Dicey records (1905: 314), 'exhibited two special weaknesses of its own which both provoked assault by and promised success to its assailants. The national Church was not the Church of the whole nation; the privileges of the Establishment were in many cases the patent grievances of the laity.' The Church held its rank by Parliamentary authority that required those outside the established faith to pay church rates, be married, and have their children baptized in Anglican churches. Their sons (all daughters experienced academic purdah) were excluded from the Universities of Oxford and Cambridge. Attacks upon the Church came from a virulent anti-clerical press, whilst works like John Wade's '*The Black Book*; or Corruption Unmasked! Being an account of Places, Pensions, and Sinecures, The Revenues of the Clergy and Landed Aristocracy' provided a picture in 1820 of pluralists amounting to one-third of all the Anglican clergy, of a three-to-two proportion of non-resident to resident clergy, of bishops holding livings, cathedral stalls and deaneries. The bishops' free exercise of patronage and pluralism was a method of rewarding friends and dependants drawn from the family roots of the gentry. By the early nineteenth century, critics of the Church of England saw its decrepit organization and structure as a symbol of the corrupt *ancien régime* that persisted in the new industrial landscape.

Religion was now playing a greater role in politics so that by the early 1830s 'a Whig Dissenting party confronted a Tory-Anglican one' (O'Gorman 1989). The 1832 post-Reform Act elections returned a solid Whig majority committed to Benthamite attack upon incompetence and abuse. However, the Reform Act of 1832 had not given direct political power to the urban middle class. In England almost three-quarters of the 471 seats went to either the small boroughs with under 1,000 electors or to the counties. What the 1832 Act did indicate was that previously accepted institutions had to show cause for their existence; of these, the Church of England was the most vulnerable to the political reformers' attacks. All churchmen agreed that the Established Church was in danger, but the necessity of reform was less openly accepted. High churchmen understood the appeal of Newman in *Ad Clerum*, the first of the *Tracts for the Times* (1833–4: 3–4):

> A notion has gone abroad that they can take away your power. They think they have given and can take it away. They think it lies in the Church property, and they know that they have politically the power to confiscate the property.

Newman knew the wealth of the Church had been that of bishops, deans, chapters and other ecclesiastical corporations, all of whom formed the Established Church. The Ecclesiastical Revenues Commissioners appointed in 1832 to inquire into the financial condition of the Establishment noted the evils of distribution of Church wealth which resulted in the Archbishop of Canterbury and the Bishop of Durham each receiving £19,000 a year but the Bishop of Llandaff had only £900 a year. The newly formed Commissioners were to act as trustees for the surplus revenue of the bishops and chapters and use the money to carry out necessary reforms. The demand of Bentham and the Utilitarians that Church revenues should be used towards the end of public utility and administrative efficiency had now been partially accepted. The Ecclesiastical Commissioners' extensive financial reorganization averted the threat of disestablishment. Bishops' property and privilege had been largely taken away without compensation (as owners of slaves had received in 1833); so that, by the 1840s, Gladstone could hold: 'It is now impossible to regulate the connection between Church and State in this country by reference to an abstract principle' (Brose 1959: 210–11). The Church of England, by accepting limited reform, was able to preserve its links with the state. As Dicey observed in 1905, 'In all ecclesiastical matters, Englishmen have favoured a policy of conservativism combined with concession.' Signs of this concession were recognizable in 1854 when Oxford University allowed the entrance of students who were not members of the Church of England and in 1868, when the Church Rate Abolition Act abolished means of compelling payment of such rates. 'Concession' was also apparent in the eclipse of the ecclesiastical courts. Their virtual demise of power has to be studied within this setting.

DISSATISFACTION WITH ECCLESIASTICAL COURTS

The presence of the Courts Christian in medieval times had been justified on the basis that its jurisdiction was governed to the spiritual guidance and betterment of Christian society. The ecclesiastical courts of the early nineteenth century still functioned on the principles laid down in the 1076 Ordinance of William I. Continuing existence of their judicial authority over secular matters had become outdated long before the nineteenth century, but anachronisms are more often extinguished than corrected. Ecclesiastical courts had been unable to reform themselves, while governments of the day were wary of interfering with the powerful interests centred in the Established Church. The history of ecclesiastical courts since the Reformation shows a slow but steady eroding of their past powers and jurisdiction.

Increasing pressure to reform the ecclesiastical courts came as a result of the publication of three Parliamentary Reports between 1832 and 1834. The Ecclesiastical Commissioners, under the chairmanship of the Archbishop of Canterbury, had shown in their Report of 1832 how half the court cases were of a testamentary nature. These figures clearly indicated that the courts' secular work had little to do with their original function, the government of souls. Testamentary matters formed a very lucrative part of ecclesiastical jurisdiction for, without such work, the Doctors' Commons could not survive as an independent body. But the 1833 recommendation of the Real Property Commission – headed by Sir (later Lord) John Campbell – that the testamentary jurisdiction of the spiritual courts should be abolished, was a major portent of the dangers ahead. The common law lawyers desired to incorporate the civilians' monopoly and profit.

Criticism continued from many quarters. The church courts had been described by the radical politician Joseph Hume as a 'nest of sinecures'. In 1828 Lord Chancellor Brougham gave rebuke to the installation of these judges by the Archbishop of Canterbury and the Bishop of London. Church dignitaries now appreciated that the old system of appointments would have to be overhauled if their courts were to remain unmolested by Parliament. But realization of the need for change had come too late and, in 1832, Parliament transferred the power of the ecclesiastical appellate court – the High Court of Delegates – to the civil authority (Duncan 1971).

Pressure mounted to abolish, rather than reform, the ecclesiastical courts. The legal profession increasingly felt that, even for matters of law, the traditional ways of the ecclesiastical courts were now obsolete. This barrage of common law criticism was not entirely from a neutral camp; their legal ranks now had sight of the lucrative prize of testamentary profit. Such opinion was summarized by the *Law Times* of 1853:

The ecclesiastical courts have usurped a jurisdiction over wills and marriages which they cannot be permitted to retain under any pretence or with any promise of reform. But then they say, you must have tribunals for these questions. Why not the regular Courts of Law and Equity? . . . And why should not the regular courts try a divorce as well as the validity of a marriage?

(*Law Times*, vol. 20: 159)

Dissatisfaction was also mounting over three basic weaknesses in the ecclesiastical system for dealing with matrimonial relief. First, the clergy themselves had little interest in the highly secularized proceedings. Second, ecclesiastical court proceedings were slow and costly, and successful resolution did not give even the innocent spouse the right to remarry during the lifetime of the other. Dr Phillimore had unsuccessfully tried to introduce a Bill in the House of Commons in 1830 that would have allowed ecclesiastical courts to grant divorce *a vinculo*. Parliamentary divorce, he reported to the 1832 Ecclesiastical Courts Commission, 'is liable to grave and obvious objection' (Report 1832: 152). But the Commission's Report ducked the question of remarriage, leaving it 'to the wisdom of the legislature' (Report 1832: 43). The ecclesiastical divorce *a mensa et thoro* had become by now little more than a necessary prerequisite to support a divorce petition to the House of Lords. The third and main incongruity was the claim of the Courts Christian to judge all matrimonial disputes within the realm. This exclusive claim had been acceptable to the great mass of English people when they had all acquiesced to the Roman faith and practice. But from the seventeenth century an increasing number of Dissenters and other minority religious groups who did not subscribe to the religious beliefs of the Church of England had come to resent the privileges which the Established Church enjoyed. Partial recognition of the Nonconformists' and Catholics' claims came with the Marriage Act of 1836, when they were allowed to solemnize their own marriages. Their fight for equal legal and social status was reflected in a struggle for reform of the ecclesiastical courts' jurisdiction in all secular matters. But the ecclesiastical courts were unable to satisfy their critics' desire for a judicial system in line with the utilitarian needs of the mid-nineteenth century. Such piecemeal reform as the transfer of actions for defamation from ecclesiastical to civil courts in 1855 was not sufficient to prevent the abolitionists' aims being virtually accomplished in 1857. That year saw the civil courts' aquisition of testamentary and matrimonial matters, and the dissolution of Doctors' Commons. The common law lawyers were rewarded by the newly established Court of Probate gaining authority over testamentary business. The ecclesiastical courts' matrimonial jurisdiction, as well as the peculiar legislative power of the House of Lords to grant divorce *a vinculo*, was transferred to the equally new Court for Divorce and Matrimonial Causes. Divorce as a civil process was about to begin.

3   Parliamentary divorce

In 1540 a law of Henry VIII either reduced or removed many of the existing abuses that had allowed annulment of existing marriages. The previous loose impediment rules concerning consanguinity and affinity were now restricted to the Levitical degrees presented in the Book of Common Prayer. Reducing malleable canonical loopholes meant divorce *a mensa et thoro's* importance increased as a legal easement for shattered marriages. But the remedy brought no relief for those wishing to marry anew.

Though now Protestant, the English church courts did not seek new powers allowing them to grant divorce *a vinculo*. Consequently the courts designated for handling marriage disputes could not provide what we understand today to be divorce. But the absence of divorce was not sustainable in post-Reformation England. Instead there developed a peculiar compromise that required the petitioner to proceed eventually to Westminster and seek individual remedy by a private Act of divorce. The granting of dispensations to marry again had become the prerogative of Parliament by means of its legislative authority. This chapter examines some of the facets of this unusual procedure that exempted annually a few individuals from the rigidity of lifelong marriage bonds.

SURVEY OF PARLIAMENTARY DIVORCE

A survey of Parliamentary divorce Acts was undertaken in 1970 to obtain information about the legal facets of this peculiar procedure, and knowledge of petitioners' social and demographic characteristics. Examination of the annual House of Lords' *Journals* provided names of petitioners and the year when the Bill was presented. Parliamentary proceedings over each Bill are to be found mainly in the respective *Journals* of both Houses, though occasionally *Parliamentary Debates* and *Hansard* provide a record of the Bill's progress. The reason why Parliamentary sources contain this information was explained by Lord Westbury: 'This proceeding was in spirit a judicial, though in form a legislative act' (*Shaw v. Gould* [1868] L.R. 3H.L.55).

Table 3.1 records how exceptional Parliamentary divorces were before the accession of George I in 1714, with only seven Acts preceding the Hanoverian ascendancy. Henceforth their numbers increased considerably, with Parliament

Table 3.1 Number of Parliamentary Acts of divorce between the Reformation and 1857

Act passed	No.	%	Annual average
Before 1715	7 ⎫	10	
1715–59	24 ⎭		0.5
1760–99	102	31	2.5
1800–57	194	59	3.3
Total[1]	327	100	

legislating an annual average of three divorce Acts in the hundred years before the abolition of this procedure in 1857. The explanation for this latter finding is found largely in a rapidly transforming social structure that reflected changes in both normative expectations and demographic patterns. For instance, the post-1800 rise in the annual rate of Parliamentary divorce reported in Table 3.1 is in demographic rate terms a decline. The population of England and Wales experienced a threefold rise in the hundred years following 1760 (6.6 million: 100 per cent). In 1801 it was 8.9 million (135 per cent); the 1831 Census reported 13.9 million (211 per cent) and by 1861 it had increased to 20.9 million (317 per cent). The married population rose accordingly. This increase helps to explain why almost a third of all the 327 Acts occurred in the twenty-five years preceding 1857.

This legislative remedy always remained an exceptional exemption from the supremacy of the Church's doctrine of marital indissolubility. The procedure was never intended to be anything other than a peculiar corrective for a small minority of those husbands who were maritally chained to adulterous wives. But the cost of unlocking the matrimonial bond was a willingness to ascend a lengthy, complex and slippery legal ladder that began in the civil court, continued to the ecclesiastical court and finally ended in the House of Lords. Few aggrieved husbands had both the stamina and the financial means to contemplate, let alone surmount, such burdensome obstacles.

DEVELOPMENT OF PARLIAMENTARY PROCEDURE

The Court of Star Chamber, in their significant judgment of 1602 in *Rye v. Fuljambe* (3 Salk.138), held that only divorce *a mensa et thoro* could be granted for adultery and that such a decree did not allow husband or wife to enter a second marriage during the lifetime of the other spouse. The Star Chamber verdict, as MacQueen in his authoritative *Practical Treatise on the Appellate Jurisdiction of the House of Lords* (1842: 470–1) explains, 'has ever since been considered the law of the land. This important decision was in effect a re-assertion of the doctrine of matrimonial indissolubility; a doctrine exploded in other Protestant countries of Europe, but retained in England, and still held sacred and inviolable in all our courts of justice.' Parliament was the only authority with power to overrule the ecclesiastical judgment that marriage was for life.

Parliament, with increased authority resulting from the Civil War (1642–9), was now prepared to circumvent ecclesiastical law by passing, in an exceptional few cases, a private Act allowing divorce. The first private Act of divorce in 1670 allowed Lord Roos, who enjoyed the special favour of Charles II, to enter a second marriage. For almost another two centuries private Act procedure was the only legally prescribed course by which a husband, inconvenienced by an existing valid marriage, could be made free to marry again though the first wife was still living.

Lord Roos had earlier obtained an Act bastardizing the two children of his adulterous wife, and then proceeded to obtain a divorce *a mensa et thoro* from the ecclesiastical court. But Roos needed to marry again and have heirs; as his petition recorded 'there was no probable expectation of posterity to support the family in the male line, but by the said John Manners Lord Roos'. The petitions of Lord Macclesfield (1698) and the Duke of Norfolk (1700) were to make similar special pleading; it was the justification for granting a Parliamentary divorce to each of these three peers. These very early Acts were generally concerned with the danger that a wife's adultery posed to a nobleman lacking a son to inherit title and wealth. The landed aristocracy required certainty of progenitor if the orderly transference of property, rank and authority within the family was to be achieved. The breakdown of marital consortium within a valid first marriage, without the possibility of a second, was an intolerable situation for ill-yoked but eminent husbands with titles and large estates to protect. Hence Parliament devised a method whereby the landed gentry and peerage could, by invoking the ancient public right of petitioning the Crown to redress a private grievance, be protected against spurious offspring disturbing legitimate claims of paternal kin. But each exemption from the rule of indissoluble marriage created a precedent for future aggrieved petitioners.

Aristocratic monopoly of Parliamentary divorce soon disappeared. One of the first petitions to succeed without first establishing special circumstances was submitted by Mr Box in 1701. Box, a London grocer, argued that his wife 'had lived in adultery, as he hath fully proved in the Court of King's Bench, and obtained a definitive sentence in the Arches Court of Canterbury'.

It was not until 1798 that Parliamentary divorce procedure was regularized by the action of Lord Chancellor Loughborough in persuading the House of Lords to accept a series of Resolutions. The new standing order (141) required that all divorce applications to the Lords should be supported by a decree of divorce *a mensa et thoro* together with a copy of evidence received by the ecclesiastical court. This meant that the Lords had a great deal of knowledge about the case before the hearing formally began.

The ecclesiastical courts' antiquated procedure of allegations, articles, objections, interrogatories and compulsories, made the process very slow and costly. Their decree of divorce *a mensa et thoro* could be given for either adultery or cruelty by the respondent, though evidence was inevitably directed towards proof of the former charge, as this was the only ground acceptable to the House of Lords. The exclusive nature of the divorce system required the petitioner to secure the services of a London-based specialist common law lawyer and a Parliamentary agent to draft and channel the Bill through Parliament. The petitioner living away from London had to incur the additional expenses of witnesses' fares to London, board and incidental expenditure, as well as the usual lawyers' fees, court and Parliamentary expenses.

As well as an ecclesiastical court decree against the adulterous wife, Parliamentary divorce procedure normally expected the petitioner to have attempted to obtain compensation from the seducer. This requirement established that the husband had used the available redresses but found them inadequate compensation for the infamy suffered. The civil criminal conversation trial for damages normally preceded the ecclesiastical hearing; this was the case for 88 per cent of all Acts passed between 1800 and 1857 for which the dates of both successful actions could be recorded.

A successful plaintiff verdict allowed damages but also recorded the jury's opinion that the husband was acting genuinely and without collusion, and that his conduct had not contributed to his own dishonour. But even if damages and an ecclesiastical decree had been obtained, the Lords were not bound to pass the Bill if they felt the standard of proof was unsatisfactory. Examples of the Lords rejecting positive verdicts of both the ecclesiastical and the secular court hearings are the dismissed petitions of Downes (1781), Nash (1787), Barthelot (1798), Crewe (1801) and Bland (1808).

The divorce Bill was first presented to the House of Lords, who insisted on examining each case afresh. At the Parliamentary hearing the parties were liable to cross-examination by counsel and by peers. Collusion would cause the petition's rejection: as Mr Chisim, a drysalter, experienced in 1778. The co-respondent – 'a man of property' – did not oppose the criminal conversation suit, nor the wife the petition, but the Lords discovered that the wife's wealthy father was paying for the divorce in the hope of a more profitable new marriage for his daughter. Thomas Chisim was unlucky, for the evidence shows that only a minority of petitions were rejected.

The second reading of the Bill normally took place next day fortnight following the first reading in the Lords. The second reading was essentially the trial of the case. The petitioner had to attend unless the House gave permission of absence, as they did in the case of Major Cunliffe (1820), who was stationed in India. Thus Baron de Robeck (1828) – who had been awarded, but had not received, £2,500 damages from Lord Lennox – was ordered to attend to see if any collusion had occurred between him and his wife or other persons, and also:

> whether at the time of the adultery of which such petitioner complains, his wife was by deed or otherwise, by his consent, living separate and apart from him, and released by him, as far as in him lies, from her conjugal duty; or whether she was, at the time of such adultery, cohabiting with him, and under the protection and authority of him, as her husband.

This case reflects the House of Lords' distaste of petitions complaining of adultery after the couple had separated.

Witnesses whose testimony supported the petitioner's allegations of adultery had to be present at the second reading. An exemption to this rule was allowed after 1820 for witnesses living in India. They could be examined there, and the evidence sent to Westminster. Eleven per cent of all known petitioners' addresses were recorded as being either in India or Ceylon. The ingredients of these conjugal curries were heat, isolation and codes of honour.

A copy of the marriage registration and a witness to the ceremony also had to be produced. After the Bill had been read a second time, it passed to a committee of the whole House who could then amend it if they so wished. Following its third reading, the Bill was sent to the House of Commons. If the Commons passed it, the royal assent followed as a matter of course, and the petitioner was now free to enter a second marriage. As MacQueen (1858: 26) critically observed, 'everything was satisfactory except the delay, the expense and, in many hard cases, the terrible exposure'. These delays were far more a consequence of prior ecclesiastical and civil court action, for the Parliamentary process was reasonably prompt, with almost three-quarters (72 per cent) of the Acts being obtained within three months of petitioning. Parliamentary procedure could be accelerated to meet compelling circumstances, as in the case of the Honourable Pownoll Bastard Pellew. The cuckold commander of HMS *Impregnable* returned to find his wife's affair with an army officer had created rumour of a pregnancy. An Act was passed within a month of obtaining a divorce *a mensa et thoro*. This speedy resolution was facilitated by the presence of the petitioner's father, Viscount Exmouth, in the Lords.

The case of Baron de Robeck (1828) indicates the Lords' unwillingness to allow Acts where separation agreements had been entered into, holding that such agreements repudiated the very basis of the marriage contract. A voluntary deed of separation made before the wife's adultery meant that no injury was done to the husband who had voluntarily released his wife (his property) from consortium. Similarly, the Lords were unsympathetic to husbands whose offensive behaviour had contributed towards their wives' misconduct. For this reason the Bills of Captain Barthelot (1798), Mr Downes (1781) and the architect John Nash (1787) were rejected.

The published Act specifically declared the marriage to be dissolved. But the spreading influential creed of evangelical morality was beginning to be reflected in the House of Lords' wish to make divorce a more shameful experience. It was felt that the wronged but virtuous husband should continue to receive proper justice, but evangelicalism's rigorous reasoning was disturbed that the adulterously sinful wife should also be rewarded by a similar licence to marry afresh. Attempts were made in 1771, 1779 and 1800 to legislate 'no marriage' clauses against the divorced wife marrying the co-respondent. These Bills, though passing the Lords, were always rejected by the Commons.

THE QUESTION OF MAINTENANCE

Financial provisions were generally made for the wife when the Bill was in the Committee stage of the House of Commons. In the earliest cases Parliament provided by enactment that the wife should not be left destitute. Later the House of Commons came to have a functionary called 'the Ladies' Friend', an office generally filled by some member interested in the private business of Parliament, who undertook to see that any husband petitioning for divorce made suitable provision for his wife (Clifford: 1885: 414). It was well understood that the Bill would not pass the Commons Committee stage unless the husband had entered into a bond that provided at least a moderate income for his wife.

The Commons' principle was that, however shameful the wife's misconduct may have been, the husband was not entitled to throw her penniless into the world. This was not to the liking of the Lords, who agreed with Lord Chancellor Thurlow that it was 'an encouragement to immorality'. But the Commons insisted on the old practice of not leaving the wife destitute. The wife who brought wealth from her family to the husband at marriage normally received financial support to reflect the size of her fortune. For instance, Mr Howard (1794) recorded that he would invest an appropriate sum (£7,000) for the benefit of his wife who would otherwise be destitute, though his generosity is diminished by knowledge that the bride, Lady Elizabeth Bellasis, had brought Howard a dowry of £12,600.

Divorce meant that the marriage had come to an end without the possibility of future reconciliation. The cold logic of the Commons' approach was therefore to insist on secured maintenance for the divorced wife rather than follow the ecclesiastical court practice of periodical alimony only to the virtuous separated wife. The Commons expected the husband to settle an assured income for his wife by putting aside such fixed assets as under the terms of the deed would provide the annual sum agreed upon. This settlement was made upon the husband's property and not upon current or future income. The husband's financial circumstances might deteriorate, but the Commons' insistence upon secured maintenance at divorce assured the wife of future payment. Parliamentary divorce practice had been designed for male petitioners drawn from a wealth-owning élite rather than a wage-earning society.

ENTICING DAMAGES

By the end of the eighteenth century the husband's successful claim for damages against his wife's seducer had been established as providing beneficial, though not essential, supporting evidence towards a successful Parliamentary outcome. The new Parliamentary stringency led to nine out of ten (86 per cent) of divorcing husbands in the period 1780 to 1839 providing the Lords with a positive verdict from the common law courts. The period between 1840 and 1857 witnessed a less rigid Parliamentary stance together with increasing public distaste for such litigation and its prurient reporting. Changing attitudes in this latter period are reflected in the lower proportion (74 per cent) of divorcing husbands with previous awards of damages; a finding that is confirmed in Wolfram's analysis (1987: 102).

Proof of a successful verdict from the secular court was intended to remove Parliamentary fear that either the spouses, or husband and co-respondent, might be colluding to deceive them. Parliament expected the seducer, through fear of damages or adverse publicity, to have defended the allegation and presented evidence detrimental to the husband's character and complaint. The authenticity of the husband's subsequent divorce petition was underlined by the fact that judge and jury had already found the allegation of adultery proved. Yet the Campbell Commission of 1853 (Report 1853: 18, 19) was unconvinced by the validity of the civil action as a deterrent against collusion. The majority of defendants neither attended nor were legally represented at the trial, which meant that the witnesses were not cross-examined nor the alleged facts properly tested. Nor could anyone stop the husband returning the damages once the Parliamentary divorce had been obtained. The Commission might have added that the wife had no right either to challenge the evidence or defend her reputation, as she was not a party to the proceedings.

Marriage for the expanding upper and middle classes of eighteenth-century England had become more a matter of personal choice and individual love than their grandparents would have felt prudent. Public opinion came to expect the marital concomitants of companionship and commitment. These familial changes helped transform male feeling as to the appropriate remedy against the injury of a wife's infidelity. In earlier times the cuckold aristocrat turned to the duel to assuage wounded ego and satisfy besmirched honour. Now, a wider circle of similarly aggrieved husbands were beginning to turn to the more profitable compensation offered by the courts within the setting of a developing commercial and industrial landscape.

Damages were intended to compensate the husband for two separate but overlapping forms of marital injury. In the first situation there was the wrong created by the seducer enticing the wife to leave home and husband, thereby causing the loss of her society and services. The second type was the action for criminal conversation against the seducer, whose discovered adultery had caused the marriage consortium to end. It underlined the male fear that the wife's unknown infidelity might deceive the husband into accepting illegitimate children as his own. The mistress was not a threat to a property-owning class; she could never conspire to present her spurious offspring as those of the marriage. This was the formal justification for such tort actions, but there were also more subliminal male fears. Behind it all lay the overriding notion of the wife as property, and patriarchal wrath at the illicit venture into forbidden territory. The adulterer's trespass undermined the master's sexual assurance and monopoly provided by marriage. The courts were willing to give generous compensation for such a wrong.

The double standard debarred a wife from bringing a similar loss of consortium suit against her husband's paramour. How could she have sued successfully! The law insisted that the wife's legal identity was subsumed within that of her husband. There was no question of whose rib it was.

The amounts awarded were often generously large, and it seems likely that juries intended to punish the seducer as well as provide compensation to the wronged husband. Damages in the period 1780 to 1819 were particularly high, with one in five (19 per cent) of all divorcing husbands who had brought actions in the common law courts being rewarded with orders of £5,000 or more. The two largest awards were £20,000 to Lord Valentine Cloncurry (1811) against Sir John Bennett Piers, and to the Honourable Henry Wellesley (1810) against Lord Paget. The Earl of Rosebery (1815) received £15,000 damages against Sir Henry Mildmay, and a further six husbands had sums of £10,000. What such amounts meant in those times is shown by Colquhoun, who estimated that in 1803 the wealthy élite of some 300 peers had average incomes of £8,000 a year, whilst that of 2,000 eminent merchants was put at an average of £2,600 a year. The seduction of a wife appears to have been an expensive pursuit, especially if the cuckold was of rank and the seducer of suitable means.

If high damages were normally awarded to wronged husbands, then sexual intercourse with a married woman by a wealthy seducer was indeed a severely punished matter. A more likely explanation is that in many cases the jury's generosity was a symbolic public rebuke of the seducer, in which case payment was not expected to be paid nor even enforced by the court. And collusive agreement between husband and seducer concerning repayment remained a strong possibility. Certainly Lord Chancellor Eldon's opinion in 1800 was that 90 per cent of these civil actions were collusive, making the law 'a farce and a mockery'. It was never part of standing orders that damages should have been recovered. On the other hand, Parliament after 1809 required the husband to show that he had made some effort to retrieve both damages and costs awarded against the adulterer and 'that they have been *bona fida* retained' (MacQueen 1842: 493). This policy was intended to be a safeguard against the risk of collusion.

The requirement could be waived if the petitioning husband could show that it was impossible to collect the award. For instance, the Bill of Mr Lindham (1829) shows that £5,000 damages awarded against the Reverend Mallock had not been paid. Nor did there seem much chance of Mr Larking (1792) or Mr Talbot (1856) ever receiving even a tenth of the £2,000 damages each was awarded against their respective servants. Evidence for the period 1801 to 1857 from the findings of Anderson (1984: table vi) – when reworked – suggest that some 45 per cent of all divorcing husbands who obtained an order did not recover a penny of their award. In some of these situations collusion between the parties meant that the husband would not seek to collect his due, in other cases the husband's upright morality deterred him from accepting tainted pimp money, whilst fear of bankruptcy caused some seducers to flee the country. The award of damages was often a hollow financial victory.

The courts were likely to reduce the amount sought if the husband's conduct was seen to be morally at fault. This was the case in the criminal conversation action brought by Charles Sturt in 1801 against George Spencer Churchill, the Marquis of Blandford, later fifth Duke of Marlborough, which is described in Mary Soames's agreeable biography, *The Profligate Duke*. The plaintiff sought damages of £20,000 from Blandford after Lady Mary Ann Sturt bore the Marquis a child. Sturt's lawyer asked the jury to award compensation for 'the greatest injury which it was possible to receive of another – the seduction of his wife'. The only evidence of adultery lay in the intercepted letters written by Lord Blandford to Lady Mary Ann that included acknowledgement of paternity. The mitigatory plea of Blandford's defending lawyer, the Attorney-General Sir Edward Law, was that the husband had encouraged the admitted liaison. However, Law turned the tables and demonstrated that Sturt himself had been living with a mistress who was the mother of his child.

The jury awarded Sturt only £100, a risible sum that reflected their distaste for his two-faced behaviour. (The lovers never met again, the Blandfords amicably separated, and the Duke's eventual bankruptcy forced the sale of his personal property that included 200 pairs of leather breeches! In his fifties the Duke, in true aristocratic Whig style, took a sixteen-year-old mistress who kept him and their large family happy for more than twenty years.)

With the introduction of civil divorce in 1857 came the formal abolition of suits for criminal conversation. But in practice little changed except the merging of damages and divorce actions into one lawsuit. The newly formed Divorce Court was instructed to utilize its authority to award damages to wronged husbands on 'the same principles, in the same manner' as before. The old practices and habits were not to be lost or amended readily.

INHERITANCE AND THE NEW MORALITY

At first sight, Parliamentary divorces appear to be an anachronism when it is remembered that ecclesiastical courts had been allowed to retain their pre-Reformation authority over matrimonial matters. Many churchmen agreed with the author of *Essay on Divorce Bills* in his criticism in 1824 that:

> As things now stand, the judicial and the legislative authorities proceed on opposite principles, and the legislative assumes judicial functions for the express purpose of doing what, according to the general law of the land and according to scripture as expounded by that law, ought not to be done at all.
>
> (Quoted in Morgan 1826: 256)

Why was it then that the legislature allowed these private Acts, each one of which was a denial of the Established Church's teaching of the indissolubility of marriage?

The safeguard of Parliamentary divorce was essential in a society where family wealth was held in the form of land, and family prestige was recognized by the antiquity of the name residing in the country estate. Large landowners wished to ensure that the esteem and financial worth attached to the family name was securely transferred to future kin. The approved method was to lock the estate into subsequent generations by successive settlement. This reduced the danger of realty being dissipated by a profligate heir, such as the Marquis of Blandford. Regulated settlement gave assurance that title successors retained substance to support honour.

Family settlement was ensured by a customary rule of succession known as primogeniture. The practice allowed the great landowners to transfer their undivided estate to the chosen heir, who almost invariably was the eldest son. This system of regulating family property was recognized by Brodrick (1881: 356) as the 'keystone of the English land system'. The landed aristocracy and those, in Brodrick's words 'struggling to enter its ranks', accepted primogeniture 'almost as a fundamental law of nature'. The ability to perpetuate family property within the male line was buttressed by the combination of the family lawyer's conveyancing skills and the traditional values of the landed classes.

The majority of early divorce Acts were passed to ensure the landed gentry's untroubled and unquestioned continued direct line of male succession. The heads of wealthy estates were aware of the risk of spurious offspring offending the purity of the family tree. The heirless Duke of Norfolk could legitimately complain to Parliament that the Duchess's adultery with John Germain could 'bring a bastard into the family, and then the estate does not go according to the law of God and nature'. For within a system of customary primogeniture the arrangements of inheritance allowed the first-born son the major portion of the estate. At the same time, transference of the family estate within future generations of the male line was encouraged by the lawyer's device of strict settlement (the heir became tenant for life) and entail (the order of succession of life tenants), which helped to reduce the risk of a future ill-considered disposal of the freehold land. But the English law of real property had traditionally allowed alienability, especially at times of marriage, death and the heir's majority – the last of these being a legal cleft in the complex web of secure settlement and succession, for the wayward son now had power to bar the entail. Danger that the heir might refuse to continue the prescribed pattern of resettlement to his own son was in practice largely neutralized by the training, tradition and financial inducements that encouraged conformity to the ancestral ways of the landed gentry (Pollock 1883: 8). All of this, legal shield and habit of class, was there to guard the family estate from being dissipated by a system of partible inheritance. A practice in which all the children had an equal claim posed a threat to the powerful landowning families. Deviation down this crumbly path could rapidly dissolve a once noble estate into a residue of small holdings. Such was the apology of the landed gentry of the mid-eighteenth century to justify their established system of inheritance. It was a practice that bolstered the eldest son, in Newman's description (1867: 96), to the position of 'a magnificently fed and coloured drone, the incarnation of wealth and social dignity'. The custom of primogeniture and strict settlement allowed a freedom of sexual habit and practice among the Whig aristocracy which was to be in sharp contrast to the rigid puritanical display of respectable Victorian middle-class society.

The upper ranks of the nobility and the wealthy landowners did not attempt or pretend to lead a life of solemnity and restraint. Maurice Quinlan (1941: 11) records: 'It was a notably calloused and cynical age. ... The best society, despite its wit, elegance and learning, was much preoccupied with drunken routs, foppery and seduction.' The illegitimate offspring of the noble and wealthy were acknowledged and maintained by their parents without comment or rebuke from society. Lord David Cecil, in *The Young Melbourne* (1939: 10–11) provides a kaleidoscopic sketch of 'the free and easy habits of the English aristocracy'. Lord Carlisle, when complaining of gout to a friend, could write: 'I believe I live too chaste: it is not a common fault with me.' To which Cecil added the postscript, 'It was not a common fault with any of them.' Nor were such faults confined to men: 'Among married women the practice [of having lovers] was too common to stir comment.' Even this audacious society's indulgence was stretched by the Duke and the Duchess of Devonshire jointly falling in love and forming a *ménage-à-trois* in 1782 with Lady Elizabeth Foster, the tale of which is retold in Brian Masters's biography of the Duchess, entitled *Georgiana*. The family consequences were that 'the Duke of Devonshire had three children by the Duchess and two by Lady Elizabeth Foster, the Duchess one by Lord Grey; and most of them were brought up together in Devonshire House, each set of children with a surname of its own' (Cecil 1939: 11). The Duke's (Canis) progeny was extended by Charlotte Spencer's child. This parental miscellany was tolerated by all concerned. Of Charlotte's child the Duchess could lovingly write to Lady Foster, 'Dear, dear Bess, . . . You are Canis's child's guardian angel' (Stone 1977: 533). Such natural children were accepted into the household nursery; they often took their father's name. As Trumbach (1978: 162) records, 'there were illegitimate Berties, Cecils, Fitzgeralds, Fitzroys, Gordons, Manners and Walpoles'. These children of the mist constituted no threat to the succession and inheritance of the legitimate heir.

This generosity of sexual freedom, and its forbearance of the consequences, depended upon the presence of a male heir; the family estate without a son lacked the certainty of continuation. Sexual waywardness by the wife who had not provided an heir was a threat to the purity of family succession. With a settled paternal heir, each spouse could afford to display a worldly tolerance to the other's extra-marital alliances.

The breezy, opportunistic morality of the traditional Whig ruling class was being replaced by the dry wind of puritanical sobriety and respectability. The spiritual righteousness of the evangelical movement gave a code of conduct that reinforced the traditional moral superiority of the middle classes. Submission to the tenets of Protestant faith required constant self-examination of temporal habit and behaviour if heaven's gates were to be unlocked at the expiration of earthly travail. As the industrial landscape of England spread, so increased the number of those whose respectability and worldly success were clear signs of their ordained ascendancy. Within this fellowship of propriety the Evangelicals mingled with the Dissenters and the Benthamites: all guarding against earthly temptation by a display of rectitude within the home and profitable endeavour at work. These new social attitudes led to the establishment in 1802 of the Society for the Suppression of Vice. The same rectitude caused Thomas Bowdler to publish in 1818 his *Family Shakespeare* in which, by 'judicious' expurgation of the bard's 'blemishes', and by paraphrase, he aimed to provide a text that a father could read to his family without risk of perverting their minds. Secure in his castle, the husband was guardian of the family virtue against the corruption that lay outside. This was a chaste morality that the Whigs such as Lord Palmerstone despised and the indigent could not afford.

The upper classes were not opposed to the enhancement of these rigid new attitudes and values. The shock of the French Revolution and its aftermath of the Napoleonic Wars had caused them to fear for their wealth and possessions. The new wind of virtue produces the principled Lord Auckland persistently attempting to ban the marriage of a divorced wife and her lover, and the worthy Bishop of Chichester desiring five years' imprisonment for adultery. The pattern, and enforcement, of morality was being reshaped by propriety's chisel.

The pleasures, satisfactions and rewards of companionship and affection became increasingly focused on the home. The patrician conjugal habits of compromise and toleration displayed by households like the Devonshires were not conventions of the expanding middle classes. Individualism and romanticism were combining with propriety to expurgate earlier standards and spawn new codes of acceptable behaviour. The new mores of domesticity no longer tolerated unchaste wives; her virtue was now the linchpin towards family happiness, while misconduct was an unpardonable iniquity. This sensorous attitude increasingly became the common form. Lady Charlotte Wellesley's judgement upon her own elopement with Lord Paget records this changing mood. When requested to return to her husband and four children, Lady Wellesley replied this was impossible 'after the Iniquitous Act she had been guilty of with Lord Paget' (Lewis 1986: 47).

The changing morality and conventions entwined with modifications to the practice and form of inheritance. At the same time inheritance patterns were themselves linked with changes in the patterns of wealth. Between the mid-eighteenth and mid-nineteenth centuries the predominant form of capital moved from real property to that of capital stock. Agriculture in 1760 still formed three-quarters (74 per cent) of Great Britain's national capital; by 1860 it had more than halved to 36 per cent (Feinstein 1981: table 7.1); such was the decline of agriculture and the growing importance of industrial and commercial wealth. This period of change witnessed the children of the bourgeoisie and the landed gentry becoming the beneficiaries of a more equitable inheritance policy. Each child now had some claim to the family wealth, although primogeniture remained the normal practice for those with land (Stone 1977: 654). The major part of the estate, including the family seat, might be settled by will or deed on the elder son, but the other children were provided with settlement of about one-third of the estate as compensation (Stone and Stone 1984: 82). By the mid-nineteenth century the middle class and 'the landless members of the upper orders' had recognised partible inheritance as a proper duty towards their children (Brodrick 1881: 97).

Industrial wealth in the form of stocks and shares allowed all children to have a ready and equitable slice of their father's wealth. Adultery by the wife now created a potentially wider and more threatening horizon of both legitimate and spurious family claimants. As the Lord Chancellor argued to Parliament in justification of the proposed 1857 divorce legislation's double standard, a wife could not be damaged by her husband's adultery and could forgive him 'without any loss of caste' but 'no one would venture to suggest' that he could condone her adultery because 'it might be the means of palming spurious offspring upon the husband' (*Hansard* 1857, vol. 145, col. 813).

CHANGING SOCIAL BACKGROUND OF PETITIONERS

The new industrial system and the accumulating industrial wealth of middle-class families encouraged the growth of partible inheritance. Alongside these changes came a severer morality that imposed even higher standards on women than on men. These social and attitudinal changes form a setting against which the changing background and social status of Parliamentary divorce petitioners can be analysed. This same backcloth also helps to explain why Parliamentary divorce did not remain a prerogative of the aristocracy.

Information extracted from the divorce papers filed in the House of Lords Library allowed the husband's status and occupation – when provided – to be recorded. Altogether, 13 per cent of the husbands were men of title. (Wolfram has a similar proportion.) Among the 12 per cent of commoners not designated 'esquire' or 'gentleman' by either their occupational status or sufficient ownership of land there appeared such miscellaneous occupations as portrait painter (1827, Grahame), chemist (1772, Hanckwitz), farmer (1766, Mathews), cabinet manufacturer (1832, Smith), linen draper (1847, Brooks) and piano maker (1839, Allison).

The peers (7 per cent) and knights (6 per cent) who successfully petitioned would almost certainly be landowners. But, at the same time, some of the great landowners were commoners who enjoyed far larger incomes than the less wealthy peers. The landed gentry were far from forming a homogeneous group. Table 3.2 suggests Parliamentary divorce procedure was predominantly used by upper and middle-class husbands, and that the latter had an increasingly important presence after 1760. Altogether nearly half (48 per cent) of all divorces were obtained by husbands occupied in some form of work activity.

As the middle class developed in numbers and power, and as evangelical morality became dominant, so one might expect an increasing resort to Parliamentary divorce. An indicator of such a movement would be an increasing proportion of petitioners who had occupational income. Divorce was seldom resorted to before 1750, then there was an increase to fourteen divorces in the decade 1750–9. In the years before 1760 nine out of ten successful petitioners were from the upper classes. Their strong association with the aristocracy is suggested by the finding that 30 per cent of all the husbands were titled.

The demographic characteristics of the pre-1760 divorcing husbands also

Table 3.2 Occupation of petitioner, by period of Divorce Act (per cent)

Occupation	Period				
	Pre-1760	1760–99	1800–39	1840–57	All divorces
Army, Royal Navy		12	22	19	17
Clergymen	4	5	6	7	6
Professional, bankers		11	12	17	12
Merchants	4	8	4	10	7
Clerks, artisans, other	4	11	5	4	6
Sub-total: occupationally active	12	47	49	57	48
No occupation recorded (gentry)	88	53	51	43	52
Total %	100	100	100	100	100
No.*	23	100	117	77	317

Notes: *Cases for which information was available.

(Occupation is, when shown, recorded in preference to status, i.e. a lawyer designated 'esq.' would be classified under 'professional'.)

differ from those of later periods in that the former group's *de facto* length of marriage was shorter and they were less likely to have sons. Thus, 44 per cent of the former couples separated within five years of marriage compared with 27 per cent for divorces occurring between 1760 and 1857. One explanation would be that these earlier divorces comprised mainly landowning husbands who were unprepared to countenance a wife's adultery if a legitimate son and heir had not yet been born. This was so for Acts before 1750, with only one of the fourteen divorced wives having a son of the marriage. But with the change in the form of wealth and inheritance all children became claimants, and a wife's adultery became an unforgivable sin. In moneyed circles such behaviour was thought to undermine the foundations of her family by fraudulently conspiring to place a cuckoo among the rightful nestling claimants to her husband's wealth. This helps to explain why by the period 1780–1819 the number of couples with sons had increased to 50 per cent. The latter finding suggests that from the mid-eighteenth century lack of an heir was no longer a characteristic of divorcing husbands.

The proportion of husbands who had earned incomes increased during the eighteenth and early nineteenth century, so that by the period 1800–39 they formed 49 per cent of all private Act divorces. A selection of cases in this period reflects the diversity of occupation; piano maker (Allison), clergyman (Blenkinsop), Navy lieutenant (Coode), butcher (Ellis), portrait painter (Grahame), barrister (Malpas) and Army captain (Shawe). Yet the remedy of Parliamentary divorce was a trickle that never exceeded ten Acts a year due to a combination of cost, legal barriers, judicial deprecation of Lord Chancellors and the social stigma discriminatingly attached to divorced women. The nineteenth-century petitions record the high proportion (21 per cent) formed by serving officers; also the surprisingly numerous appearances of clergymen, who clearly did not believe they contradicted their faith by seeking divorce. This analysis leads to the conclusion that 'by the beginning of the nineteenth century Private Acts of divorce were far from being a monopoly of those whose wealth and status came directly from real property' (Gibson 1972: 41). The work of Anderson (1984: 435) provides support for this view: 'it is striking how the ratio of upper to middle-class applicants remained roughly one to one during the century (1760–1857) under consideration'. The conclusion of Stone (1990: 356) largely agrees with the evidence of this chapter: 'Parliamentary divorce was the privilege of a plutocracy, composed half of members of the landed elite and half of rich professionals and businessmen.' (Table 3.2 suggests that between 1760 and 1857 there was a movement towards middle-class petitioners, but there are immense problems of classifying and coding occupation and status in this period.)

This section has attempted to present a broad canvas of the intertwining features that led to an increase in Parliamentary divorces after 1750. Some of these major social components were the new forms of wealth and the changing manner of inheritance that blended with the upper and middle classes' belief that all their children should have some slice of the inheritable cake. At the same time the middle classes increased in both numbers and influence, allowing their mores of sobriety and respectability to become the hallmarks of Victorian family virtue. Within the home, married women were their husband's subordinates, subjected to an Old Testament morality of submissiveness and unimpeachable chastity. The upholders of this code were more forgiving towards their own sex.

WIFE PETITIONERS

Discrimination was underlined by the Lords' attitude and practice towards women petitioners for divorce. There is record of only eight such wives, and they all petitioned between 1800 and 1857. Perhaps the most surprising aspect of this procedure is that petitions from married women were accepted at all and that four were favourably received.

As well as the expected proof of her husband's adultery, the wife had to provide additional evidence of his flagrant conduct. In the four successful cases the husband's adultery was compounded either by incest or bigamy. These latter two offences became the narrow Parliamentary perspective by which a husband's unacceptable matrimonial behaviour was judged. The first Act was granted to Mrs Jane Addison in 1801 after proof of incestuous adultery by the husband Edward with her sister Jessy Campbell. (Jessy's husband James Campbell, a doctor residing in Bengal, obtained a divorce a few months later naming Edward as co-respondent, having obtained damages of £5,000 against him in 1798.) Under the pre-Reformation rules of carnal affinities, it was legally impossible for the Addisons to renew a marital relationship, for this would be incestuous following the adultery of Edward with his wife's sister. Such concern caused Mrs Addison's petition to record that 'aggravated circumstances precluded every possibility of reconciliation in so much that your petitioner would consider herself morally guilty of the crime of incest'. The Lords were moved by the canonical logic of this plea to grant a divorce, have the son and daughter removed from Mr Addison and made wards of Chancery (though custody of the daughter was given to the mother), and to forbid the future marriage of Edward and Jessy. The next divorce obtained by a wife was that of Mrs Turton in 1831. Her petition recorded similar grounds and circumstances to those of Mrs Addison, namely that her unmarried sister Adeline had borne two children by Mr Turton. Mrs Ann Battersby's Act of 1840 and Mrs Georgina Hall's Act of 1850 both similarly followed their respective husband's conviction for bigamy.

It was not simply legal disparity that caused only a minute number of wives to seek redress. Married women were financially dependent on their husbands. Few women had the independent means to pay the very high expenses required for private Acts. Wives with property at marriage had no protection against unscrupulous husbands until the end of the eighteenth century when the granting to women of separate estates in equity became a more generally accepted family practice. But at the same time the development of restraint upon anticipation spread so that even a married woman with property settled for her separate use could only receive the current income it produced. This revenue alone might be an entirely insufficient sum to pay the costs of a Parliamentary divorce. Nor could wives look to awards of damages as a means of covering legal costs and fees.

The rejected wives' Bills underline the biased Lords' weighting of sex. Mrs Teush's petition of 1805 complained of husband Frederick's 'shameful profligacy' that had led to his mistress's three children. The petition was rejected on the convoluted grounds of public morality, as were her next two attempts. When Frederick and his mistress acquired a Scottish home, the tenacious Mrs Teush seized her opportunity and petitioned the Edinburgh court. This time her perseverance was readily and properly rewarded. Mrs Moffat's Bill of 1832 failed in the Lords by sixteen votes to nine, following Lord Chancellor Brougham's criticism that successful wife petitions must be 'extra-ordinary in their enormity'. The Lords also rejected Mrs Ann Dawson's plea in 1848, and on five other occasions, 'because in their opinion it would have tended to relax neccessary safeguards' (Clifford 1885: 418). It was of no consequence that the dissolute husband had coerced Ann into a clandestine marriage when she was fifteen, frequently flogged her, beat his son and fathered children on two other women. None of this evidence restrained Lord Campbell from believing that Mrs Dawson's Bill did not show anything which 'would prevent the parties once more living together as good Christians' (*The Times*, quoted in Horstman 1985: 43). It was never a procedure intended to benefit wives.

CRITICISM OF PARLIAMENTARY DIVORCE

The efficacy of Parliamentary divorce came under increasing attack from Utilitarian critics. They believed the procedure to be an awkward and grossly partial expedient creating grave injustice for the great majority denied benefit. Similar complaint had been directed towards the outdated ways of the ecclesiastical courts, though the common lawyers – ever on the lookout for new business – had a vested interest in hastening their closure. The related questions of cost and access to legal remedy were some of the issues directed towards the Royal Commission formed in 1850 with the directives to 'enquire into the present state of the Law of Divorce . . . and more particularly into the mode of obtaining a Divorce *a vinculo matrimonii*, in this country'.

The Commission, under the chairmanship of Lord Campbell, reported in 1853 that when the costs and fees of ecclesiastical and civil litigation had been included, the cheapest divorce 'can hardly be less than £700 or £800; and when the matter is much litigated, it would probably reach some thousands'. They concluded: 'The great expense and the long delay of these proceedings is a grievous hardship and oppression to individuals, and they amount in many cases to a denial of justice' (Report 1853: 21). Their evidence suggested that an unopposed church court suit cost a minimum of between £120 and £140, while Parliamentary proceedings were at least £200 with an additional £50 to £100 for lawyers' fees and witnesses' expenses.

There is reason to believe that the Campbell Commission was not always as separated from the interests of the reformist common lawyers as judicious detachment required. The Commission may also have overstated the cost of the average divorce suit, partly because no allowance was made for the damages and costs that a husband might obtain from the civil court. Anderson (1984: 442) takes this latter factor into account in his calculations for the period 1821–57, and concludes that 'about half the petitioners can be estimated to have paid less than £475 for their divorce Act'. Wolfram (1987: 81) similarly believes the 1853 Commission exaggerated the cost of divorce. But it needs to be remembered that husbands did not always enforce payment, or increasingly after 1830 even seek damages. Yet even if the overall net cost of divorce is lowered to around £450, the amount is still more than most middle-class men could earn in a year. A brief review of that period's income pattern supports this argument. Eighty per cent of the population in mid-nineteenth century England and Wales were classified as working class, with average earnings of less than £100 a year. At this time entry into the middle class might still be acquired for as little as £60 a year (Burnett 1969: 247, 234).

The next objection to Parliamentary divorce came from those who wished for a wholly secular jurisdiction to handle all matrimonial disputes. It was the aristocracy who, unknowingly, had already helped to clear the path to secular divorce by being the instrumental group behind the state's insistence in 1753 that celebration of marriage could take place only in an Anglican church. The Marriage Act of 1753 forced Catholics and Dissenters to flout either the law or their consciences, and led finally to the Marriage Act of 1836 which broke the Church of England's exclusive control over marriage by establishing an alternative and wholly secular rite.

The attitudes and opinions of advocates of secular divorce were expressed by Hector Morgan: 'There is a partiality in the law, in giving to the rich man a means of redress which the poor cannot obtain; and which, if it were dispensed at all, should be dispensed equally and fairly before the legal tribunals' (1826: 261). The middle class understood who 'the poor' were in this matter.

Seventeen years before the Report of the first Royal Commission on divorce was published, Lord Campbell (then Sir John) had declared his views on private Acts of divorce.

> It was a disgrace to the House of Commons, and to the House of Lords, and to the whole country, that whilst marriages by the law of the land were indissoluble, they could be dissolved by prerogative. When the case of a divorce Bill was before either House, and witnesses were examined at the Bar, the whole proceeding was a mere farce – a most expensive farce, it was true – but a farce that brought no credit at all to any party.
>
> (*Hansard* 1836, vol. 26, col. 915)

This was to be the majority opinion within Parliament in 1857 when the Church of England's control over matrimonial jurisdiction was transferred to the secular courts, thereby abolishing the necessity for private Act divorces in England and Wales.[2]

4   The coming of judicial divorce

The two centuries between the Restoration in 1660 and the introduction of civil divorce in 1857 was a period within the history of England and Wales when validly contracted marriages remained judicially indissoluble. Parliament did not make any attempt to change this policy until the latter end of this period but, instead, directed its attention towards the evils connected with the formation of marriage. Until the Marriage Act of 1753 it had been the Church's prerogative to declare what were the acceptable ways of contracting a recognizable and valid marriage and to judge upon the lawfulness of disputed marriages. Intervention by the state in 1753 challenged the Church's former monopoly. This new legislation would eventually force Parliament to be equally concerned about providing a more rational legal route out of a calamitous marriage than that offered by the existing costly and protracted itinerary that led to the House of Lords and a private Act of divorce.

Towards regulated marriage

At this stage it becomes necessary once more to examine briefly the history of the English law of marriage and its intimate relationship with canon law. A consequence of the Church's view that marriage was a counterbalance to man's natural tendency towards promiscuity and sin had led canon law to adopt a presumption in favour of marriage. The clerical shepherds tolerated liberal admission into the matrimonial fold for fear of the Devil's embrace upon their flock.

Marriage had by 1700 become a formless contract whose variations of matrimonial ceremony created a problem of readily knowing whether the couple were married, espoused or still formally single. Uncertainty became the cost of accepting a variety of forms of private marriage.

The retention of unreformed ecclesiastical marriage law led to the continued existence of clandestine marriages. Areas of London became notorious for the ease with which a marriage could be contracted; the service, such as it was, being conducted by those passing as clerics. The most celebrated area in London for such marriages was around the Fleet. Sometimes over a hundred couples were married in this manner by one clergyman in the same day. An exponent of such work was the Reverend Alexander Keitt who, between 1709 and 1740, is recorded to have 'solemnized' some 36,000 marriages, while another Fleet parson earned £75 in October 1748 for his services. The keeping of the registers recording clandestine marriages was a scandal. They were easily falsified; bribery would result in the marriage being predated, or the record being lost or destroyed. The ease of contracting marriage and the absence of formal records created doubt around the legality of individual clandestine marriages and the legitimacy of their offspring. Though the trend of the law had been to make matrimony easy to contract, the Tudor curtailment of a liberal annulment policy had now made the institution almost escape-proof.

Marriage was a means by which the diffusion of capital, status and title between two families could be beneficially cemented together. But the proprietary interests of the wealthy were endangered by the dubiety of valid, though irregular, marriage processes. The eighteenth century was beginning to witness the challenge to patriarchal authority; individualism was spreading, and more young people had opportunity to read or view romantic works. Such spirit caused the eighteen-year-old Lord Tankerville to elope with Camilla Colville, the daughter of a butcher; the Bennett family failed to break the marriage and the new Countess eventually became a Lady of the Bedchamber to Queen Caroline (Cannon 1984: 75). A marriage process that admitted children's mercurial emotions of the moment rather than the consideration and settlement of paternal approval put family wealth and prestige in jeopardy. Unsanctioned alliances could readily dissipate and even destroy the diligence of earlier generations. The heir or heiress could find a carousing evening transformed into a more sober morn, wedded to yesterday's stranger.

The nature of property and its method of transmission were changing to meet the needs of an industrializing society. Wealth was increasingly contained outside realty; such personalty could be in the form of money, company stock or leasehold investment. Developing usage of strict settlements and partible inheritance gave all children an allotted share of the family wealth. This portion could not be reduced later even if children displeased their father.

The concern of the nobility and upper middle class, fearing loss of the family fortune by the clandestine marriage of an heir or heiress, resulted in increasing pressure upon Parliament to regularize the marriage laws of England. The desired legislative bridle was secured by Lord Hardwicke's Marriage Act of 1753 for 'the better prevention of clandestine marriages'. Critics in the House of Commons feared that the cost of the proposed obligatory church service would deter marriage and thereby cause depopulation. A further fear was that curtailment of heirs or heiresses eloping with their straitened lovers would reduce social mobility and lessen the opportunity for the wealth of the rich to find its way into the pockets of the poor. Even eugenicist reasoning came into Parliamentary debate, with one MP declaring:

> If this Bill passes, our quality and rich families will daily accumulate riches by marrying only one another; and what sort of breed their offspring will be, we may easily judge: if the gout, the gravel, the pox and madness are always to

wed together, what a hopeful generation of quality and rich commoners shall we have amongst us?

(Hansard 1753, vol. xv: 15)

The passing of the 1753 Act meant that a variety of modes of marriage were replaced by one constituted form. Marriages were now to be valid only if celebrated by an ordained priest of the Church of England in a church or a chapel. The only exceptions were Jews and Quakers who were permitted to celebrate their own marriages. The Act forbade the solemnization of marriage without banns or licence; those under the age of majority – then twenty-one – required parental consent. The benefits of the legislation were that marriage was now recognized as a public contract subject to a formal process of authentication set by state regulation and enforced by secular courts. But the price for bureaucratic certainty was the rekindling of community divisions; everybody, including Dissenters and Roman Catholics, had either to marry according to the ritual of the established religion or remain unmarried. In essence the marriage ceremony was (and remains) a civil act contracted before a licensed clergyman (or registrar – as permitted today), but its spiritual significance was internal and personal only to the faithful. Critics were expected to take a pragmatic view but, instead, saw the Act's observance as another example of the intolerable intrusion of the Church of England's authority into community life and family affairs.

The stringent provisions of the Marriage Acts of 1753 and 1823 led to defiance by those whom the law aimed to control. Growing pressure, especially from an increasingly vocal body of Dissenters, eventually led to the removal of this grievance by the Marriage Act of 1836. Non-Anglicans, in addition to Jews and Quakers, were permitted to conduct marriage ceremonies in their own places of worship. Of greater significance was the establishment of a civil marriage ceremony conducted by state officials in register offices. English law now recognized the validity of a marriage ceremony which was purely civil in character and completely divorced from any religious element. Those wishing to marry now had the choice of either religious or secular vows of marriage.

The needs of a Malthusian era imbued with Utilitarian ideals required demographic facts to service the efficient administration of an expanding urban population. Such an outlook had contributed to the formation in 1801 of a national census programme. Against this backcloth came the Marriage Act of 1836, to be followed immediately by the Births, Deaths and Marriages Registration Act. The two Acts brought into being registrars and superintendent registrars, and with them bureaucratized central collation of the new civil registration requirements. The registration of marriages had now become a civil act rather than an ecclesiastical exercise.

Parliament had partly conceded the rational consequences that followed its breaking of the exclusive dominion of old canon law principles in 1753. But logically it also followed that if the state insisted it control the formation of all marriages, then jurisdiction for their subsequent regulation should also be in its hands. The question which then arose was, if marriage was now permitted to all at a nominal cost in civil registry offices after 1836, then why should not divorce also be made readily available in the civil courts? Yet at this time matrimonial law was still administered primarily in the ecclesiastical courts even though the parties may not have been members of the Church of England or even Christians. Reformers and conservatives alike appreciated that a civil contract was contrary to the ecclesiastical theory of marriage. By the mid-nineteenth century such problems and paradoxes were becoming an increasing embarrassment which Parliament was hard put to justify.

A SOCIETY WITHOUT DIVORCE

Until 1753 marriages could be dissolved under the old canon law of nullity, which accepted that pre-contract to another person prior to this marriage created a bigamous, and therefore void, union. But this exit for disaffected couples disappeared with Lord Hardwicke's Act, and so between 1753 and the coming of civil divorce in 1857 it was legally impossible to sever the bonds of an unhappy marriage except by the costly private Act procedure or the now limited law of nullity, or through mortality. We know the poor were very poor. Low wages made it impossible for working men to provide their families with anything other than the bare necessities of life. Families were often left destitute by unemployment, desertion, sickness or death of a parent. It is clear that the great majority of the unhappily married did not have the money necessary to attempt legal action in ecclesiastical courts, let alone contemplate going on to seek a private Act of Parliament.

The harsh family life-chances of pre-industrial times are underlined by the unusually precise demographic record of parishioners kept by William Sampson, the rector of Clayworth village in Nottinghamshire. Sampson's evidence for Clayworth in 1688 leads Laslett (1977: 165) to conclude that a good two-fifths of all the village's unmarried dependent young persons were bereaved of a parent. Remarriage was an appropriate solution to widowhood, so that up to one-third of all marriages in Stuart England were second, or later, marriages for one of the partners. The marital experience of John Brason, the Clayworth village butcher in 1688, illustrates this hard family world. Brason, by the age of forty, had buried three wives and was married for a fourth time. But not all marriages were concluded by death. Only a recluse could imagine that the practical impossibility of divorce enforced a state of matrimonial attachment for all those who had vowed lifelong affiliation.

What, then, did the great majority of these married people do when a marriage broke down through incompatability or desertion? Unfortunately we cannot answer with any certainty for there is little sound empirical evidence upon which to base reliable conclusions. All that can be done is to make generalizations based upon the subjective evidence of eighteenth- and nineteenth-century writers. Such material provides the best indicator of the nature of marriage breakdown in past times. This evidence suggests that dishonour of marriage vows was not stifled by the *de facto* impossibility of divorce.

The social unreality of describing England and Wales as a 'divorceless society' is corroborated by Randle Lewis. He records in 1805: 'It is a lamentable truth that scarcely a week passes without advertisement in some of the daily prints, publishing the parting by elopement, adultery, agreement or otherwise of some unhappy pair. A much greater number separate without that unnecessary step' (Lewis 1805: 63). Some of the reported separations and desertions were a result of the harsh labouring conditions and debt pressing down on some men, provoking the husband to abandon his family and disappear. The needs of deserted, destitute wives had caused Joseph Massie to propose (1758: 3) the establishment of charity houses (workhouses). Almost a century later the Poor Law officers in London's Shoreditch district were placing in newspapers the description of fifty-four men charged with deserting their wives and families, and offering rewards for their apprehension (Menefee 1981: 26).

It seems likely that wives did not often leave their husbands unless marital conditions were so unbearable as to make desertion the only solution. A woman alone and with children to maintain was in danger in the society of that time. The only remedies for destitute wives were resort to the Poor Law with all its known miseries, prostitution, or finding another man willing to support her. Men were more able to find new work and so husbands were better placed to leave their wives. The restrictive marriage laws together with the economic disparity that existed within the population, and also between the sexes, resulted in some strange customs. Some of these were disregard of marriage formalities, desertion, wife sales and bigamy.

Informal remedies

The 1753 legislative trespass on popular habit curtailed the previously recognized clandestine marriage ceremony. Marriage regulation and the denial of divorce together encouraged popular resort to existing alternative informal arrangements acknowledged and accepted by local custom and lore as constituting a marriage form even though these practices lay outside the legal framework. Those who had grown up with these modes, or who disliked the established marriage ceremony and its cost, or who lived some distance from an Anglican church, had especial reason to disregard official rules in favour of private ordering. For much of this time official records either do not exist or are weak in content, and there is danger in accepting the evidence of anecdotal antiquarianism. Yet when the available sources are examined there does appear to be some disregard of marriage from within the lower-income population. Evidence for the century following the 1753 Act leads Gillis to suggest some 15 to 20 per cent of couples lived outside legal marriage. Characteristically such irregular unions were contracted by popular local customary ceremony. The popularity of these rites in rural areas is seen in the Ceiriog Valley, Wales, where the parish baptism registers from 1768 to 1805 indicate 60 per cent of all recorded births were attributed to non-marital conjugal arrangements (Gillis 1985). These informal rituals incorporated some public token of each partner's free acceptance of the other within a relationship accepted as one of marriage by the local community. The union was symbolically legitimated before friends and relatives through such folk traditions as the exchange of rings, offering the key to the door, or the couple 'jumping the broom' over a besom brush.

Within the new factory landscape of industrial Britain Victorian moralists recorded their deprecatory vision of inner-city tenement cohabitation that disregarded both official and unofficial ceremony. One contemporary account of Manchester working girls' behaviour records: 'It is true; many of the factory girls consider themselves chaste, because they do not live unchaste, but "tally" [that means young people living together without being married] with some young men' (Shaw 1843: 28). Many of them were not aware of the officially prescribed formalities. This disregard of formal marriage was prevalent among the railway navvies of the 1840s (Coleman 1965: 187, 194). The number of officially recorded illegimate births in 1851 led the Registrar General (*Census* 1851: XLIV) to conclude that one in thirteen of the unmarried women of England and Wales were 'living irregularly'. It is hardly surprising that the absence of available and effective legal relief led to the formation of other informal remedies for treating matrimonial ills within England's divorceless society. In the late eighteenth century a number of working men believed that they had the right to sell their wives. It was supposed by some that the disposal of the wife as a chattel with a halter round her neck in the market-place legally severed the marriage. Others recognized both the legal sterility and the folk acceptability of the sale. The presence of a halter was a symbolic gesture intended to deprive the husband of any future right to sue the purchaser for criminal conversation damages. The wife no longer had any further claims on her husband for support as, so the folk belief went, all rights and duties had passed to the purchaser. In law the husband did not commit an offence if the wife consented (as she usually did) to be sold but, as he had connived at her adultery, he would still be held legally liable for maintenance. A fabricated sale acted as a community *rite de passage*, whereby the marketplace provided public witness to the parties' willing agreement to the exchange of rights and duties. The halter's association with cattle firmly establishes the wife's worth within the property table gauchely presented by Petruchio in *The Taming of the Shrew*:

> She is my goods, my chattels; she is my house,
> My household stuff, my field, my barn,
> My horse, my ox, my ass, my anything.

The husband's 'anything' could still be described in Sir William Blackstone's *Commentaries* (1783) as 'the inferior [who] have no kind of property in the company, care, or assistance of the superior as the superior is held to have in those of the inferior; and therefore the inferior can suffer no loss or injury'. And, like Petruchio, the 'superior' could sell 'what is my own'.

These sales were, whatever the intention, humiliating experiences for women. The extensive study by Menefee (1981: 211–59) records that between the mid-eighteenth and nineteenth centuries there were almost 300 references to wife sales in England. It is a relief to note that there is no account of an Englishman being sold by his wife! This commerce occurred in a society where labour was bought and sold, and indenture and apprenticeship were often only a few rungs above slavery – which itself was only officially abolished in 1807; in which children were sold by parents and where servants would be engaged in the marketplace at the time of mop fairs.

Thomas Hardy's *The Mayor of Casterbridge* could shock Victorian sensibilities by its graphic narrative of Michael Henchard's drunken disposal of his wife at Weydon-Priors fair. It was not only fiction that provided accounts of wife sales. The urbane wit of *The Times* of 1779 extended itself to comment:

> By some mistake or omission, in the report of the Smithfield market we have not learned of the average price of wives for the last week. The increasing value of the fair sex is esteemed by several eminent writers as the certain criterion of increasing civilisation. Smithfield has, on this ground, strong pretensions to refined improvement, as the price of wives has risen in that market from half a guinea to three guineas and a half.
>
> (Mueller 1957: 568)

On a similar sale in 1797 the same newspaper unctuously observed: 'Pity it is, there is no stop put to such depraved conduct in the lower order of people', while a year earlier it had recommended that 'It would be well if some law was enforced to put a stop to such degrading traffic.' The sale of a wife at Knaresborough in 1807 for sixpence and a quid of tobacco was reported by *The Morning Post* as 'one of those disgraceful scenes which have, of late, become too common' (Ashton 1886: 66).

However offensive the practice may have been, the parish administrators of the Old Poor Law were not beyond using such customary habit to rid themselves of unwanted financial liability. In the bizarre case of Henry Cook, whose wife and child were in the Effingham workhouse, the husband was persuaded by the parish officers to sell his wife. The master of the workhouse took Mrs Cook to Croydon market and sold her for one shilling, while the parish officers, relieved to be rid of their charge, paid the expenses of the journey and the cost of the 'wedding' dinner (Pinchbeck 1930: 83). (The unfortunate Mrs Cook was later deserted by her second 'husband' when he realized the invalidity of their marriage. The parish officials appealed unsuccessfully to the magistrates to get Henry to maintain his wife and her now larger family.) The treatment of Mrs Cook underlines the state to which wives were reduced by their inferior economic position, legal status and social condition.

The continuous nineteenth-century reporting of such auctions and sales within plebeian society indicates that the practice met a folk need. The custom acted as a safety valve socially by legitimating the breakdown of old and the formation of new relationships within a state that severely restricted access to divorce. It was a popularly sanctioned ritual that provided *de facto* divorce and remarriage in one speedy transaction. Both legislator and judiciary turned a blind eye as long as there were no outrageous transgressions from the informally established pattern. There had developed a twofold system for dealing with matrimonial casualties: the lower income groups fabricated informal and unapproved measures, the wealthy had the means to face the formal but costly Parliamentary procedure. But the majority in the middle received little assistance from either route.

Committing bigamy was one possible method by which the already married person could clothe a new liaison with social respectability. Those who were detected and prosecuted often received judicial clemency. William Hawes, whose wife had been cohabiting with another man for sixteen years, received one week's hard labour in 1855. The judge commented that 'this was one of those cases which showed the present defective state of the law . . . and the consequence was that, owing to the enormous expense of obtaining a divorce, it amounted to an absolute denial of relief to the mass of society' (Menefee 1981: 25). But in an age in which centralized checking of marriage certificates was not attempted, the true extent of 'successful' bigamous marriages remains unknown. But official statistics show that though England had a population six times larger than that of Scotland, it had forty-three times as many court proceedings for bigamy. MacQueen (1858: 34) associated this difference to the availability of divorce in Scotland and prophesied the crime would decline in England 'because when divorce is available the temptation to commit bigamy will no longer arise'. At this point it becomes necessary to examine the system of Scottish divorce: first, because of its very existence over the period of time when Parliament effectively prohibited divorce to all but the wealthy citizens of England and Wales, and secondly, as the only means of entering a second marriage open to married English persons other than by a Parliamentary divorce.

Scottish divorce

A comparison between the two countries shows how different their respective divorce procedures had turned out to be. When papal supremacy was thrown off in 1534, Scotland came out of the schism far better than England and Wales. Calvinism held that the sin of adultery was such as to dissolve the innocent spouse's contractual obligation to lifelong partnership. Consequently, since 1560 both the ecclesiastical law and the civil law of Scotland had permitted the remedy of divorce *a vinculo*. The difference in legal costs between the two procedures was highlighted by the Campbell Commission which reported (Report 1853 54–5) that: 'The average cost of rescinding a marriage in Scotland is £30. Where there is no opposition, £20 will suffice. . . . The parties litigant [the ninety-five petitioners granted a divorce in the five-year period November 1836 to November 1841] were almost all of the humbler classes.' In more than one-third of these ninety-five cases the wife succeeded in obtaining a divorce against her husband. In short, the Scottish process was open to all classes and the law made no distinction between the sexes on the usage of the acceptable grounds of adultery or malicious desertion for four or more years.

The cost of transport to Scotland, together with the necessary period of residence there, meant that the possibility of Scottish divorce was out of the question for the majority of the population. The opening of the railways intensified the fear of some in the south that the remedy of Scottish divorce might be made too common. The general availability of civil divorce in Scotland compared with our restrictive Parliamentary procedure was one of the factors that led critics to discuss the efficiency of the English practice.

Need for reform

One of the principal factors leading to the Matrimonial Causes Act of 1857, as Chapter 2 noted, was increasing middle-class discontent at the working and procedure of the ecclesiastical courts. The law reform movement was led by Utilitarian thinkers like Sir Samuel Romilly and Jeremy Bentham. Such men were motivated by a wish to rationalize the legal process rather than a desire to assist the poorer classes greater access to civil courts. Utilitarian advocates of divorce reform observed with approval the system of civil divorce operating in Scotland and European countries such as France and Germany.

In post-Revolutionary France, rejection of the old ecclesiastical regime led to the introduction of unimpeded divorce in 1792. This new liberal attitude towards the family allowed some 20,000 divorces to occur in the nine main cities of France in the eleven years 1792 to 1803 (Phillips 1988: 257). Though consensual divorce in France was severely restricted in 1803, the influence of such radical Continental legislation was brought to the attention of the middle class by the writings of Utilitarian reformers. The realism of Bentham led him to observe (1789: 225) that, 'The rule of liberty would produce fewer stray families than the law of conjugal captivity. Render marriages dissoluble and there would be more apparent separations but fewer real ones.' Bentham went on to argue that the number of broken marriages need not necessarily increase with the introduction of judicial divorce, though immorality would be reduced. Consequent history of divorce in this country shows that the theme of 'immorality' has always remained in the forefront of divorce law reform debate.

The fundamental principle of legislation for Bentham was that 'the public good ought to be the object of legislation'. In comparison with the divorce laws of France and Germany the choice of legal redress available in England seemed most unsatisfactory, especially in the treatment of wives. Here the only *de facto* remedy available to a wife whose husband was guilty of adultery or cruelty was the ecclesiastical courts' decree of divorce *a mensa et thoro* which, as Lord Lyndhurst informed the House of Lords in 1856, put her,

> almost in a state of outlawry. She may not enter into a contract, or, if she does, she has no means of enforcing it. The law, so far from protecting, oppresses her. She is homeless, helpless, hopeless, and almost destitute of civil rights. She is liable to all manner of injustice, whether by plot or by violence. She may be wronged in all possible ways, and her character may be mercilessly defamed; yet she has no redress. She is at the mercy of her enemies. Is that

fair? Is that honest? Can it be vindicated upon any principle of justice, of mercy, or of common humanity?

(*Hansard* vol. 142: 410)

The danger of the separated wife's impoverishment was intensified by the law that still allowed her property, possessions and even earnings to be the right of the husband.

Behind the criticisms of the existing legal framework lay the overtones of those who argued that the wrong done to a spouse – especially the husband – could only be remedied by divorce *a vinculo*. Hector Morgan (1826: 257) believed that 'if justice require that the wrongs of the husband should be redressed by a divorce, the redress should be more expeditious, more within the reach of every man'. (Morgan was no different from the majority of fellow legal writers in refusing to acknowledge that the rights of the wife should be considered in any future divorce reform.) The Reverend Martin Madan writing in 1781 saw no reason why divorce should not operate for all husbands as a remedy for the innocent and punishment for the guilty: 'Why is such a one to be forced to live with an adulteress; to maintain by the sweat of his brow the children of other people; to suffer all the miseries and inconveniences which a profligate wife may bring upon him?' Such critics felt that the sanctity of family life required an accessible remedy to punish the transgressor (man's failure could be more readily forgiven) and buttress the virtuous.

Books by notable writers, such as Disraeli's *Sybil* in 1845 and Dickens's *Hard Times* in 1854, described working-class life and conditions as it actually was, with all its hardships and financial impoverishment. Stephen Blackpool, the poor factory labourer in *Hard Times*, was informed that there was a law to help break the marriage bonds holding him to his drunken wife but, as Mr Bounderby observed, 'It [a Parliamentary Act] is not for you at all. It costs money. . . . I suppose from a thousand to fifteen hundred pounds, perhaps twice the money.' The existing financial barriers to the possibility of a second marriage following breakdown of the first had resulted in sections of the working classes developing over the years a sub-culture which allowed deviancy from the expected code of behaviour of their betters. The resultant wife sales, desertion, disregard of marriage formalities and bigamous marriages have already been described. The criminal court records showed a number of cases in which bigamous husbands were brought to trial even though the evidence clearly proved that their original wives had deserted without cause or justification. Such husbands saw bigamy as the only course if they wished to set up home with another woman and provide her and any children of the liaison with the socially and legally expected aura of marriage to cover their cohabitation.

In sentencing the luckless Hall for bigamy at Warwick Assizes in 1845, Mr Justice Maule gave vent to a classic piece of sustained irony, the report of which gave an impetus to the movement for a change in the law. (There were many versions of this trial: the account is Lord Campbell's.) The prisoner was informed about the procedure he should have undertaken before marrying again.

'You ought to have brought an action for criminal conversation; that action would have been tried by one of Her Majesty's Judges at the Assizes; you would probably have recovered damages; and then you should have instituted a suit in the ecclesiastical court for divorce *a mensa et thoro*. Having got that divorce, you should have petitioned the House of Lords for a divorce *a vinculo*, and should have appeared by counsel at the bar of their Lordships' House. Then, if the Bill passed, it would have gone down to the House of Commons; the same evidence would possibly be repeated there; and if the Royal Assent had been given after that, you might have married again. The whole proceeding would not have cost you more than £1,000.' The prisoner: 'Ah, my Lord, I never was worth a thousand pence in all my life.' Mr Justice Maule: 'That is the law, and you must submit to it.' Hall's final comment was, 'That is a hard measure to us who are poor people, and cannot resort to the remedy which the law has afforded to the rich.'

(*Hansard* 1856, vol. 142: 1985)

The grave sarcasm of the judge represented a state of things wellnigh intolerable, and reform of the law was felt to be inevitable. There was a disparity of matrimonial justice, not only between the rich and the poor, but also between the very rich and the increasingly powerful middle class. The 1832 Reform Act had given the urban middle-class male the vote; it resulted in aristocratic rule by consent rather than by prescription. Aristocratic politicians had no wish to see a basically middle-class party created to oppose them, and so it was essential for their continuing control of power that attention should be paid to the most independent and rapidly growing section of the electorate. The middle classes, as the Whig Prime Minister Earl Grey acknowledged, formed 'the real and efficient mass of public opinion, and without them the power of the gentry is nothing'. The latter's self-imposed contraction of its previous power and privilege resulted in reforms within the Church, the Civil Service and the Universities of Oxford and Cambridge, as well as the abolition of both church rates and the landed property qualifications for MPs. Mr Kennedy, Whig MP for Ayr, appreciated it was 'of the utmost importance to associate the middle with the higher orders of society, in the love and support of the institutions and government of the country' (Gash 1953: 15). The middle class were no longer prepared to accept anything less than that which had been available to the aristocratic and governing classes for the previous 200 years.

The authority of the Established Church in both spiritual and secular matters had weakened since 1800. At the same time, the numbers of Dissenters had increased, forming a fifth of the country's population in 1811. By the mid-nineteenth century half of those attending church were non-Anglicans composed mainly of dissenting Nonconformists. The increasingly powerful influence of the latter is reflected by the general election of 1847 which returned twenty-six MPs from the middle-class Dissenting party, with Church disestablishment among its objectives; while a further thirty-four MPs were pledged to the same aim. Their supporters detested the power of the Established Church in all fields of social and political life. Its patronage in the administration of the laws of marriage and divorce was only one aspect of the Church of England's linkage with the Roman Church which the Dissenters disliked so intensely and wished to see abolished. Largely due to middle-class criticism of the outmoded divorce procedure, the Whig government formed a Royal Commission in 1850, under the chairmanship of Lord John Campbell, to inquire into the state of the law relating to matrimonial offences.

Establishing judicial divorce

Lord Campbell, as Chairman of the Commission, diligently followed the advice he gave his brother: 'For God's sake do not become a radical.' But the urgent legal and social problems facing the Commission needed investigation and solution. If it was decided that the ecclesiastical courts had outlived their usefulness, then what type of secular court was to replace the old system? The Commission recommended in their Report of 1853 that a 'new tribunal shall be constituted to try all questions of divorce'. But if they were finally to recommend transferring the divorce jurisdiction to a secular court, then should the House of Lords' tradition of allowing divorce *a vinculo* only upon the suit of the husband be the new practice? The Commission's recommendation was that no change should take place and 'that divorces *a vinculo* shall only be granted on the suit of the husband and not (as a general rule) on the suit of the wife'.

Concerning the most important social question of whether the poor and lower income groups should have reasonable access to secular divorce, the Commissioners gave no view. After noting that the likely cost of divorce *a vinculo* was never less than £700 or £800 in England, they observed that 'in Scotland divorce was a right for all'. But the idea of Scottish practice coming southwards was not to the Commission's liking. They quoted with approval Sir James Mackintosh's belief that: 'To make the dissolution of marriage in the proper case alike accessible to all, is one of the objects to which, in great cities, and in highly civilized countries, it is hardest to point out a safe road' (Report 1853: 15). Lord Redesdale, in dissenting from the majority recommendation of a constrained system of judicial divorce, foresaw the likely outcome of his colleagues' proposals was to be that:

> These divorces will thus be opened to another and numerous class, but a still more numerous class will be equally excluded as at present. Once create an appetite for such licence by the proposed change, and the demand to be permitted to satisfy it will become irresistible.
>
> (Report 1853: 28–9)

It proved to be a remarkably accurate prediction.

The Commission does not appear to have inquired into the advisability of adding to the grounds for divorce, and the Bill which resulted from their Report did not attempt to alter existing law. The Matrimonial Causes Bill was passed upon its fourth attempt in 1857 after the first Bill had been presented to

Parliament by Lord Cranworth, the Lord Chancellor, on behalf of the government, in June 1854. Parliamentary debate provides insight into the minds of the legislators as they set the legally prescribed divorce procedure for the next eighty years. Parliamentary advocates of reform argued that over the previous two centuries divorce had been recognized by English law, and the grounds had already been established. They claimed that the Bill was basically a utilitarian inspired measure aiming to do no more than present a plan for the efficient procedural reorganization of divorce. It would transfer the exercise of judicial responsibility from the legislature to the judges.

The most active opposition came from a minority of bishops led by Wilberforce of Oxford and Kerr Hamilton of Salisbury, who upheld the sacramental nature of marriage, and who consequently believed that the Christian faith did not allow dissolution of marriage. Such a view was in direct contrast to the past attitude of bishops who, when sitting in the Lords, had neither protested against nor opposed private divorce Bills as being contrary to either secular or divine law. Lord Redesdale continued his criticism of the Bill's proposals, arguing that family stability was being threatened by such legislation: 'It was perfectly well known that a legal divorce was an impossibility, and to that circumstance might be traced the sacredness of the marriage tie among the lower orders of the English people which was so remarkable' (*Hansard* 1856, vol. 142: 410). Though the language was of the Victorian conservative, the argument against easing the divorce laws remained remarkably similar over the following century. Lord Redesdale was incorrect in his analysis of the 'lower orders' family habits, for they had long been forced into an acceptance of unofficial folk ways which, of necessity, bypassed the prescribed legal channels that dealt with marriage breakdown.

In a later Lords debate (*Hansard* 1857, vol. 145: 531), the Bishop of Oxford made a criticism that was to remain valid until the 1940s: believing that the Bill 'professed to give relief to persons to whom it would never reach'. A supporter of the Bill, Lord Lyndhurst, a former Lord Chancellor, argued with clear, forceful logic for a more drastic revision of the law in conformity with the practice of other countries. In refuting Lord Redesdale's prophesy that the Bill's legislation would lead to increased immorality and family breakdown, Lord Lyndhurst maintained:

> The direct tendency of the present law is to demoralise and degrade the lower classes. A man finds his wife committing adultery; he has no remedy; he cannot apply to a court of justice to dissolve his marriage; he therefore continues to live on with her, committing acts of brutal and degrading violence on her – or he turns her out and she goes to live with the adulterer. What is the effect of such a scene upon the lower orders of the people? . . . What, I should like to know, can be more destructive of the morality of the lower orders?
>
> (*Hansard* vol. 145: 500)

Like other Victorian and later reformers, Lord Lyndhurst appreciated that successful transformation of our laws governing divorce could best be achieved by showing that the victims of injustice were in moral danger.

When the Bill reached the Commons it was strongly attacked by Mr Gladstone for both its ecclesiastical and social wrongs, especially the sexual discrimination over grounds acceptable for divorce, which he regarded as immoral. Gladstone argued that divorce legislation would bring about the end of family life.

> At no time have the middle and lower classes of the English people known what it was to have marriage dissoluble. Take care, then, how you damage the character of your countrymen. You know how apt the English nature is to escape from restraint and control; you know what passion dwells in the Englishman.
>
> (*Hansard* vol. 147: 854)

Whatever sympathy might have been felt by members of the House of Commons for such views, they knew the opportunity of divorce had to be made available to at least the middle classes. After three months of acrimonious Parliamentary debate the objective of Prime Minister Lord Palmerstone was achieved. On 21 August 1857, the fourth Matrimonial Causes Bill passed its third reading in the House of Commons, receiving the Royal Assent one week later, and became law on New Year's Day 1858.

The Matrimonial Causes Act of 1857

The Act, as the Attorney General, Sir Richard Bethell, explained to the Commons in 1857,

> involved only long-existing rules and long established principles, and it was intended to give only a local judicial habitation to doctrines that had long been recognized as part of the law of the land, and for a century and a half administered in a judicial manner, although through the medium of a legislative assembly.
>
> (*Hansard* vol. 147: 718–19)

The adoption of adultery as the only ground acceptable for divorce underlined the new statute's familial links with private Act procedure. The legislation of 1857 was about procedure and process, the substantive law of divorce remained unchanged. As before, the husband could petition on the ground of his wife's adultery alone, but the wife had to prove her husband had been guilty of adultery, with the additional aggravation of either bigamy, rape, sodomy, bestiality, incest, cruelty or desertion for two years or more. Yet when it came to judicial separation – which replaced the ecclesiastical decree of divorce *a mensa et thoro* – the remedy was equally available to the husband or wife on the previous grounds of either adultery or cruelty, or the new ground of desertion for two years or more. But the double standard continued for divorce, and adultery remained the Victorian supreme marital sin. A spouse might desert home and family or be an alcoholic; such marriage-destroying behaviour did not equal adultery –

especially if it was the wife's infidelity. Thus the first main criticism of the Act was that both the ground and the double standard between husband and wife established by the House of Lords for divorce *a vinculo* were left unchanged. It was no wonder that Lord Campbell wrote in July 1857: 'I am very glad that the Divorce Bill finally passed the Commons framed almost exactly according to the recommendations of the Commission over which I had the honour to preside – preserving the law as it has practically subsisted for two hundred years' (Hardcastle 1881: 421).

The second imperfection was the legislators' unwillingness to break away from the ecclesiastical hold upon our matrimonial laws. The principles and procedures of matrimonial law as practised in the ecclesiastical courts were transferred into the new statute. Canon law had been converted, moulded and formed into a statute which could be dealt with by the courts dealing with the new procedure. By section 22 of the 1857 Act the new civil Divorce Court had, in suits other than divorce, to 'proceed and act and give relief on principles and rules which in the opinion of the said Court shall be as nearly as may be conformable to the principles and rules on which the Ecclesiastical Courts have heretofore acted and given relief'. Parliament remained unwilling at the inception of the new scheme to annex the new law from its pedigree of ecclesiastical court pre-Reformation canon law. The legislators were so successful in confining the Matrimonial Causes Act to canon law that an American scholar, Professor Howard, could still write fifty years later (1904: 109): 'It is, indeed, wonderful that a great nation, priding herself on a love of equity and social liberty, should thus for five generations tolerate an invidious indulgence, rather than frankly and courageously to free herself from the shackles of an ecclesiastical tradition!'

Because the 1857 legislation was no more than a continuation of private divorce Act practice, the legislators were impelled to codify those circumstances which had led to the rejection of private Bills. The new Act made connivance, condonation and collusion absolute bars to presenting a petition (section 30), while the petitioner's own adultery, delay, cruelty, desertion or conduct conducing to adultery were to become discretionary bars (section 31) in which 'the Court shall not be bound to pronounce such a decree'. Such wording was meant to give the judge an unfettered discretion in this matter. However, judge-made law was soon superimposed on the will of Parliament. In 1869, Lord Penzance laid down rules which were to govern the Divorce Court for many years. The Judge Ordinary held (*Morgan v. Morgan* and *Porter* (1869): L.R.IP & D.644) that 'a loose and unfettered discretion of this sort upon matters of such grave import, is a dangerous weapon to entrust to any Court, still more so to a single judge'.

Behind all this lay the belief that the sanctity of marriage required that the new divorce procedure continue to be a degrading process. Success was to be achieved only after a lengthy adversarial trial in which fault was proved against the respondent spouse. Either spouse could insist on contested matters of fact being tried by a jury (section 28); such was the trial process. This right was utilized, for 13 per cent of all divorce hearings in the period 1858–87 came before a jury (calculations upon *Judicial Statistics* for 1898, table G). In a salacious divorce trial of 1864, the jury's verdict in favour of the petitioner, Blanche Chetwynd, against a husband 'who had made his house a brothel, whose life was adultery, whose language was obscenity', brought applause from the courtroom spectators (quoted in Horstman 1985: 93). To the Victorian public, the successful petitioner was innocent, blameless and good; the convicted respondent was guilty, depraved and bad.

The possibility of the spouses' mutual consent to divorce was disallowed. In 1860 a new official, the Queen's Proctor, was appointed to ensure that the rules were obeyed. Part of his duties was to investigate cases of suspected spousal agreement or collusion in petitioning; these were practices that were abhorrent to the accusatorial process. Up to 1893 the number of instances of intervention were 426, or an annual rate of about thirteen. The Proctor's work was helped by the requirement that there would now be a statutory three-month delay – extended to six months in 1866 – before the divorce could be made absolute. These procedural barriers help to explain why some fifth of all petitioners between 1858 and 1887 failed to obtain a divorce.

The Act gave little encouragement to those Parliamentary members who had urged that the localized County courts should be given matrimonial jurisdiction. But the Attorney General was not willing to see the County courts 'charged with the duty of trying the question of adultery'. As he explained, divorce should be accessible but not too accessible. This meant that the parties, their lawyers and witnesses still had to proceed from their home area to the newly created Divorce Court in London. All these restrictive conditions were intended to discourage divorce and thereby, so it can be argued, buttress the respectability and unity of the conventional Victorian family. Both the unreformed but now statutory divorce law and the attached new process for seeking divorce remained powerful government instruments for social control. The governing classes' beliefs and values were reflected and reinforced by judicial judgments concerning expected standards of marital conduct.

Professor Dicey was too optimistic in his belief (1905: 347) that the 1857 Act 'did away with the iniquity of a law which theoretically prohibited divorce but in reality conceded to the rich a right denied to the poor'. In reality the only principle discarded was the propriety of providing divorce for the few able and willing to confront the circuit of civil, ecclesiastical and Parliamentary trial. Matrimonial relief was now to be dispensed in a more attainable civil court to a larger number of injured spouses; but for many the prescription's cost remained prohibitive. As a sardonic journalist explained to the readers of *Blackwoods Edinburgh Magazine* in November 1857 (p.594): 'Divorce is possible now, but very select indeed. Repudiation for the million will never do. Saturday-night wife-beaters would be divorced on Monday as regularly as Monday came, and remarried as regularly the next Sunday three weeks. The wives want protection and not Free Trade.' The incomes of the lower-middle and working classes did not put them in a position to contemplate petitioning for divorce. This was the third and most important weakness of the 1857 Act.

Civil divorce and its consequences

From 1 January 1858, dissolution of marriage became the prerogative of the Divorce Court. The issues surrounding divorce had become a public matter. Further Matrimonial Acts which were passed in the fifty years after 1857 dealt mainly with ancillary questions relating to property and maintenance, custody of children, and various procedural matters. The divorce law of England had not been changed in any meaningful sense by the 1857 Act; nor was it to be modified until 1923, and more fundamentally by the Herbert Act of 1937.

Though *The Times* of 4 August 1857 was correct in its belief that the 1857 Act was 'not in the form of an isolated boon to an influential nobleman', it was certainly not 'a general measure of relief for all'; in practice the availability of divorce was still very restricted. Discrimination existed against both the poor and women. Working-class couples with oppressive marriages were not able to afford the high legal costs, and so separated without resort to the divorce courts. Wives were severely restricted by the additional wrongs they had to prove against their husbands, while economically they were normally dependent upon husbands for support and general well-being. Over the next century there was a slow but steady blunting of both forms of discrimination. The remaining section of this chapter, and the next three chapters, develop the story of how the unwarranted barrier to divorce for these two groups has been largely removed.

Wives had to wait for nearly seventy years before the Matrimonial Causes Act of 1923 gave them equality of treatment in the grounds for divorce. Legislative sexual discrimination was strongly criticized by opponents of the Bill who argued that if divorce was going to be granted by the civil courts then, on Christian principles, wives should have the same rights as husbands, holding, as Mr Gladstone did, that the Bill was 'a measure which . . . would lead to the degradation of women' (*Hansard* 1857: vol. 147, col. 393). The traditional justification for such indiscriminate justice was expressed by *The Times*, (4 August 1857): 'In the conjugal relation, at least, the laws of nature have produced a dissimilarity of position between husband and wife, whatever may be their respective claims to superiority. It is only on one side that spurious offspring can be introduced into the family.' The harsh Victorian double standard of morality is also exemplified by the judgment of Sir Cresswell Cresswell – the first Judge Ordinary of the Divorce Court – in *Seddon v. Seddon and Doyle* ([1862]: 2 Sw. & Tr.640), that: 'It will probably have a salutary effect on the interests of public morality, that it should be known that a woman, if found guilty of adultery, will forfeit, as far as this court is concerned, all right to the custody of or access to her children.' This rule, which was never deemed applicable to a man, was not altered until 1910. Whatever the discrimination displayed by legislature and judiciary, there had been one benefit for women. Divorce, though circumscribed, was now available to them as of right and not by stinted condescension of the Lords. But it was not until 1891 that the courts decided, in the case of *R. v. Jackson* ([1891] 1Q.B.671), that a wife had a right to her personal liberty and with it the consequential right to live apart from her husband. The law of England no longer allowed the husband to bar or to restrain his wife's freedom of movement by means of imprisonment. A consequence of the judgment was, in the words of Judge McCardie, that: 'the shackles of servitude fell from the limbs of married women and they were free to come and go at their own will' (*Place v. Searle* [1932] 2K.B.497). Yet the Court of Appeal's decision in 1891 had no significance for the majority of working-class wives without money or assets but with children to feed and clothe. They remained unable to utilize their middle-class sisters' newly won freedom of movement, for such action rendered them homeless and destitute.

At first the new Court for Divorce and Matrimonial Causes was reluctant to order maintenance for an adulterous wife, though Parliamentary private Act divorce practice had allowed this. Now the guilty wife would receive financial provision only in very exceptional circumstances, though by the 1880s occasionally the Court began to exercise its discretion in favour of a 'guilty' wife. But even by the 1930s there were only a few exceptions to the overall policy of dismissal. Further moral censure was displayed in 1861 by Sir Cresswell Cresswell who warned that the petitioning wife would receive no more maintenance than was sufficient for her support, and that it should be assessed on a much more moderate basis than for alimony in cases of judicial separation (*Fisher v. Fisher*: 2 Sw. & Tr.410). Judge-made law was an effective deterrent to wives seeking divorce.

Initially a decree of dissolution would be given only if (section 32) the husband settled sufficient property to produce an income for his wife's support. The right to maintenance was not a personal right against the ex-husband, but a right against the property settled for her. The power that Parliament had formerly exercised in private Act procedure had simply been transferred to the new Divorce Court. Thus, maintenance would still be secured by the husband's property; but such a remedy gave no thought to a petitioning wife whose husband lacked assets though he had a regular income. This weakness was largely corrected by the Matrimonial Causes Act 1866, which allowed the courts to order weekly or monthly sums of maintenance without the need of security.

The work of Rowntree and Carrier (1958: 221–2) shows that some three-quarters of divorcing husbands in 1871 could be broadly classified as having middle- or upper-level incomes. Generally they would have been able to provide secured maintenance. Wives, without this financial security of certain regular payment, formed only a small proportion of all divorced wives between 1857 and the end of the century. The Parliamentary legislators of 1857 had never envisaged that, as the twentieth century advanced, divorce would become available to all and be utilized by many, though few husbands would have the means to provide secured maintenance. It was not until the Second World War that post-divorce maintenance became a pressing legal and social problem. In such roots lies the current maintenance dilemma.

By legislative vote, divorce had become a judicial matter for the newly established Divorce Court. Consequently, Parliament's provision of statutory divorce meant that it would have to review, regulate and control the efficacy of rules and conditions governing the law's operation. Divorce was now a Parliamentary affair that henceforth could not be readily dismissed. The logical outcome of the Marriage Act of 1836 had materialized; family matters – as witness the Custody of Infants Act of 1839 – were very slowly being regulated by government intervention.

The first year of the Act's operation saw 253 petitioners seeking dissolution in 1858; this was a considerable increase on the annual resort to the old-style Parliamentary divorce. The next thirty years did not provide the copious increase in petitions which critics had forecast. The fear that libertine husbands would rush to discard vulnerable wives proved false. Legal barriers and the social stigma helped to produce a divorce rate that was one of the lowest in Western Europe. Petitions in England and Wales in 1887, expressed as a rate per 1,000 marriages, were one-eighth the French experience and two-thirds that of Scotland. In 1900 divorce petitions still only totalled 606, of which wives provided 41 per cent.

Wives were able to form a significant minority of petitioners. The period from 1858 to 1889 had seen a steady rise in the average yearly number of petitions for dissolution filed by wives, from 84 (37 per cent) in the years 1858–9, to 214 (42 per cent) in the years 1880–9, making an average of 150 per year for the thirty-two years after 1857. Whatever the rigours of harsh divorce rules upon women, this was an improvement on the previous two centuries' record of four successful petitions. But the great majority of unhappy wives locked into failed marriages remained debarred from divorce by the high cost of access, the restrictive legal double standard, and their subordinate condition within Victorian society.

Part II
Divorce or separation

5   Constraints of poverty and gender

When the hearing of divorce suits was transferred to a civil court in 1857, a notable authority on the law observed: 'There are two ways of withholding divorce from the poor. One is to say so in words; another is to erect an unapproachable tribunal' (MacQueen 1858: 129). The working of the new divorce procedure had been forecast with remarkable accuracy, for only a small number of broken marriages could contemplate the high legal cost of presenting a divorce petition to the newly formed Court for Divorce and Matrimonial Causes in London. All divorce petitions had to be heard in London; though section 12 of the 1857 Act clearly stated that 'The Court . . . shall hold its sittings at such place or places in London or Middlesex or elsewhere as Her Majesty in Council shall from time to time appoint'. But the clause was very soon a dead letter, for the judges decided to restrict the legislator's intention that an issue of fact might be tried before an Assize judge in any county. This judicial fettering of the power given by Parliament remained unaltered until 1920. The rule that all divorce petitions had to be heard in London continued from the period of Parliamentary divorce to 1922 when the new legislation of 1920 was implemented.

The need to proceed to London added to the already high legal fees payable by those resorting to divorce. This financial obstruction to divorce is reflected in the evidence that working-class people constituted four-fifths of the population of England and Wales in 1871; but only 17 per cent of the petitioners in that year were from the manual classes, the latter being mostly skilled artisans or their wives (Rowntree and Carrier 1958: 222). At this time the earning ability between skilled craftsmen and labourers was considerably wider than it is today. Then, skilled men such as carpenters or masons could earn around £1.50 a week compared with an unskilled labourer's wage of 75p. The former's earnings allowed the possibility that if the marriage failed, enough might be saved by thrift and perseverance to pay for a divorce. Skilled labourers were aware that the gulf between them and their unskilled brothers was not only displayed in earnings but also in ways of life that accepted the habits and ideals of the middle classes. Respectability did not allow broken marriages to be resolved by the formation of new family bonds outside the status of marriage. This explains why the 1871 'manual' divorcing population was almost without exception from the skilled artisan class. Such divorces did form a surprisingly high proportion of all petitions when one considers the legal and economic barriers that had to be successfully surmounted. The only means by which the lower-paid working classes could seek a divorce was by the *in forma pauperis* procedure. But, as the next section shows, this supposed aid gave no practical help to the poor.

DIVORCE AND THE POOR

The law allowed very poor litigants to apply for certain limited forms of free legal assistance by the *in forma pauperis* procedure which dated from the fifteenth century. Until 1914, this procedure was the officially provided avenue for would-be divorce petitioners who were unable to pay their own legal fees. To qualify for assistance the petitioner had to be worth less than £25 with an income of under £1.50 a week.[1] No special department or formal machinery existed to assist poor persons to obtain the required court permission to proceed as an *in forma pauperis* petitioner. Such persons had neither the financial means to engage a lawyer nor the ability to prepare their own application for hearing in the Divorce Court. Poor litigants who were determined to get a divorce had to find altruistic solicitors and counsel willing to assist them free of charge. The solicitor had to prepare and present grounds for the divorce suit before counsel who, in turn, produced an opinion as to the reasonableness of the proceedings. If counsel's opinion was favourable, an application was made to the court for leave to petition *in forma pauperis*. All this had to be successfully completed before the petitioner could proceed. As the solicitor and barrister helping the petitioner to present a successful application were themselves likely to be selected by the court to conduct the subsequent divorce petition free of charge, it is not surprising that only a few poor petitioners found it possible to present an application.

In the twenty-five years from 1858 to 1882 the number of *in forma pauperis* applications averaged five a year. During the next quarter of a century the average rose to thirty-two applications a year, forming 4 per cent of all annually filed matrimonial petitions. However, the number of applications that proceeded to the stage of filing a petition were even fewer. The judge might dismiss the application; for instance, in 1911 a quarter of the thirty-nine applications were rejected. If successful, the applicant was merely released from the obligation to pay court fees amounting to about £6, but he would still have to pay the cost of witnesses' fares to London, hotel expenses and any other 'out of pocket' expenses of his solicitor and counsel. This meant that in an undefended pauper suit the petitioner had to pay a minimum sum of £10, though it would be considerably more if the case was defended or the petitioner lived some way from London. But generally the average sum required from the 'pauper' petitioner to meet such expenses varied from about £12 to £21.

Poverty remained a major barrier to divorce in England. The separate investigations of Booth in London and Seebohm Rowntree in York showed that some 30 per cent of the population of these cities was living in poverty due to the combined factors of large families and low wages. Rowntree's study (1901: 133) revealed that 'the wages paid for unskilled labour in York are insufficient to provide food, clothing and shelter adequate to maintain a family of moderate size in a state of bare physical efficiency'. By 1913 the average weekly wage was: £1.20 for unskilled labourers, £1.32 for semi-skilled manual workers and £1.90 for skilled manual workers (Routh 1965: 104). Many of the unskilled and semi-skilled male workers therefore must have earned a weekly wage below the limit of £1.50 a week set by the *in forma pauperis* requirements. It was not that large numbers of the working class were too wealthy to qualify, but that they were so poor that petitioners had nothing left over from their slender financial resources to pay lawyers' out-of-pocket expenses. Aggrieved wives had even less scope than their husbands to save the minimal expenses incurred in petitioning. Married women had the double disadvantage of fewer opportunities to earn, and considerably lower wages than those of a man.

The small proportion of divorce petitioners in England and Wales receiving assistance from the *in forma pauperis* procedure, when compared to the sizeable effect of the generous system of legal aid operating in France, highlights the paltry help given to the poor in this country. In 1891, when the thirty-eight *in forma pauperis* applications formed under 5 per cent of divorce petitions in this country, 7,834 petitions for *assistance judiciaire* were admitted in France, forming 44 per cent of the 17,867 divorce petitions in that year. But it was not only more generous financial assistance towards the cost of divorce that led to France having 26 divorce petitions for every 1,000 marriages in 1891, as against England's comparable ratio of 2 per 1,000 for the same year. French law also allowed a judicial separation to be converted after three years into a judgment for divorce.

The divorce laws of England in 1900 severely restricted the availability of divorce both to the poor and to wives. Consequently, this country had one of the lowest rates of divorce in the Western world. This denial of justice is underlined by evidence for the period 1900–10 that though there were some 9,000 separations annually – consisting of court separation orders (7,000) and solicitors' deeds of separations (2,000) – yet the number of *in forma pauperis* divorce petitions were some 35 annually (Report 1912b: 208, 217). Barriers to divorce caused unhappy couples formally to separate at a rate of 27 for each 100,000 of the population; in more liberal Scotland the comparable proportion was fewer than 1 separation per 100,000 population. A reliable indicator of the extent of marital breakdown within Victorian and Edwardian England needs to look beyond the rate of divorce.

The impediments that restricted access to the Divorce Court were well understood by the County Courts Procedure Committee, under the chairmanship of Lord Gorell, when they reported in 1909: 'Without doubt, there is a practical denial of justice in this matter to numbers of people . . . who belong to ranks in life in which the relief to be obtained under the Divorce Acts is probably more necessary than in ranks above them'. The 1912 Report of the Royal Commission (Gorell) on Divorce and Matrimonial Causes estimated that an undefended petition brought by a person living in or near to London would entail a minimum cost of between £40 and £45, though this figure increased by £12 or more if witnesses were required. About one-third of divorce petitions were defended, and in these cases the costs varied between £70 and £500. The cost of divorce has to be set against the estimate that only one in ten of the population earned more than £3 a week (Money 1911: 50). The Majority Report (1912a: 48) of the Gorell Commission quoted with approval evidence given by Mr Fitzsimmons, the Court Missionary at the Thames Police Court, observing it was 'weighty'.

> It is not so much a question of demand. I think the poor should not be denied the benefit of any law by reason of poverty. Respecting the question as to whether there is any demand for it, it ought to be remembered that the poor have known that the question of divorce was so far out of their reach that the idea of asking for the thing never occurred to them.

In addition, many of the poor would not consider the *in forma pauperis* procedure because of its association with the workhouse and the Poor Law. Judge Parry, writing in 1914, well understood the reality: 'the self-respect of working men in many cases hinders them from applying for assistance rendered nominally distasteful by the pauper taint' (Parry 1914: 184). A similar view was expressed by the Gorell Commission.

The evidence collected by the Gorell Commission provided an overwhelming picture of justice denied. Such were the stringent conditions attached to the *in forma pauperis* procedure that *The Times* in a leading article (30 December 1912) called them 'prohibitive' whilst *The Law Journal* (1912: 48–50) spoke of the system as 'next door to worthless'. Considerable agitation for reform of the outdated and now almost inoperative procedure in the years 1912 and 1913 led to its replacement by the Poor Persons' Procedure in 1914.

High cost, legal severity and social stigma explain why the yearly number of divorce petitions in the period immediately before the Great War was under a thousand (1910–13: 919). But this figure in no way reflected the extent of broken marriages, for nine out of ten such casualties resorting to the matrimonial courts in this period turned to the summary jurisdiction. The outcome was permanent separation rather than judicial dissolution. The next section explains how the summary courts came to aquire a matrimonial jurisdiction.

FORMATION OF THE MAGISTRATES' MATRIMONIAL JURISDICTION

The state of married society in early Victorian England had been curtly proclaimed in 1840 by Mr Justice Coleridge in *Re Cochrane* (8 Dowl.633): 'There can be little doubt of the general domination which the law of England attributes to the husband over the wife.' The degrading condition of women in the mid-nineteenth century was being challenged by the women's rights movement. A leading advocate of the political emancipation of women was John Stuart Mill, who gave the cause a foremost place in his election campaign of 1865. Four years later, in *The Subjection of Women*, he exclaimed: 'Marriage is the only actual bondage known to our law. There remain no legal slaves, except the mistress of every house.' Though the women's rights movement aimed mainly at a greater reorganization and improved status for the middle-class woman, its resultant pressures extended down to the working-class woman. The need for political pressure was well understood by a leading feminist, Miss Frances Power Cobbe (1878: 80) in her protest against the physical cruelty experienced by working-class wives: 'We live in these days under Government by pressure and the office must attend first to the claims which are backed by political pressure; . . . were women to obtain the franchise tomorrow, it is morally certain that a Bill for the Protection of Wives would pass through the legislation before a session was over.' Parliament's apology for the exclusion of women from the right to vote was provided by the view that feminine interests and wants were best left to the all-male Parliament, who would ensure that these needs were not neglected. Enfranchised male voters had already been increased fivefold by the Acts of 1832 and 1867, to two and a half million in 1870. But governments of this time had no desire to extend voting rights to meet the intellectual appeal of the middle-class feminist women's movement or the pressures of the unskilled male worker. To justify the limited franchise it became necessary for the legislature to remedy some of the more pressing social evils and legal injustices that could be observed in Victorian society, especially those concerning women. It was still true to record that marriage a hundred years ago turned a woman into 'a mere nonentity in point of law' (Lush 1901: 349). One aspect of the legal subjection of wives was reflected in the right of the husband to chastise his wife. Such authority had been declared by canon law in the twelfth century, holding 'a man may chastise his wife, and beat her for her correction, for she is of his household and therefore the Lord may chastise his own'.[2] There is abundant evidence that working-class husbands knew their legal 'rights'. At the beginning of the nineteenth century, Randle Lewis (1805: 86–7) could record: 'The lower rank of people, however, still claim and exert their ancient privilege; yet some of the men outstep all reasonable bounds; and some women undeservedly and patiently endure it.' The practice of wife-beating was not readily forsaken: a century later the observations of Lady Bell (1907: 238) on Middlesbrough working-class life showed it was 'not so entirely a thing of the past as some of us would like to think'. All this was within a setting in which family violence all too readily occurred, and in which institutional brutality was gratuitously imposed upon husbands.[3]

Male drunkenness was the factor influencing much reported brutality. Public houses were the centres of social life for many a working man seeking comfort and company away from the over-crowded, dank tenements; and solace by drinking away the reality of today's and tomorrow's toil. Such demand caused Manchester in 1850 to have one licensed premises for every eighty adults; the result was that being drunk and disorderly formed one-third of all summary convictions in England and Wales for 1871. This intemperate spending caused even greater hardship for many wives and children already deprived of the basic necessities of food and clothing. But more disturbing to Victorian conscience were the accounts provided by social workers, police court missionaries and official reports describing violence and cruelty to wives and children unable to defend themselves against drunken husbands and cruel fathers.

The law offered no practical form of legal relief to ill-used working-class wives. Indignation that the state of the law was ineffective was reinforced by both the lurid newspaper reports of appalling cruelty and the campaigns of such reformers as John Stuart Mill, Frances Power Cobbe and Sergeant Pulling. The latter argued in an address to the National Association for the Promotion of Social Science at Liverpool in 1876:

> The lesson taught to the ruffian is, that if he ill-uses his dog or his donkey he stands a fair chance (thanks to the Society for Preventing Cruelty to Dumb Animals) of being duly prosecuted, convicted and punished; but that if the ill-usage is merely practised on his wife the odds are in favour of his entire immunity, and of his victim getting worse treatment if she dare appear against him.

By the mid-1870s violence within the family had become a public and political issue.

Parliamentary action

The need for a Parliamentary Bill to protect working-class wives from the assaults of their husbands was raised in 'an appeal for women' by Colonel Egerton Leigh in the House of Commons in 1874. Empirical justification for Parliamentary intervention was provided in the following year by a Home Office Report entitled *The State of the Law Relating to Brutal Assaults*. Miss Cobbe estimated from evidence contained in the Report, and the reports of chief constables, that approximately 1,500 brutal assaults were committed yearly by men on women, the great majority being that of husband on wife. For Sergeant Pulling, the judicial answer to wife-beating was that of flogging and imprisoning the convicted husband. But Miss Cobbe appreciated that assaulted wives needed financial provision as well as protection from brutal husbands. Her remedy was that (1878: 83):

> A Bill should, I think, be passed affording to these poor women by means easily within their reach, the same redress which women of the richer classes obtain through the Divorce Court. They should be enabled to obtain from the Court which sentences their husbands a Protection Order, which should in their case have the same validity as a judicial separation. In addition to this, the custody of the children should be given to the wife, and an order should be made for the husband to pay the wife such weekly sum for her own and her childrens' maintenance as the Court may see fit.

Due to the intervention of Lord Penzance, a vital change was made to the applicability of a Bill dealing with maintenance in the Divorce Court. Lord Penzance had already shown sympathy for the plight of the ill-used wife when Judge Ordinary in the Divorce Court from 1863 to 1872. In the case of *Kelly v.*

Kelly (1869, L.R.2 P.& D. 31), where a clergyman had attempted to force his wife into complete subservience, Penzance had held that: 'The health and safety of the wife is, no doubt, the leading consideration of the law.' Upon the Lords' third reading of the Bill, Lord Penzance proposed an additional clause that gave assaulted wives the relief which had been proposed by Miss Cobbe. It was passed without opposition and provided that a wife whose husband had been convicted of an aggravated assault upon her should have the right to obtain a separation order, together with maintenance from the magistrates court. In this incidental way Parliament gave a matrimonial jurisdiction to the criminal courts.

Under section 4 of the Matrimonial Causes Act of 1878, working-class wives had acquired for the first time a statutory right to financial support from their husbands. However, maintenance was ancillary to the granting of a separation order. The former matter had been a secondary consideration in the legislators' minds, and for this reason there was no statutory limit as to the amount of maintenance that might be ordered. The court also had discretion to give the wife the legal custody of the children of the marriage under ten years of age. But adultery by the wife disqualified her from maintenance unless such adultery had been condoned, conduced or connived at.

The sponsors of the 1878 Act had wished to see available a quick and cheap legal remedy providing protection for wives of brutal husbands. But the Act did not effectively achieve its purpose because wives were unwilling to complain when they knew that maintenance was unlikely to be paid regularly and a non-cohabitation order could not be effectively enforced against a ruffian husband. Nor did the 1878 Act help wives who had been deserted. In such a situation, the wife's need was for maintenance not protection. A deserted wife without financial means was forced to enter the workhouse before the parish authorities could take action against the husband. The two other available remedies were of no practical benefit to a working-class wife. The common law right of pledging her husband's credit for necessaries was an ineffectual remedy in practice. The remaining possibility was to petition for financial provision to the Divorce Court by way of a decree of restitution of conjugal rights, judicial separation or dissolution of marriage. The remedies of the Divorce Court involved legal fees and court costs beyond the pocket of the housewife without means of her own. Such criticisms were to be partially remedied by more sweeping reforms in 1886 and 1895.

The Married Women (Maintenance in Case of Desertion) Act 1886 gave a more direct and economically useful remedy to wives. Magistrates were enabled to award the wife maintenance up to a maximum limit of £2 a week, if she could show the Bench that her husband was able to support her and their children but had refused or neglected to do so and had deserted her. No maintenance provision was made for children. Unlike the 1878 Act, it did not provide for the wife's protection by way of a non-cohabitation order; indeed, the 1886 Act, by implication, reinforced the wife's duty to live with her husband by declaring that she was bound to give her husband consortium if he wished to re-establish cohabitation. A further weakness of the 1886 Act was that it did not allow maintenance for the wife forced to leave home because of the husband's maltreatment. Wives who left their husbands under such conditions were usually unable to provide for themselves or their children, and were forced to return to the degradation from which they had attempted to escape. The succession of wife cruelty cases coming before the London courts in 1900 caused one magistrate to exclaim: 'The sight of this domestic misery completely appals me. I can bear it no more' (Holmes 1900: 61). To which Thomas Holmes, a police court missionary, added: 'Every magistrate in London has the same experience'.

Until the legislation of 1886, the only practical remedy for the great mass of deserted wives and mothers left destitute was to turn to the Poor Law guardians. A consequence of the new summary matrimonial legislation was that wives began to exercise their new rights, with the result that there was a decline in the orders made under the Poor Law offence of 'deserting or neglecting to support the family' from some 5,300 annual orders in the 1880s to 3,056 in 1894.

The Acts of 1878 and 1886 did provide practical help to battered or destitute wives; maintenance orders were made to 3,631 wives in 1894.[4] The scope of this legislation was further broadened in 1895 by the Summary Jurisdiction (Married Women) Act, which provided the nucleus of grounds for complaint that were to appear in subsequent summary court legislation. A wife could now obtain a maintenance order from the magistrates courts if she could show her husband had committed one of the following matrimonial offences:(a) he had deserted her; (b) he had been convicted of an aggravated assault, or had been sentenced to pay a fine of more than £5 or to two months' or more imprisonment for assault; (c) he had been guilty of persistent cruelty that caused her to leave home; or (d) he had wilfully neglected to provide reasonable maintenance for her or their children, causing them to live separate from him. The cruelty clause aimed to remedy the weakness of the 1886 Act by allowing magistrates to order maintenance against a husband whose behaviour had caused the wife to leave him. Thus, at the beginning of this century, the wife could obtain orders from the summary courts that authorized separation, financial support not exceeding £2 a week, and custody of a child under the age of sixteen.

The 1895 Act's implementation at the beginning of 1896 resulted in an immediate 60 per cent increase in the number of wives from that of 1894 turning to the magistrates courts. A further 30 per cent rise in the number of complaints took place between 1896 (7,428) and 1900 (9,553). A matrimonial jurisdiction had been created, in the words of the Lord Chancellor, to benefit 'the poorer classes'.[5]

The summary jurisdiction at work

The trenchant evidence of witnesses to the 1909 Royal Commission on Marriage and Divorce makes clear many of the practical and moral problems attached to the working of this summary jurisdiction. Many of these issues still have a contemporary relevance. Wives whose husbands had disappeared without a known address were unable to serve the court summons. Those who did successfully bring their husbands to court might find the amount ordered was totally inadequate for the needs of the family. Magistrates varied in their approach to the assessment of maintenance. The evidence of a clergyman was that 'the magistrate takes rather a lenient view of the man and rather a large view of the man's necessities, and says the man must be able to keep himself respectable; and if he is to be at work he must live well; those things are taken into consideration and dwelt upon too largely' (Report 1912b: 440). Failure to receive maintenance, together with a lack of acceptable and adequately paid employment, forced many wives to find another man who could provide for them. The ensuing adulterous relationship could then be seized upon by the husband to absolve him from any maintenance obligation.

Problems of ensuring regularity of payment and enforcing arrears were just as common then as now. In Newcastle-upon-Tyne, of the 512 husbands who had been ordered to provide maintenance over the previous eight years, only 16 per cent were still paying. Many witnesses pointed to the futility of the situation in which the wife could not enforce her rights without means of finding the whereabouts of her husband, and to the slenderness of the hope of enforcing maintenance even if he were traced. Wives who pursued their defaulting husbands had to pay for the summons and the cost of enforcement. The summons was costly and gave the wife no advantage, for the ultimate sanction of imprisonment cancelled the arrears, and removed the possibility of ongoing payment. At the same time a husband, who through unemployment or poverty could not pay the maintenance order nor get the amount reduced, might find himself continuously in and out of prison if a vindictive wife repeatedly obtained a fresh summons.

Destitution and hopelessness caused by the inability to enforce maintenance forced many deserted wives and children into the cold charity of the workhouse. Consequently a large proportion of the workhouse population in Edwardian times consisted of deserted wives, though it was 'the most humiliating experience of her life' (Report 1912c: 291), and carried a 'stigma which attaches permanently' (Report 1912b: 318). The granting of outdoor or workhouse relief allowed the Poor Law guardians to issue a warrant authorizing the police to arrest and bring the husband to court. Thus, the one effective enforcement method available to a separated wife was only activated by becoming chargeable to the rates, thereby ensuring the stigmatization associated with the workhouse. As a result of the Gorell Commission's recommendation, the Criminal Justice Act of 1914 (section 30(1)) allowed magistrates to order that maintenance should be paid into the court and not, as previously, directly to the wife. In this way the summary court collection service was conceived out of the abjection of the workhouse.

Thus, England at the beginning of this century had two systems of legal remedy for similar matrimonial difficulties. Those able to pay the legal costs brought their broken marriages to the Divorce Court in London. There the matter would be determined by a judge of the civil High Court girdled within the Royal Courts of Justice, supported by the advocacy of counsel expert in family law. The matrimonial disputes of the poor were handled within a summary jurisdiction by an untrained lay magistracy sitting in courts created to try petty crime. A comparison of the two systems of judicature, High and summary, in 1901, shows that for every one wife seeking a divorce, forty sought the cold comfort of a maintenance order. Both the working classes and women had reason to dislike our matrimonial laws and their administration.

THE DOUBLE STANDARD

The Victorian family cannot be readily stereotyped; the variance of its habits and customs reflects the width of social patterns and expectations within a rapidly changing society. Yet the experiences and realities of the Victorian age have to be compressed in order to allow an observable canvas. Women's role was held to be that of wife and mother. *The Ladies' Cabinet* of 1857 cloyingly explains to its middle-class readers that woman was,

> given to man as his better angel, to dissuade him from vice, to stimulate him to virtue, to make home delightful and life joyous . . . in the exercise of these gentle and holy charities, she fulfils her high vocation. But great as is the influence of the maiden and wife, it seems to fade away when placed by that of the mother. It is the mother who is to make the citizens for earth . . . and happy are they who thus fulfil the sacred and dignified vocation allotted to them by Providence.
>
> *(The Ladies' Cabinet*, 1857: 156)

In the same year as this exhortation to motherhood, providence gave Queen Victoria and Prince Albert their ninth – and last – child. Their marriage presented the nation with the virtuous and emotional symbol of the stable and respectable family household, even though the Prince Consort could complain that his constitutional lot was to be 'only the husband, and not the master in the house'. Victorian society expected women to obey man's command; the Poet Laureate, Lord Tennyson, held 'all else confusion'. In this manner the legal and social subordination of women was justified; as Lord McGregor (1957: 67) observes, 'outside the family married women had the same legal status as children and lunatics; within it they were their husbands' inferiors. . . . The legal powers of husbands over their wives reflected the personal status of women in the family.' The husband had right to his wife's current and future possessions, even her children, in the name of marital harmony.

The 1857 legislation followed earlier practice by allowing an aggrieved husband to petition for divorce on the wife's single act of misconduct, and additionally to seek damages against the man committing this trespass. The law did not work in reverse: the wife never had a comparable right of damages against the woman with whom the husband had committed adultery, nor of divorce against her husband. Indeed, a husband's adultery with an unmarried woman was not an offence at all, for no man's rights had been violated. This was all part of the wife's legal disability for, having no legal identity apart from her husband, she was unable to sue alone during marriage until 1883 (as a consequence of the

Married Women's Property Act, 1882). And, even if the wife had been allowed damages against the other woman, the husband would only have transferred the award from his right to his left hand.

The mid-Victorian's double standard of morality was rooted in the sexual fears, ignorance and power of men. William Acton, the then leading authority on sexual matters, could reject the thought that women might possess sexual feelings as 'a vile aspersion'.

The daughter was expected to be chaste, the wife equally virtuous. Differing standards upon sexual habit and behaviour is exemplified in Victorian discussion of, and legislation upon, prostitution. The informal code of conduct for men was far more tolerant of their sexual needs and habits; widespread prostitution was one consequence. Metropolitan London alone had 3,325 brothels operating in 1841. Liverpool was believed to have some 9,000 prostitutes, 500 of whom were under thirteen. It was this unsavoury backcloth that buttressed much of Victorian family life. All this lay behind William Lecky's apology that the prostitute was 'ultimately the most efficient guardian of virtue. But for her, the unchallenged purity of countless happy homes would be polluted' (1869: 283). The prostitute's function was, by this reckoning, a sexual conduit for man's lust, though the risks for both were high.

Evidence of the unacceptably high rate of venereal disease among soldiers and sailors and its debilitating effect on the defence of the Empire led to the first of the Contagious Diseases Acts being passed in 1866. Parliamentary sanctioning of this double standard authorized compulsory medical examination of suspected prostitutes, and the enforced treatment and containment of those found infected; but their male clients were ignored. The sexual degradation of women in a male-dominated Victorian society is reflected in the work of a Royal Commission appointed to investigate the outcry from campaigners led by Josephine Butler against the pain and humiliation sanctioned by the Contagious Diseases Acts. The Report of 1871 held there was 'no comparison to be made between prostitutes and the men who consort with them. With the one sex the offence is committed as a matter of gain; with the other it is an irregular indulgence of a natural impulse' (Report 1871: 177). Sexual hypocrisy and cruelty is one facet of venerated Victorian values.

This hypocrisy was evident in the summary matrimonial jurisdiction, for the husband's adultery by itself was not sufficient for the magistrates to order maintenance. Though a working-class wife had no redress against her husband's infidelity, a maintenance order obtained on some other ground had to be revoked upon proof of her subsequent misconduct. Another grievance was that a wife could not obtain an order while still living under the same roof as her husband. As one magistrate explained to the Gorell Commission (Report 1912b: 93): 'I say to the wife, "Have you left him?" She says, "I have not left him". I say, "But you must leave him for his cruelty or failure to maintain". She says, "How can I leave him? I have my children; where am I to go?"' The only place for many such wives was the workhouse with all its squalid associations.

SEPARATION ORDERS AND ILLICIT UNIONS

Justices had powers under the 1895 Act (s. 5(a)) to order that the wife 'be no longer bound to cohabit with her husband'. The non-cohabitation clause in a magistrate's matrimonial order, alternatively known as a separation order, was the main remedy for wives who had been cruelly treated by their husbands. Although the award of a separation order was discretionary, magistrates in the ten year period 1903–12 attached separation orders to 85 per cent of all maintenance orders made. Magistrates did not understand that they were misusing their powers by inserting a non-cohabitation clause to most orders for maintenance. This exclusive focusing of magisterial attention upon giving the wife a separation order received a sharp jolt from the judiciary. In 1906 Sir John Gorell Barnes, then President of the Probate, Divorce and Admiralty Division of the High Court, in *Dodd v. Dodd* (P.203–7) condemned the widespread use of separation orders, reminding magistrates that the 1895 Act intended that a non-cohabitation clause was to be used only in cases of cruelty and habitual drunkenness, where protection as well as maintenance was required. He went on to observe:

> Those who were concerned with it [the 1895 Act] appear to have their minds, if not entirely yet mainly, on the protection of women rather than on the general effects of the Act and its probable influence on the morality of the country. . . . Permanent separation without divorce has a distinct tendency to encourage immorality and is an unsatisfactory remedy to apply to the evils it is supposed to prevent.

Spouses were being judicially separated without the opportunity to enter a new marriage, the result being the formation of illicit new unions and illegitimate offspring.

This involuntary repudiation of the institution of marriage caused many observers to query whether a more satisfactory and permanent solution was required for the great mass of broken marriages than that offered by the summary courts. The latter's remedy of enforced separation was seen by critics such as Basil Tozer (1909) as a harbinger to immorality. Middle-class opinion had been moving towards a concern with the reported imperfections of working-class sexual behaviour and to a recognition that environmental and social influences were obstacles to the acceptance of the approved familial code.

Observations of the daily life of the poor produced in Victorian reformers a moral revulsion that prevailed in a good deal of their pressure to ameliorate working-class family life. Charles Booth thus commented on attitudes in parts of East London at the end of the 1890s:

> With the lowest classes premarital relations are very common, perhaps even usual. Amongst the girls themselves nothing is thought of it if no consequences result; and very little even if they do, should marriage follow, and more pity than reprobation if it does not. . . . This peculiar code of morality is independent of recognised law, and an embarrassment to religion, but it is intelligible enough and not unpractical in its way. . . . I do not know exactly

how far upwards in the social scale this view of sexual morality extends, but I believe it to constitute one of the clearest lines of demarcation between upper and lower in the working class.

(Booth 1902: 55–6)

It would be a mistake to conclude from these and similar statements that 'underclass' family life in 1900 was completely at variance with expected practice. The male hierarchy of status and class within the working class ranged from skilled artisan and foreman down to the unskilled labourer. Reports of supposed working-class immorality are largely describing the depressed *lumpen proletariat* or – in contemporary jargon – the underclass. They record an accepted sub-culture of informal 'marriage' among a segment of the population which was at odds with the proclaimed norms of society. Cause must be largely attributed to the unchangeable bonds of marriage prescribed by English law for those who could not afford to pay the high costs of judicial divorce. For a minority of the poor, marriage remained an alien institution that need not be contemplated. For others, the lottery of marriage became a sanctioned gamble within a society which supressed formal second chances until death formally indemnified the losers.

The governing establishment were embarrassed and disturbed by the reality that for all the power and wealth contained within English industrial society a quarter of their countrymen were permanently exposed to physical and material degradation. Social and military anxieties were still further aroused by fears for the Empire following the large percentage of army recruits rejected for the Boer War due to physical defects. Uneasiness over their declining birth rate was also felt amongst the higher income groups when reading eugenicist claims by writers such as the Whethams (1909) that 'this systematic depletion of the best blood of the country is a new phenomenon in the history of England'. The remedy was felt to be provision of a better environment for the mass of the population to work and live in. Such an outlook led to the introduction in 1909 of income tax rebates for those with children. These same influences led Winston Churchill, as President of the Board of Trade in the Asquith government, to defend the social policy of the Liberal Party. *The People's Rights* in 1909 was an eloquent plea for social legislation.

People talk vaguely of the stability of society, of the strength of the Empire, of the permanence of a Christian civilisation. On what foundation do they seek to build? There is only one foundation – a healthy family life for all. . . . The object of every constructive proposal (which the Liberals are making) is to buttress and fortify the homes of the people.

Similar considerations, too, had led Sir Gorell Barnes to present his decision in the case of *Dodd v. Dodd* as a call to reform:

This judgement brings prominently forward the question whether . . . any reform would be effective and adequate which did not abolish permanent separation, as distinguished from divorce, place the sexes on equality as regards offence and relief, and permit a decree being obtained for such definitive grave causes of offence as render future cohabitation impracticable and frustrate the object of marriage.

([1906] P.207–8)

The President of the Divorce Court was providing much more than a warning against objectionable summary court practice; it was a general condemnation of the two-tier system of divorce and separation.

There was an immediate response of approval from the press.[6] The *Daily Telegraph* (7 May 1906) was outright in its opinion: 'It is not and it cannot be denied to be a fact, that a law exists which is declared to be contrary to the interests of public morality by the highest authority concerned in its interpretation upon the bench. A law of that kind ought not to remain upon the Statute Book for twenty-four hours after a declaration of that character.'

The animated correspondence in The *Daily Telegraph* during August and September 1908, on the subject of separation orders and divorce for the poor, provides evidence of public disquiet with the existing divorce legislation. Its editorial comment on 6 August expressed the views felt by many leading persons on the unsatisfactory nature of the law:

It is difficult to believe that in a Christian and civilised country there is permitted to exist by statute an intermediate condition, neither that of matrimony nor divorce, which leaves to the woman nothing of marriage but its harshest fetters, and yet leaves the man free in everything but name. The situation created by the rapid increase of separation arrangements is not even remotely realised by the average person. But a profound moral evil is there. It has been created by artificial and irresolute legislation.

Foremost in the mind of critics was the aspect of sexual morality. The *Guardian* (14 April 1909) declared:

We think it exceedingly probable that these orders are responsible for far more immorality than divorce itself. Whereas divorce recognises and registers the civil results of immorality actually committed, separation orders facilitate and encourage its future commission by placing thousands of married men and women in a position of enforced celibacy.

Divorce injustice to the poorer classes resulted in *The Standard* (8 April 1909) observing:

Thus it comes about that the magistrates find themselves engaged with increasing frequency in dissolving marriages by a kind of legal fiction. Ill-assorted couples of the working classes, unable to go to the High Court, appear before the stipendiary and obtain a separation, which enables them to live apart, but does not give either party the right to marry again.

Lord Gorell once again judicially reminded public and legislators alike by his fresh judgment in *Harriman v. Harriman* ([1909] P.123) of the hardships of the poor to which he had already drawn attention three years earlier. Our laws neither insisted upon permanent marriage nor allowed free divorce, whilst the compromise of a legal separation satisfied few. In 1909, Lord Gorell tried unsuccessfully to persuade Parliament to allow County courts to hear the divorce petitions of poor persons. The high cost of divorce had led many poor people to write to him when he was President of the Divorce Court 'urging reform in this matter, and protesting against the injustice to them of the present system' (*Hansard*, HL, 1909, vol. II, col. 473). By this time legislators were growing more humane and less rigidly disposed to regard the institution of marriage simply from ecclesiastical presuppositions.

APPOINTMENT OF A ROYAL COMMISSION

Growing demand for divorce law reform secured the appointment by the Asquith Government in 1909 of a Royal Commission on Divorce and Matrimonial Causes, sitting under the chairmanship of Lord Gorell. The Commission's terms of reference were 'to inquire into the present state of the law of England and the administration thereof in divorce and matrimonial causes and applications for separation orders, especially with regard to the position of the poorer classes in relation thereto . . . and to report whether any and what amendments should be made in such law, or the administration thereof'. The Commission's Report, which was published in 1912, continues to 'impress by a quality of vision and humanity' (Finer and McGregor 1974: 108). The four published volumes of factual evidence meticulously gathered from 246 witnesses made clear the vast amount of preventable matrimonial misery then existing in England and Wales.

Many women's associations provided the Commission with evidence urging reform of the existing divorce laws. It was not only the middle-class feminist and women's suffrage movements that sought equality of treatment. Much of the pressure for reform came from the women's labour movement representing the views of large sections of working-class women. One of the reasons was that the reforming Liberal government had introduced non-contributory old age pensions in 1908, and health and unemployment benefits through the contributory National Insurance Act of 1911. There was a growing realization that because of restrictive divorce laws, many women living in illicit unions would be deprived of the benefits and allowances payable to their married sisters. Miss Margaret Llewelyn-Davies who, as General Secretary of the Women's Co-operative Guild represented some 26,000 artisans' wives, informed Lord Gorell that 'feeling was extremely strong – unanimous as regards an equal standard for men and women, and equal facilities for rich and poor – and all except about five or six were of the opinion that serious incompatibility should be a ground for divorce' (Report 1912d: 150).

The Majority Report made a strong plea that Parliament should 'act upon an unfettered consideration of what is best for the interest of the State, society and morality, and for that of parties to suits and their families' (Report 1912a: 37). Considerations of morality led the Commission to argue that adultery by the husband was no less excusable than if committed by the wife, and that therefore the grounds of divorce should be similar for both sexes. This recommendation was a victory for the sanitizing evangelical standards of single-male celibacy, husbands' faithfulness and family respectability.

On the broader front the Commission could not find any general consensus of Christian opinion on either the propriety of divorce or the acceptable grounds for dissolving a marriage. The Majority Report argued that there was no logical reason why adultery should remain the only recognized offence for divorce. It therefore recommended an extension of the matrimonial offence to include the following new grounds: cruelty, desertion for three or more years, incurable insanity and incurable drunkenness. A quarter of a century later Parliament legislated this extension; meanwhile adultery was to remain the sole ground for divorce.

Poor persons' inability to pay the expenses necessary to obtain a divorce or to obtain assistance from the *in forma pauperis* procedure was a matter of considerable concern to the Commission. Provision of pauper suits in this country, compared with either Scotland, Germany, France or the Netherlands, showed 'how fallacious it is to consider that a small number of divorces in England is indicative of a high state of morality in the country'. It was largely upon questions of morality that the Commission focused its deliberations. The authority to make separation orders (which were the equivalent of the High Court decree of judicial separation) gave justices, who were practically all laymen, nearly all the powers possessed by High Court judges; except actual dissolution of marriage. The fact that magistrates usually, as a matter of course, made separation orders in conjunction with an order for maintenance, regardless of whether the former was necessary for the immediate protection of the wife, had placed 200,000 persons in a position of 'potential immorality' in the fifteen years since 1895 (Report 1912b: 212). Many witnesses felt that matrimonial legislation had ignored the moral consequences of separation orders which condemned 'the parties obtaining them either to a life of celibacy, or immorality, both of which states are against public policy and the general welfare of the nation' (Gates 1910: 7). Dr Ethel Bentham told the Commission of the likely undesirable consequences when a home was broken up by the wife's desertion. 'A man left with children is forced to have a housekeeper and, in the small houses of the poor, decent sleeping arrangements are not possible, and disaster nearly always ensues' (Report 1912d: 31).

The Commissioners observed that 'as a general rule it will be found that the home once definitely broken up is not re-formed' (Report 1912a: 98). Evidence showed that return of a spouse to the matrimonial home was more often out of economic necessity than any sign of genuine reconciliation. As Lord Gorell explained to Mrs E. Hubbard of the Mothers' Union: 'The reconciliations which have been spoken of in so many cases are not reconciliations in fact at all; the necessities of the parties make them come together'(Report 1912c: 193). The Commission was unimpressed with the argument that separation orders hindered reconciliation; they were critical of separation orders for the reverse reason that they led to the formation of illicit unions. The Report (1912a: par. 142) held that the consequences of permanent separation without divorce were 'in many cases disastrous; in the case of men, leading in numerous instances to adulterous connections and general immorality, and in the case of women, but to a lesser extent, to the same result'.

The inadequacy of the lay magistracy was a recurrent theme of the evidence to, and content of, the Commission's Report. Lay magistrates did not have the knowledge or legal training to deal adequately with domestic hearings. Mr Hay Halkett, the stipending magistrate for Hull, told the Commission that 'the reason why the Act (1895) has an unsettling influence is that it is not understood by, I am afraid, many of the justices of the peace in the country to be permissive – that the court may, but it is not necessarily obliged to separate people' (Report 1912b: 298). Sir John Macdonell, the editor of the *Civil Judicial Statistics* from 1894 until his death in 1921, gave evidence 'that these powers given under the various Acts are exercised somewhat differently by magistrates throughout the country' (Report 1912b: 22). This and other like evidence showing the misunderstanding and misuse of separation orders led the Commission to the conviction that criminal courts were inappropriate settings for the handling of grave family issues affecting women and children. Because permanent separation was unsatisfactory and led to immorality the Commission recommended that, ideally, the power of magistrates' courts to make such orders should be abolished. If permanent separation was a necessary remedy then it should be through a simplified process in the High Court. But total abolition of magistrates' matrimonial powers was unrealistic, being 'at present the only remedy within the reach of the very poor' (Report 1912a: 69). Therefore the summary courts' powers should be limited so that separation orders 'should only be granted where they are necessary for the reasonable immediate protection of the wife or husband, or the support of the wife and the children with her'. The Commission went on to recommend (Report 1912a: 73) that separation orders should have an upper time limit of two years, 'partly because that period gives ample time for the exercise of the magistrates' powers to produce its effect', after which time the wife should be required to turn to the High Court.

Only a quarter of petitioners seeking divorce in 1908 came from the working-class population.[7] The limited opportunities for divorce among the poor meant that the existence of this remedy was either not known or, if known, not sought because of inability to meet the cost. A Stepney Council alderman, who was a railway clerk, informed the Chairman that he had never met a poor person who wanted divorce. Similarly, a Church Army welfare visitor to prisoners' wives and families had during her eleven years' experience never heard any of her 3,000 clients desiring divorce. Yet official statistics showed that some 11,000 working-class broken marriages annually came before the magistrates. This type of evidence suggests that within the sub-culture of the very poor divorce was something so alien to their knowledge and practice that it was never considered when a marriage broke down. It was the skilled worker, or his wife, who desired the prior approval of the law before establishing a new relationship. The Majority

Report (Report 1912a: 95) concluded: 'The remedy of divorce is at present . . . practically inaccessible to the poorest classes and the evidence before the Commission shows that this state of things does not tend to develop due regard for marriage, but the reverse'. It was therefore proposed that divorce should be made more accessible to the poor. One suggested way of reducing the cost for those with low incomes was to decentralize the London Divorce Court and allow petitions from those with joint incomes of less than £300 per year and assets of under £250 to be heard in the provinces by specially appointed commissioners having the powers of High Court judges. Nothing was done to implement this recommendation until after the Second World War.

The basic tenet of the Majority Report was to 'recognise human needs, that divorce is not a disease but a remedy for a disease, that homes are not broken up by a court but by causes to which we have already sufficiently referred, and that the law should be such as would give relief where serious causes intervene, which are generally and properly recognised as leading to the break-up of married life' (Report 1912a: par. 242). This principle is reflected in the core of their recommendations that, first, working-class people should have the same chance of divorce as the more wealthy and, second, that women should have the same rights to divorce as men. But the government did nothing to implement the recommendations due to the priority given to the Kaiser War. With the return of peace, Lord Buckmaster in 1920 introduced a Bill, based upon the Majority Report, that required wives with separation orders to proceed after two years to the High Court and petition for divorce. The Bill, though passed by the House of Lords and backed by a petition with over 100,000 signatures, was unacceptable to the Conservative government, as was a similar Bill a year later. These Bills show the concern felt by many over enforced separation without divorce. This was to be a problem increasingly discussed over the next fifty years.

6 Between the wars

The ideals of the female suffrage movement had gained support during the First World War through women's contribution to the war effort. As a reward, Parliament provided in 1918 a limited form of enfranchisement for women aged at least thirty. The following year the Sex Disqualification (Removal) Act gave women the right to serve on a jury or as a magistrate and, in theory, opened almost all professions to women. The gradual movement towards sexual equality was reflected in the field of family law by the Matrimonial Causes Act of 1923. This Act implemented the Gorell Commission's recommendation of female equality with men in divorce by allowing a wife to petition upon the grounds of her husband's adultery without the previous necessity of proving an additional aggravating offence. Wives were now placed on par with their husbands. The result was a rise in the proportion of divorce petitions that were filed by wives from 41 per cent in 1921 to 62 per cent in 1924.

The legislation of 1923 was also intended to remove an increasingly apparent and embarrassing manipulation of the existing divorce law. The Matrimonial Causes Act of 1884 had allowed a deserted wife with a decree for restitution of conjugal rights to petition immediately for divorce if the adulterous husband remained recalcitrant to this frigid juridical entreaty. The wife openly committed perjury by petitioning for the return of her truant husband; the real intent was to obtain financial support and a speedy divorce. Securing the restitution decree bypassed the statutory two-year waiting period needed to prove desertion as an 'aggravation' under the 1857 Act's divorce requirements. As Lord Gorell shrewdly observed in 1907: 'It is not too much to say that the restitution part of the proceeding is a farce, because their true object is not the object which appears on the face of them' (*Kennedy v. Kennedy* [1907] P.51).

For thirty years the 1884 Act's provision had made no impact on divorce numbers. Then, in 1914, the rules governing the Poor Persons' Procedure were eased, and the Kaiser War began. Marriages were broken by the disintegrating effect of regiments of husbands being consigned to the slaughter fields of France while their wives left home to man the factory and till the land. With the return of peace, an increasing number of wives petitioned for restitution as a quick method of circumventing the legal handicap placed upon them by the 1857 legislation. More wives sought restitution in 1919 (491 petitions) than during the decade 1901 to 1910 (453 petitions). The proportion of wives petitioning for restitution in 1919 was almost half (45 per cent) the number seeking dissolution.

The decree of restitution had at all times been sought almost exclusively by wives. An annual average of three husbands similarly petitioned between 1891 and 1920. Wives increasing usage of this convenient loophole was now causing discomfort to the legislature. When the divorce double standard was removed in 1923 the restitution decree's utility disappeared with it; wives' resort accordingly fell sharply to an annual average of 38 petitions over the next decade.

The reformed divorce law of 1923 now said that on all matters other than adultery, however serious the disagreement, unacceptable the behaviour, or alienated the affection, the marriage must still continue. Without proof of adultery the only legal remedy remained permanent separation by order of the High Court or the magistrates court.

The first significant divorce law amendment to the 1857 Act had removed legislative sexual inequality but could not do anything directly to remedy the basic injustice that most married women were financially dependent on their husbands. Opportunity to divorce continued to be restricted by legal limitation, gender and class.

THE POOR PERSONS' PROCEDURE: 1914–40

The cost of bringing a divorce action continued to provide a major barrier to divorce. Limited improvement did, however, occur within the established machinery for providing financial help. The redundant *in forma pauperis* procedure was replaced in 1914 by the Poor Persons' Procedure. It was run until 1926 by the newly formed Poor Persons' Department, within the Office of the Supreme Court. Although the Department was not confined to matrimonial matters, some 90 per cent of its work was related to divorce cases. From the beginning of 1914 a 'poor person' could be legally aided in the High Court if they had a reasonable cause of action or defence, and their means did not exceed £50, though this sum could be raised to £100 in special circumstances. Even if, by diligent saving, the working man could raise the necessary amount to pay for his own legal fees, there was always the additional potential liability of his wife's own costs to be remembered. These costs had to be paid by the husband regardless of whether he was successful or not, except when the wife respondent had substantial means of her own. This meant that the husband of limited means had to raise more money to petition than did his wife.

The court's granting of a certificate allowed court fees to be remitted, while the case was conducted free of charge by volunteer lawyers. But any out-of-pocket expenses incurred by these lawyers had to be paid by the applicant. What had proved to be the fundamental weakness of the *in forma pauperis* procedure still remained. In 1918 only a quarter of applicants for legal aid reached the stage of filing their petitions. The Lawrence Committee on Poor Persons' Rules observed that: 'Unless a fund is constituted out of which the expenses of the Poor Persons can be defrayed, the really poor or quite destitute persons have no chance of availing themselves of the Rules to obtain a divorce' (Report 1919: pars 7, 10).

Poor petitioners who did manage to raise the necessary divorce costs now faced the further hurdle of finding a solicitor willing to handle this work. Many solicitors firms would not undertake matrimonial cases, even for their own clients, due to the unsavoury professional image associated with divorce work. Others, who did not object to the nature of the work, hesitated 'to receive at their offices persons who are often ill-dressed and frequently ill-mannered' (Report 1925: par. 7). The result was that only a minority of solicitors and barristers were willing to undertake Poor Persons' cases and give their services free of charge. Less than a tenth of the 790 London solicitors undertaking divorce work in 1918 had handled a Poor Persons' case. Even more disturbing was the evidence that some of the supposedly willing solicitors charged Poor Person petitioners a sum of money to cover alleged 'office expenses' in addition to their actual out-of-pocket expenses. It is not surprising that with these economic and professional obstructions, few applicants, though passing the 'means and merits' test, obtained their desired divorce.

Disruption of married life by the Kaiser War resulted in 5,085 petitions flooding into the London Divorce Court in 1918 compared with an average of 965 for the years 1911–13. The two divorce judges could not cope and the only solution was to implement the Gorell and Lawrence Reports' recommendations in favour of provincial hearings. Though it was enacted in 1922 that Poor Persons' divorce cases could be heard at local Assizes (they ranked as the High Court), it was not until the Poor Persons' Department was decentralized in 1926 that such cases were heard outside London. All undefended petitions – which formed 90 per cent of all hearings – could now be filed in one of twenty-six District Registries, the hearing taking place at the nearest Assize courts. This produced a lowering of costs for provincial poor petitioners. The need for such an improvement is reflected in almost half (47 per cent) of all Poor Persons' petitions in the five years 1926–30 being filed in District Registries. The changes of 1926 helped to produce an increase of a third (31 per cent) in decree nisis between 1926 (2,859) and 1927 (3,740).

The new powers of the Assize judge gave qualified help to those outside the limits of the Poor Persons' scheme who did not have the means to pay the costs of a London hearing. But decentralization did nothing to help those persons whose low income did not give them the means to pay any contribution towards the cost of a divorce suit. Nor did it benefit those whose wages were too high to obtain a certificate but insufficient to pay their own legal fees. The plight of the latter group underlined a fundamental weakness of the scheme, for there was no system whereby a person of moderate means need pay only part of the cost.

In 1926 the running of the Poor Persons' Department was transferred from the Office of the Supreme Court to the London and Provincial Law Societies who, in turn, set up some ninety committees throughout England and Wales. Applicants now had to satisfy a selection committee of local solicitors rather than a Master of the Supreme Court that they had reasonable grounds for presenting or defending a case in court and were within the set financial limits. Impoverished petitioners normally had to present their cases without benefit of legal assistance to the local area committee. The very person who was likely to be poorly educated and unversed in administrative and legal niceties had to decide the best way to obtain and present evidence whilst avoiding the pitfalls of collusion. A weakness of the 1926 Rules was that they provided neither indication or guideline to the public, the lawyers or the local committees as to the manner in which these applications were to be decided. In performing their duties the local Law Society committees were making quasi-judicial decisions without either granting an interview to the applicant or giving reasons for their rejection. There was no appeal against the committee's decision. In certain cases the judge's function was further usurped by committees 'trying' discretion cases to the extent of refusing financial aid and thus the opportunity of divorce, though the court might well have given a decree if the case had come before it. Sanctimonious disapproval of discretion cases is shown in the moralizing censorship of one provincial committee decision that: 'the parties have obviously regarded a marriage so lightly (that it had) felt reluctant to put the court and the conducting solicitor to so much trouble in bringing about its dissolution' (A Barrister 1938: 181). The committees' screening allowed financial assistance to only the safe and dependable cases.

The Lawrence Committee's report had resulted in the introduction in 1921 of an income means test of £2 a week or, in special circumstances, £4 a week, to the existing capital limit of £50, or £100 in special circumstances. Though wages had risen during the 1920s, the upper limit remained unchanged. As a result, large numbers of low-income husbands found themselves outside the financial limits of legal aid. Social survey findings of the 1930s demonstrate how unrealistic was the supposition that those with incomes between £2 and £4 a week could afford to take legal proceedings. A random survey of 5,000 family budgets in 1936–7 indicated that 15 per cent of Great Britain's population had a weekly wage below £2.40, half of which was spent on food (Crawford and Broadley, 1938). A further 60 per cent had wages of between £2.40 and £4.80 a week. Making allowance for differences in family size within this latter group, the estimated weekly per capita income averaged £1, of which almost 40 per cent was spent on food. There was little left from this weekly wage after the additional expenditure on rent and clothing for the husband to contemplate divorce. The wife was in an even worse position than the husband in trying to find the additional out-of-court expenses.

An uncontested divorce case in the 1930s would have cost around £50, increasing to £100 upwards on each side if contested (A Barrister 1938: 176). Would-be petitioners who earned too much to be helped by the Poor Persons' Procedure yet lacked the savings to meet the likely costs had either to save diligently what little they could or find a solicitor who would allow payment by instalments. But full court and counsel fees of around £40 still had to be paid for, as well as any witnesses' expenses (A Barrister 1938: 183).

The emerging picture indicates that from 1921 until the outbreak of the Second World War the majority of working-class persons seeking divorce were

Table 6.1 The proportion of all matrimonial petitions filed with legal aid, 1921–76, England and Wales

Period	All matrimonial petitions filed* (yearly average)				Total: all petitioners (100%)	Percentage of husband/wife petitioners with legal aid		
	Husband		Wife			Husband	Wife	All
	No.	%	No.	%				
1921–5	1,367	43	1,840	57	3,207	32	19	24
1926–30	1,715	41	2,495	59	4,210	34	35	34
1931–5	2,181	44	2,766	56	4,947	40	37	38
1936–40	3,583	47	4,082	53	7,665	32	41	37
1941–5	8,938	55	7,257	45	16,195	26	19	23
1946–50	21,374	55	17,750	45	39,124	Not available		22
1950–5	14,311	44	18,026	56	32,337	46	67	58
1956–60	12,423	45	15,276	55	27,699	23	58	42
1961–5	15,706	41	22,219	59	37,925	53	78	68
1966–70	21,360	37	35,730	63	57,090	44	78	65
1971–5	41,207	34	80,319	66	121,526	32	70	57
1976	43,345	30	101,469	70	144,814	27	69	57

Source: Calculations based on annual *Civil Judicial Statistics*.
Note: * Dissolution, nullity, judicial separation and restitution of conjugal rights; the latter two categories formed 2 per cent of the total of 'all petitioners' in the years 1931–40.

barred from the usage of the Poor Persons' Procedure by the harsh £2 a week income-limit rule. There was also a minority who were so poor that, though their wages qualified them for legal aid, they could not afford the required lawyers' out-of-pocket expenses. Those who benefited by the Poor Persons' Procedure were that section of the low-income groups within the working classes who fell between the two limits of dire poverty and an average working wage.

Limited and imperfect though the Poor Persons' Procedure had proved to be, a minority of all the low-income spouses with broken marriages were now able to petition for divorce by virtue of the changes brought about in 1914. Table 6.1 records that by the 1930s well over a third of all divorces were granted to Poor Persons' petitioners, and it has been calculated that 'the granting of these facilities has raised the divorce rate over 50 per cent' (Glass 1934: 259). Against this measure of benefit has to be set the evidence from government statistics confirming that the majority of applicants seeking divorce under the Poor

Persons' Procedure were prohibited through their limited financial means and the scarcity of willing lawyers. Most of those who needed professional assistance and desired legal remedy were being denied access to these services. In the years 1921 to 1940 just over a quarter of all applicants for certificates under the Poor Persons' Procedure reached the point of filing a petition. The official divorce rates for the inter-war years were recording a fraction of the true level of marital breakdown.

Wives were more successful than husbands in obtaining a certificate for legal assistance, nearly half (47 per cent) succeeding over the period 1931–40, compared with 38 per cent of husbands. Yet only a third of the original wife applicants and a quarter of the husband applicants in 1931–40 reached the first stage in the judicial process of having their petitions filed (Gibson 1971a: tables 1 and 3). But even the filing of a petition did not imply that the case would proceed to the divorce court.

Over the twenty-year period 1921-40 more men and women (some 90,000) unsuccessfully sought divorce through the Poor Persons' Procedure than all the divorce and nullity decrees (87,209) granted by the court. The Poor Law taint attached to the Procedure meant that only those who were both qualified through poverty and prepared to ignore the associated stigma would attempt to obtain legal aid. It is reasonable to suppose that these *de jure* united but *de facto* broken marriages came from the poorer sections of the community.

The Matrimonial Causes Act of 1937 did not include revision of the Poor Persons' Procedure and so the majority of the working class remained excluded from access to the divorce court. The new grounds for divorce, however, did lead to a 60 per cent rise in Poor Person petitioners between 1936 and 1938; the increase being due to the backlog of wives utilizing the wider grounds. After 1937 the increasing numbers of petitioners revealed more clearly than ever the unwillingness or inability of solicitors to undertake Poor Person divorce suits. Dissatisfaction with the existing procedure led to the formation of another committee, this time under the chairmanship of Mr Justice Hodson, but the outbreak of war stopped their work. Even before the Second World War there were signs that solicitors were no longer willing to countenance a system which put a special burden on those practising in poorer areas. The Welsh Law Societies declared in 1939 that they would no longer deal with Poor Person cases unless, amongst other demands, their members received a reasonable fee for this work (Egerton 1946: 17). This was an open challenge to the Law Society and its belief in the voluntary system.

POLICE COURTS FOR THE POOR

A well-known London stipendary magistrate, Mr Claud Mullins, observed in 1935:

No order . . . that a Police Court can give permits either husband or wife to re-marry. If the husband is young, there is always the possibility that, sooner or later, he will embark on some other attachment. . . . Very few men that we see in Police Courts will ever be in a position to maintain two women, to say nothing of two families; our economic system, like our morals, is based on monogamy.

(Mullins 1935: 15–16)

The consequences resulting from summary separation rather than judicial divorce had been exposed by the Gorell Commission. A quarter of a century later the Establishment remained disturbed by the same moral issues, though they were unable to offer a practical solution.

Lack of divorce opportunity through low income, legal ignorance or insufficient ground, meant that justices dealt with four out of five marriages that came to the courts in the years 1921–5. It was to be the matrimonial jurisdiction of magistrates courts rather than the divorce courts on which Parliament largely focused its attention over the inter-war years.

Until 1920 a wife could only obtain a maintenance order up to the sum of £2 a week for herself and her children regardless of the size of the family to be supported. The Married Women (Maintenance) Act of 1920 introduced maintenance orders up to ten shillings a week for children under sixteen. In the mid-1920s Parliament began to direct its attention on the proper needs of and duties towards children. The Guardianship of Infants Act 1925 instructed the courts that in disputes concerning children the welfare of the child was 'the first and paramount consideration'; the Act incidentally also raised the maintenance limit for a child to £1.[1]

A further improvement for deserted wives came about when the Gorell Commission recommendation that a wife whose husband had been persistently cruel or had wilfully neglected to maintain her should not have to leave him before applying for a maintenance order was implemented with the passing of the Summary Jurisdiction (Separation and Maintenance) Act of 1925. But the order was still not enforceable as long as she resided with her husband and if the wife remained after three months the order was cancelled. The 1925 Act brought two further benefits to wives by introducing interim orders in cases where the hearing was adjourned to a later date, and by requiring husbands with maintenance orders to notify the court of any change of address. The passing of the 1925 Act reflects the change in social and legislative action moving away from physical protection of the wife in favour of providing her with financial security. But the legislature had ignored the paramount problem of separation without divorce. The existing summary legislation, in the words of J.F. Worsley-Boden, had been 'accompanied by the abuses which commonly thrive in parasitic fashion on systems which are inadequate in conception and incompetent in execution' (1932: 272).

Maintenance default

Enforcement of maintenance orders became an increasing public concern. The real source of the problem was clear to Miss Eleanor Rathbone when she explained that 'a separation, at least in working-class marriages, is always a desperate expedient, for there it involves not only the break-up of the home and the severance of the children from one parent or the other, but the splitting up into two of an income which is usually barely sufficient for the upkeep of one household' (1924: 97). The proportion of maintenance defaulters imprisoned annually compared with new orders made reached the staggering proportion of 46 per cent in 1923; in 1932 it was still 40 per cent. The 3,648 maintenance defaulters imprisoned in 1932 formed 7 per cent of all prison receptions. Between the five years 1925–9 the average yearly number of maintenance defaulters imprisoned was 3,905, of which 43 per cent were for periods of two months or more. Clearly imprisonment was not a deterrent to defaulting husbands. The reason was that many of these men simply did not have the means to pay. It is not surprising therefore that the highest rate of imprisonment coincided with the periods of greatest industrial depression. In 1931, some two million men were out of work; others were experiencing short-time wages.

Statistics provided by Miss Margery Fry to the Magistrates' Association in 1932 suggested that a large number of husbands were being imprisoned because of their poverty rather than their wilful refusal to obey the court order. The Report of a Departmental Committee on Imprisonment by Courts of Summary Juris-diction in Default of Payment of Fines and Other Sums of Money (the Fischer Williams Committee) found it disturbing that in many cases justices were unable to obtain reliable information about the man's earnings. It was essential that the court should investigate a defaulter's financial and social circumstances before committing him to prison. The Committee concluded critically that a situation where 'a court dispensing justice should have to act on less information than a society dispensing charity is an indication of one of the defects of the present system' (Report 1934: par. 125). As a result of the Committee's recom-mendations, the Money Payments (Justices Procedure) Act 1935 was passed with the intention of reducing the number of civil prisoners. The court now had a duty under the Act (s. 8 (1)(b)) to determine that non-payment of a maintenance order resulted from wilful refusal or from culpable neglect before sending a defaulter to prison. At the same time, Sir John Simon, the Home Secretary, sent a circular letter to all justices requesting, as a matter of great social importance, their co-operation in reducing the number of maintenance committals.

> This army of persons reaches prison not because offences have been committed . . . but because of failure to pay sums due under decisions of the courts . . . The presence of prisoners of this type in the same prison as those who are sentenced as a direct punishment for their offences makes harder the task of the prison authorities.
>
> (Geeson 1936: 16)

The proportion of prison committals to new maintenance orders made dropped from a quarter in 1935 to a fifth in 1936, and remained at this latter rate until the Second World War.

Rethinking summary procedure

There appeared a growing realization that the judicial process and atmosphere experienced in magistrates courts was not conducive to resolving marital discord. A typical observation came from Sir E. Marlay Samson, stipendary magistrate at Swansea and Chairman of the Magistrates' Association, who noted the need for 'remedies for the existing dissatisfaction in regard to the matrimonial procedure in Police Courts' (Mullins 1935: 8). In similar vein, Claud Mullins argued that 'matrimonial jurisdiction came to Police Courts in a most haphazard way . . . it is scarcely surprising that our methods for carrying out these duties have never been seriously examined, and that they are now thoroughly old-fashioned' (Mullins 1935: 23). A major problem was then, as now, the way by which an even balance and proper distinction could be maintained between conciliation methods and legal requirements governing evidence and procedure.

A growing unease was being expressed by stipendiary magistrates and justices' clerks about the suitability of family disputes being heard in courts which were designed to handle petty crime and which displayed a dominant police presence. Cecil Chapman, a London magistrate, had observed earlier that it was exceedingly difficult for the facts to be 'properly sifted in a court which is fully occupied with other matters' (Chapman 1925: 61). A similar view came from Mr J. Cairns, a fellow magistrate:

> Police courts do not appear to be the proper tribunal, if a tribunal at all is needed, to unravel the tangled threads of matrimonial trouble. They are concerned chiefly with the administration of the criminal law and maintenance of public order. Their business is with offences against the public order, not with domestic squabbles.
>
> (Cairns 1934: 131)

Nor were these magistrates alone in their concern. Lord Merrivale, a past President of the Probate, Divorce and Admiralty Division, informed Parliament in 1935 that 'These cases . . . are mixed up with the ordinary criminal proceedings of the courts, and they are conducted in the same way as the criminal proceedings' (Mullins 1935: 32).

Three 'Courts of Domestic Relations' Bills had been presented unsuccessfully to the House of Commons between 1928 and 1930. The pressure for procedural reform was nevertheless maintained. In 1934 the Magistrates' Association made it known that they 'would welcome the establishment of special courts for dealing with domestic relations with a panel of justices and a special time set apart for the hearing of such cases and with procedure for preliminary inquiries before the hearing'. Later in the same year Lord Listowell introduced a Summary Jurisdiction (Domestic Procedure) Bill designed to produce a 'special technique' for dealing with domestic cases. Both the Archbishop of Canterbury and Lord Reading (Rufus Isaacs, an ex-Lord Chief Justice) felt that more attention should be devoted to attempts at reconciliation. But many lawyers disliked any proposed alterations of the basic common law principles rooted in the legislation. The Bill was withdrawn upon the Lord Chancellor announcing the setting up of a government inquiry, 'to be directed to the general question of providing the courts with adequate means of carrying out the whole of these social services'.

The Committee, under the chairmanship of Mr S.W. Harris, hoped their Report would 'draw public attention to the value and growing importance of the social side of the administration of justice' (Report 1936: viii). They found that the law relating to the making of separation and maintenance orders made no provision for reconciliation, though the majority of courts did recognize the need. The Committee's recommendations tried to reconcile the fact that conciliation and the provision of legal remedies by way of judicial process did not sit easily together. Conciliation was not to be excluded; indeed it was to be encouraged. But it was not to be formalized, and should be left to the discretion of the courts.

The Report showed that far more wives approached the magistrates courts than appeared at hearings. Replies from courts indicated that only 15 per cent of the wives who approached the courts eventually obtained orders.[2]

The Committee warned that reconciliation could not be inferred 'because the partners do not appear before the court within a limited period' (Report 1936: par. 13). The men and women who resorted to the magistrates courts were the poorest and least informed members of society. Because this was so, the Committee proposed that there should be greater provision for legal representation of those who could not afford it as 'many of the parties in matrimonial disputes before Justices are not legally represented, and are of not sufficient education or ability to put their cases before the court in a proper manner, or to give all the information which may be available to them' (Report 1936: 46).

The Summary Procedure (Domestic Proceedings) Act 1937 largely enacted the Harris Report's recommendations. Implementation of the Act removed some of the prevailing criminal atmosphere of the magistrates courts and also recognized the use of probation officers to encourage reconciliation. The Bench hearing domestic matters was now to consist of not more than three justices among whom, ideally, there should be at least one man and one woman. This removed the Harris Report's criticism of matrimonial hearings in some courts having Benches of more than thirty justices. The fact that the summary courts' matrimonial jurisdiction was providing a social as well as a legal service was beginning to be acknowledged.

The introduction of the Poor Persons' Procedure had already assisted a small proportion of the poor to seek divorce, but for the majority of broken marriages there still remained a lack of practical choice between the summary and High Court jurisdictions. Differences separating the two types of court were apparent not only in the available legal remedy but also in the disparity between the quality of justice meted out to the poor and that provided for the more wealthy. A pungent 1930s court cameo is provided by Mr Geeson, the justices' clerk at Newcastle:

Those whose names appear in the Society columns of the Press would not dream of applying at, say, Bow Street for a legal separation; but the man of moderate or slender means who had suffered disaster in his married life must, with his wife, have his case dealt with amid the police court atmosphere where, in many courts throughout the country, he will find himself rubbing shoulders with a packed, ill-assorted crowd including gamblers, pickpockets and reckless motorists. . . . Dread of association with a police court is felt by all law-abiding citizens, and not less by the respectable poor than by their more fortunate fellows.

(Geeson 1936: xiv, 7–8)

Similarly, Mr Cairns described the Metropolitan Police Court as a 'miniature Divorce Court', sympathetically observing that 'complete emancipation costs money and, as in so many other things, the poor have to be satisfied with the second best' (Cairns 1934: 134). The majority of broken marriages were still being directed by costs, law and custom to the 'second-best' jurisdiction.

In the five-year period 1931 to 1935, the summary court dealt with three applications brought by wives for every one divorce petition filed by either the husband or wife. Most wives coming before justices did not subsequently experience either dissolution or reconciliation but remained separate and estranged. Such facts contradict the wishful thinking of those like Lord Merrivale, who maintained:

The success of marriage as an institution was shown by the fact that with 8,000,000 households in Great Britain, only 4,000 decrees of divorce had been promulgated last year [1934]. The remainder of the husbands and wives of the country knew better than those who gossiped about easy divorce and the facilitation of the discharge from the matrimonial tie.

Lord Merrivale unwittingly went on to dispel his own image of a maritally united kingdom:

On the other hand, during the preceding year 11,000 orders had been made by Justices under the Summary Jurisdiction (Married Women) Acts. This jurisdiction was much closer than that of the Divorce Division to the domestic lives of the people because, in the great majority of cases, separation was involved, and separation by magistrates' order practically precluded any reconciliation. About 50,000 such orders were said to be in operation.

(quoted in Geeson 1936: 54)

It was against this type of thinking that Alfred Fellows wrote: 'This ostrich policy of pretending that we have a system of Christian monogamy might be regarded as a harmless one, and a normal product of unctuous rectitude, save for the fact that it results in real and grievous hardship' (Fellows 1932: viii–ix).

The number of applications for maintenance had hardly varied in the fifteen years between 1921 (13,244) and 1935 (13,806) but the number of petitions filed for dissolution had risen by 85 per cent to 5,157 in 1935. Middle-class public opinion, in the years following the First World War, had become less willing to display censure on those who had been divorced, though there is evidence that within working-class circles divorce 'was considered a worse disgrace than drink' (Walsh 1953: 21).

REFORM OF THE DIVORCE LAW

The law allowed only one possibility for divorce: the petitioner had to come to court and prove the respondent's adulterous guilt. The need for change was given effective publicity by A.P. Herbert's amusing novel *Holy Deadlock*. Sir Alan allows Mr Boom, a solicitor, to reveal to a client the existing state of law:

> If you violently knock your wife about every night the ordinary person will conclude that you have not much affection for her; but the law requires you to prove it by sleeping with another woman. For that is the only act of a husband that the law regards as really important. It would be the same if you were certified a lunatic: or became a habitual and besotted drunkard: or were sentenced for embezzlement to fourteen years' penal servitude: or were found guilty of murder but were reprieved, and so let off with imprisonment for life. Such trifles mean nothing to the divorce laws of this Christian country. Adultery, misconduct, intimacy, or nothing – that's the rule.
>
> (Herbert 1934: 27)

Public opinion was becoming disturbed that other equally wounding and offensive behaviour were not acceptable grounds for divorce.

The legislative fallacy that supposed only sexual misconduct was sufficient a cause to justify dissolution of an extinct partnership had consequently led to the courts' insistence on demonstration of the innocent victim's 'clean hands' and the guilty spouse's irrefutable infidelity. The ensuant court rules of marital combat debarred estranged spouses from presenting an amicable divorce agreement or reaching a civilized understanding. Collusion was a bar to divorce.

Whatever may have been the formal requirements, it was commonly known that collusion did occur. In such cases the wife would be informed by her husband or his solicitors of the date and place where evidence of adultery would be available, the adultery in fact being committed in order that the petition might go through. It was this situation that caused the Report of a Joint Committee of the Two Convocations of the Church of England in 1935 to 'register an emphatic protest against the way in which it is now possible to arrange a divorce, desired for quite different reasons, under the cover of an inferred act or series of acts of adultery' (Merrivale 1936: 63). Hotel chambermaids were financially encouraged to witness such compromising night arrangements as would later allow the court to impute the committal of adultery from their evidence. Yet in many cases, as A.P. Herbert drolly showed in *Holy Deadlock*, the respondents' hands had in fact remained clean. As the sage solicitor Boom explained to the husband, one of the spouses must commit adultery – or at least pretend to commit adultery. The law was pliable for the affluent and harsh to the poor. The working of the law was described by an anonymous barrister:

A rich person seeking legal advice relating to matrimonial affairs consults the family solicitor, or some other solicitor recommended by someone who knows him well. The matter is talked over quietly and privately. ... If it is decided to apply for divorce, the guilty party is very often advised to give evidence of his or her adultery to the other party in order to minimise the unpleasantness and difficulty of the proceedings, and both parties are advised how to co-operate whilst avoiding the pitfall of 'collusion'.

(A Barrister 1938: 178)

Divorce by mutual consent was possible if one were wealthy enough to pay the costs of hotel rooms, private detectives, witnesses' corroborative evidence, and legal and court fees. Those, like Colonel Josiah Wedgewood, MP, who made it known that they had not committed adultery although they had been divorced for this reason, were not subsequently prosecuted for their temerity. However, the law showed just vengeance on a gardener who declared at his divorce hearing the tactless truth that adultery had never taken place with the woman named on the wife's petition. The petition was dismissed and the man was subsequently charged with conspiring to manufacture false evidence. Yet if he had committed adultery the court would have granted the mutually sought-after divorce rather than impose a prison sentence of four months. On the other hand, the law did not allow both spouses to admit adultery. No wonder Lord Chief Justice Hewart complained: 'Perhaps it is not vouchsafed to everybody, whether in Holy Orders or out of them, to appreciate the full sublimity and beauty of the doctrine that if one of two married persons is guilty of misconduct there may properly be divorce, while if both are guilty they must continue to abide in the holy estate of matrimony' (*Daily Telegraph*, 21 October 1935).

Public opinion began to appreciate that the circumstances leading to break-down of marriage were often more complex than proof of the only matrimonial offence the law recognized. Once again there was the feeling, as expressed by the Archdeacon of Coventry, that the existing divorce law 'had resulted in a state of affairs which was disastrously prejudicial to public morality. As the law stands at present, those who wish to bring an end to marriage are forced to take one of two alternatives – either one must commit adultery or one must commit perjury'.[3] It was within this framework of moral concern that the Matrimonial Causes Act 1937 came to be passed.

The Matrimonial Causes Act of 1937

Mr (later Sir) A.P. Herbert, following his success in a Parliamentary ballot, introduced a Private Member's Bill into the Commons in February 1936. The Bill did not receive a reading but was reintroduced by Mr Rupert de la Bère in November 1936. Largely due to a combination of Sir Alan's skill, a series of fortunate accidents and eventual government approval, the now considerably amended Bill received the Royal Assent in July 1937.[4] The feeling behind this legislation is evident in the Act's preamble:

Whereas it is expedient for the true support of marriage, the protection of children, the removal of hardship, the reduction of illicit unions and unseemly litigation . . . and the restoration of due respect for the law, that the Acts relating to marriage and divorce be amended.

The Act came into operation at the beginning of 1938. It implemented some of the 1912 Royal Commission proposals by extending the grounds for divorce to include, in addition to adultery, the two important new grounds of desertion for three or more years, and cruelty. The Act did not explain how these two new faults were to be defined and interpreted, thereby providing judges with a wide discretion. An incurably insane spouse could now be divorced upon proof of continuous confinement and treatment for at least five years preceding the petition. Acceptance of a tragic involuntary affliction was the first major inroad into the concept of fault and the matrimonial offence.

As a sop to those critics who believed these new grounds would threaten the sanctity of marriage, the Act introduced a three year restriction on petitioning from the time of marriage. The only exceptions to this brake were those cases certified by the High Court as indicating evidence of exceptional hardship to the petitioner or depravity by the respondent.

The Act brought incidental change to the summary courts' matrimonial jurisdiction by extending the grounds of complaint for a maintenance order to include adultery. The fact that desertion was now a ground for divorce made it especially important that magistrates should be careful to give a non-cohabitation clause only upon the specific request of a wife. Such an order meant that a wife could not later complain to the Divorce Court of her husband's desertion from the time of the order that had directed him to live apart from his wife.

Following the 1937 Act, no further changes in the acceptable grounds for divorce were to occur until 1969, whilst grounds for a maintenance order in the summary court remained unchanged until 1978. The reforms of 1937 did not seriously affect the long-term divorce trend. More important elements affecting resort to divorce after 1945 were the immediate impact of wartime separation and the significant post-war changes in personal expectations. Revision of individual habits combined with a lowering of the financial barriers to divorce and the development of a state structure of non-stigmatizing financial provision. The more generous availability of legal assistance and the formation of the National Assistance Scheme to replace the Poor Law were to prove of especial benefit to wives.

7 From matrimonial offence to irretrievable breakdown

War conditions tested the constancy of many a hasty marriage exposed to the cold reflection of prolonged separation. These marital casualties of the Second World War resulted in an annual average of some 43,000 divorce petitions during the three years 1946–8, husbands filing 59 per cent of the petitions. Such large numbers caused lengthy delays in a system designed to deal with an average of five to seven thousand petitions a year. A wartime Committee had already rejected the suggestion that County courts should be allowed to handle divorces; instead, recommending Assizes should hear defended as well as undefended petitions, for such matters should be heard 'in the highest court available'. The pressure on the over-burdened London Divorce Court and Assize judges was partly eased in 1946 by appointing Special Commissioners with the authority of High Court judges to sit in London and provincial towns to hear divorce petitions.

INTRODUCTION OF LEGAL AID

The return of peace found fewer potential petitioners qualified for aid under the Poor Persons' Rules. This was through the government's failure to raise the existing £4 financial limit in line with inflation. The dual effects of low limits and rising wages is reflected in the proportion of legally aided petitioners falling from 38 per cent in the 1930s to 20 per cent in 1945. At the same time higher real wages and greater overtime opportunities did allow diligent husbands to save the required £50 to £70 costs of a straightforward undefended divorce. Yet there still remained the 1930s legal aid problem of an increasing number of low-income men and women denied divorce because of their inability to pay the legal costs involved, though not poor enough to qualify for assistance.

The post-war welfare state's desire that ready access to justice should properly be as much a citizen's right as availability of educational opportunity or health care led to the Legal Aid and Advice Act of 1949. The introduction of the new procedure in October 1950 meant that, for the first time, petitioners would not be debarred by poverty. Those assessed just above the free limit no longer had to meet all their legal costs. A new class, those assessed between the 'free' and 'maximum' limits, received state help though they were expected to pay a contribution (with the protection of a known fixed upper limit) set down in the scale rates.

The new system of legal aid greatly improved poor petitioners' access to divorce. The number of legally aided petitioners rose threefold between 1949 and 1951, while there was a 9 per cent rise in the number of petitions filed. But it was a 21 per cent rise in the number of wives petitioning which accounts for this increase; the number of husbands petitioning in 1951 declined by 3 per cent over the 1949 figure. The introduction of the legal aid scheme did not reverse the downward trend in the number and proportion of petitions presented by husbands. Poverty had hindered far more wives than husbands from access to the divorce courts, and wives were the immediate and most numerous beneficiaries of the legal aid scheme.

Once the backlog of assisted petitioners had been cleared, the annual number of petitions fell back to around the 1950 level of some 30,000. The evidence suggests the introduction of legal aid did not lead to a permanent rise in the divorce rate.

FAULT TO BREAKDOWN

The law governing divorce in 1950 remained that set down in 1937. Retention of the matrimonial offence meant that the petitioner, in all but a few exceptions, had to prove the respondent's voluntary committal of either adultery, desertion or cruelty. The noticeable exception was the respondent's incurable insanity, this intrusion in to the doctrine of fault having been introduced in 1937.

The law could not accept that marriage failure was often the consequence of a multitude of factors emanating from both spouses. Redress could only be granted if the petitioner came to court with 'clean hands'; the divorce trial charade required the 'innocent' petitioner to prove the respondent's 'guilt'. The latter was expected to defend the allegation. This was a travesty of the reality in which more than nine out of ten petitions remained undefended because the respondent either equally desired divorce or accepted that the marriage had failed. As early as 1950 Lord Denning publicly acknowledged his disquiet over the conflict between statute and practice.

> I desire to say emphatically that the fact that the husband has obtained this decree does not give a true picture of the conduct of the parties. I agree that the marriage has irretrievably broken down and that it is better dissolved. So let it be dissolved. But when it comes to maintenance, or any of the other ancillary questions which follow on divorce, then let the truth be seen.
>
> (*Trestain v. Trestain* [1950] P.198)

Truth was, in theory, also elicited by means of discretion statements. Petitioners who had sexually erred were required to record such misconduct in a written statement to the judge with an attached prayer requesting forgiveness. The House of Lords in *Blunt v. Blunt* ([1943] A.C. 517) had generously extended the judge's discretionary scope to grant absolution upon hearing the petitioner's confession of adultery. All of this testified to the reality of breakdown in a legal world of fault. In commonly exercising their discretion the judges were daily recognizing the social truth of marriage breakdown.

Continued blackbook insistence upon the matrimonial offence led to increasing disquiet over the efficacy of our divorce law. It was not so surprising that Irene White received all-party support in 1950 for her Private Member's Bill allowing an additional breakdown ground to be attached to the existing matrimonial offences. The Bill proposed that either spouse could seek divorce if they had lived apart for seven or more years without prospect of reconciliation. This struck at the concept of fault, for a 'guilty' spouse now would be able to divorce the 'innocent' partner. Mrs White justified her radical proposal by the standard 'marriage and morality' argument: 'Many thousands of men and women are living apart in a state which is not marriage, in any full sense of the word, but in which they are unable legally to form another union or to establish a normal home life' (*Hansard*, vol. 485, col. 927–8). Parliamentary approval of the Bill embarrassed the government, who feared that this measure, together with the newly introduced legal aid scheme, would create a surge in marriage breakdown. Mrs White withdrew her Bill upon the government promising to appoint a Royal Commission to inquire into our laws of marriage and divorce.

The Royal Commission, under the chairmanship of Lord Morton, received evidence from those who firmly believed that any relaxations of our fault-based divorce law would undermine family stability and respect for the institution of marriage as a lifelong obligation. The 'institutionalist' belief was strongly supported by the Archbishop of Canterbury. Against this view was set the realists, who advocated change away from the principle of the matrimonial offence. They argued that a marriage was only as strong as the commitment of each spouse forming it. A sound moral matrimonial policy should reflect actual behaviour, allowing as many couples as possible to enter freely and embrace within wedlock's covenant.

The Report's inability to define and clearly examine opposing viewpoints produced a volume of preconceived convictions that did nothing to clarify the very issues the Commission had been formed to resolve. In a critical analysis of the Report, Lord McGregor (1957: 193) concluded: 'The Morton Commission has proved a device for obfuscting a socially urgent but politically inconvenient issue.' When the Royal Commission reported in 1955, all but one of the eighteen members agreed that the doctrine of the matrimonial office should be retained. The dissenting voice of Lord Walker urged the adoption of a new principle of irretrievable breakdown of marriage as evidenced by three years' separation, in place of the matrimonial offence. Lord Walker argued:

> The commission of a matrimonial offence is often the symptom or sequel of a marriage which had broken down for quite other reasons. . . . The true significance of marriage . . . is lifelong cohabitation. . . . But when the prospect of continuing cohabitation has ceased the true view as to the significance of marriage seems to require that the legal tie should be dissolved.

> Each empty tie . . . adds increasing harm to the community and injury to the ideal of marriage.
>
> (Report 1956: 341)

The argument was to be repeated a decade later by the Law Commission, eventually to become the established policy. The government quietly filed the Report, relieved that no radical change in matrimonial law or procedure had been proposed for either the High or summary court jurisdictions.

Half the Royal Commission had favoured Mrs White's proposal to make seven years' separation an additional ground for divorce. This was strongly opposed by the Archbishop of Canterbury, Dr Fisher, who believed the idea lacked moral principle and would encourage illicit relationships. Similar moral and theological concerns led the Archbishop in 1957 to warn that clergy who married divorcees placed themselves in 'spiritual peril'. A dominant pillar of Establishment thought and practice had firmly declared itself for the status quo and against divorce reform.

The Church of England had explained in evidence to the Morton Commission, that the matrimonial offence was 'entirely in accord with the New Testament'. Biblical support for the law's matrimonial offences had already been benevolently extended from that expressed by the resolution of bishops attending the third Lambeth Conference in 1888.

> That inasmuch as our Lord's words expressly forbid divorce except in case of fornication or adultery, the Christian Church cannot recognise divorce in any other than the excepted case, or give any sanction to the marriage of any persons who had been divorced contrary to this law, during the life of the other party.
>
> (Cornish 1910: 93)

The same problems of squaring theological teaching to changing common practice had faced the Church in the area of family limitation. The Lambeth Conference of 1908 strongly condemned the growing use of contraception as 'demoralising to character and hostile to national welfare'. Fifty years later, due to the unsolved problems presented by growing populations in Third World countries with insufficient resources, the Church of England declared itself in favour of family planning at the 1958 Lambeth Conference. Also in 1958 the report of the Church of England Moral Welfare Council entitled *The Family in Contemporary Society* (1958: 109) found that 'far from disintegrating, the modern family is in some ways in a stronger position than it has been at any period in our history of which we have knowledge'. This confident diagnosis of the state and condition of the contemporary English family went a long way to nullifying the Church's past support for the doctrine of the matrimonial offence as a necessary safeguard to family stability.

Following Mr (now Lord) Deedes's unsuccessful attempt in 1958 to introduce a Private Member's Bill similar to Mrs White's, Mr Abse made a similar effort in

1963 to allow divorce after seven years' separation. The proposal led to condemnation from various Church heads including the Archbishop of Canterbury, Dr Ramsey. Later in the same year, Dr Ramsey told the House of Lords:

> If it were possible to find a principle at law of breakdown of marriage which was free from any trace of the idea of consent, which conserved the point that offences and not only wishes are the basis of breakdown, and which was protected by a far more thorough insistence on reconcilation procedure first, then I would wish to consider it.

He was asking some of his fellow churchmen under the chairmanship of Dr Mortimer, Bishop of Exeter, 'to see whether it is possible to work at this idea, sociologically as well as doctrinally, to discover if anything can be produced' (*Hansard* HL, vol. 298, cols 1543–7).

The Group's report in 1966, *Putting Asunder: A Divorce Law for Contemporary Society* signified the radical change in Church opinion upon divorce. They observed that in a secular society, 'any advice that the Church tenders to the State must rest, not upon doctrines that only Christians accept, but upon premises that enjoy wide acknowledgement in the nation as a whole' (Canterbury 1966: 12). The Report condemned the continued usage of the matrimonial offence, when in practice 'both its members, however unequal their responsibility, are inevitably involved together' in the failure of the marriage (Canterbury 1966: 18). This view reflected, and supported, the public attitude which upheld the right of each spouse to examine their own matrimonial condition. Emphasis was now on private contentment and happiness; corporate support for the institution of marriage had been replaced by individualism.

The Group urged the Church of England to permit divorce if the marriage had irretrievably broken down: 'We are far from being convinced that the present provisions of the law witness to the sanctity of marriage. . . . As a piece of social mechanism the present system has not only cut loose from its moral and juridical foundations: it is, quite simply, inept' (Canterbury 1966: 32). The primary recommendation of the Report was approved by an overwhelming majority of Church Assembly members. The sacramental concept of marriage had been abandoned by the Church of England. This long-established opponent of divorce reform was now urging change. At the same time the Archbishop of Canterbury informed the legislature that the principle of the matrimonial offence existed for historical reasons and not 'for any reasons of Divine necessity' (*Hansard*, HL, 1966, vol. 278, col. 271). Parliament was free to consider anew the relevant social and legal criteria for a modern divorce law now that the Established Church had liberated itself from earlier theological assumptions. Yet the Report's proposed remedy was almost worse than the problem it was meant to cure. The Church's historic opposition to divorce by consent was maintained. The courts were to hold an inquest in every case to judge if the marriage had irretrievably broken down, or whether reconciliation was still possible. But the judicial process was never designed for this costly and time-consuming inquisitorial role, nor was there the infrastructure to establish these new tribunals adjudicated by judges who would be assisted by 'forensic social workers'.

This period also witnessed further Parliamentary and court encroachment into the concept of the matrimonial offence. The senior appellate court was radically revising its judicial attitude towards the doctrine of fault. The Law Lords' two case decisions in 1964 (*Gollins v. Gollins* [1964] A.C.644: and *Williams v. Williams* [1964] A.C.698) were instrumental in taking the moral sting out of the matrimonial offence of cruelty. Judges now had to look at the individual relationship and the behaviour's impact upon the petitioner, even though the respondent did not intend such results. Lord Denning informed Parliament in 1966 that cruelty could now be established 'if an intolerable situation is created. . . . We really have, in fact, divorce because of the breakdown of marriage' (*Hansard*, HL, vol. 278, col. 310).

It was because admission of joint agreement or consent to divorce was unacceptable to an adversary procedure requiring the parties to be hostile, that collusion remained an absolute bar until the passing of the Matrimonial Causes Act in 1963. The Act gave judges the discretionary right to grant divorce to a colluding petitioner. This change meant that financial arrangements as part of a bargain for divorce could be disclosed to the court without fear that this collusion would automatically block the decree. Sanctioned by Parliament, these arrangements made divorce by consent a social reality. It was also the case that by the mid-1960s some 30 per cent of all petitioners were seeking the court's discretion in respect of their adultery. Judges almost invariably exercised discretion realistically in the petitioner's favour; only three applications failed among the 3,850 similar petitions coming before the Principal Registry in London during 1965 (Law Commission 1966: 12, 15). In consequence the demarcation between 'guilty' and 'innocent' had become blurred. All this meant that Parliamentary and judicial intervention had together radically eased the divorce mainstay of the matrimonial offence by allowing important exemptions from its doctrinal rigidity.

The Lord Chancellor, Lord Gardiner, referred *Putting Asunder* to the newly established Law Commission, which was already engaged upon an examination of matrimonial and family law. The Law Commission published their brilliantly incisive analysis *Reform of the Grounds of Divorce: The Field of Choice* in November 1966. The report agreed with the Archbishop's Group that the present system was no longer satisfactory. The objectives of a good divorce law should be:

(1) To buttress, rather than to undermine, the stability of marriage; and
(2) When, regrettably, a marriage has irretrievably broken down, to enable the empty legal shell to be destroyed with the maximum fairness, and the minimum bitterness, distress and humiliation.

(Law Commission 1966: 10)

If the marriage was dead then 'the object of the law should be to afford it a decent burial' (Law Commission 1966: 11). The Commissioners rejected breakdown with inquest as 'procedurally impracticable', lengthy and expensive, and likely to be humiliating and distressing to the parties. The three other alternatives considered were: divorce by consent, a period of separation, and breakdown without inquest. The latter was judged to be the most practical for a revised divorce law.

The Law Commission's report set down many of the expected social, moral and legal consequences for the family if the existing fault-based law of divorce was reformed. Some 180,000 illegitimate children of stable extra-marital unions could be legitimated by the subsequent marriage of their parents, and 'in each future year some 19,000 children who would otherwise be condemned to permanent illegitimacy might be born in wedlock or subsequently legitimated' (Law Commission 1966: 19). Discussion between the Law Commissioners and the Archbishop of Canterbury's Group resulted in the former publishing divorce proposals that were a consensus of opinion between the two bodies. Their recommendations were the basis of William Wilson's Divorce Reform Bill making breakdown of marriage the sole ground for divorce. In attempting to accommodate differing shades of opinion and reach a consensus, the sponsors of the Bill had produced what *The Times* (16 January 1968) labelled as an 'uneasy compromise'. Instead of substituting the criteria of marriage breakdown for that of the matrimonial offence the Bill allowed the two to stand unhappily side by side. The second reading was passed on a free vote on 9 January 1968, and the Bill went on to complete its Committee stages in the House of Commons. Then, due to lack of Parliamentary time, the Bill lapsed. Later in the same year a slightly amended Private Member's Bill was reintroduced by Alec Jones.

The Labour government had a generally favourable attitude towards the reformers' proposals but, as is Parliamentary policy towards Bills concerning individual conscience, refused formal sponsorship. Authoritative legal backing was nevertheless effectively provided by Lord Gardiner, a liberal and reforming Lord Chancellor who had been instrumental in establishing the Law Commission in 1965 and appointing Sir Leslie (now Lord) Scarman as its first chairman. Further legal strength came from John Silkin the government Chief Whip and a solicitor, and Leo Abse, a divorce lawyer who was the principal promoter and Parliamentary driving force behind the Bill. The Law Commission's *The Field of Choice* proved a catalytic document, presenting MPs and public alike with a factual, clearly reasoned and neutral examination of the issues. The report's dissection of the controverial aspects of divorce helped to persuade undecided minds towards a partiality for change. Similar depth of knowledge and technical skill was again evident when the Law Commission assisted the reformers by drafting their Bill.

Reformers argued that divorce occurred to victims of breakdown, but was not the ailment itself. Opponents replied that easing the law would cause a rise in divorce which would undermine the institution of marriage and thereby destroy the basic foundations of family life. Some thirty womens' organizations protested their concern that unwillingly divorced wives remained unprotected against financial hardship and distress (Lee 1974: 139, 150–1). Bruce Campbell, QC, a leading critic of the Bill, derided the proposed safeguards for wives as 'quite inadequate. . . . We are not talking about millionaires but the millions of ordinary men and women, who live on a tight budget which simply does not permit maintaining two households (*Hansard*, HC, 1968, vol. 774, col. 2043).

The debate was set in a Parliament sympathetic to liberal reform, controlled by a Labour government returned in 1966 with a safe majority of ninety-nine seats. The same individualist-orientated legislature – reflecting society's liberal 1960s moral outlook – had already agreed to Mr Abse's Homosexuality Bill (1966) and Mr Steel's Abortion Bill (1967), and was now about to accept Mr Jones's Divorce Bill. Campaigners had effectively created a majority of public opinion, as reflected in the press and the opinion polls (see p.108), favourable to the Bill's aims. Public feeling was echoed by the Commons voting 185 to 108 at the crucial second reading.

The most controversial family matter of the previous twenty years had been debated in and out of Westminster. Now MPs had been given the responsibility of deciding for change or the status quo. For this reason, party voting patterns are informative of Parliamentary accountability. Almost half (47 per cent) of all Labour MPs voted for, as against 6 per cent who opposed the Bill; voting among Conservative MPs showed 9 per cent for and 35 per cent against the proposals (Lee 1974: 133). The government's overall encouragement and vital Labour backbench support had been crucial factors in the Bill's Parliamentary progress and successful completion. Marriage and the family had been in the nation's spotlight, the debate had aroused passion and controversy, but 53 per cent of all MPs (Labour 47 per cent; Conservative 56 per cent; women MPs 50 per cent) did not feel strongly enough on the issue to vote. The Bill now passed through twelve sittings of the Standing Committee before moving to the House of Lords. The Royal Assent was granted in October 1969.

THE DIVORCE REFORM ACT OF 1969

The Divorce Reform Act forms the basis of current divorce law. The petitioner is required to show that the marriage has irretrievably broken down instead of, as prior to 1971, proving the respondent's committal of a matrimonial offence. The divorce courts cannot find that irretrievable breakdown has occurred unless they are satisfied that there exists at least one of five 'facts'. But the old theory of fault has not been removed from the divorce courts, for three of these facts – adultery, intolerable behaviour and desertion (for two years or more) – make use of matrimonial misconduct to prove the existence of breakdown. The two other facts for presuming that the marriage has broken down were new. Divorce by agreement was allowed if the couple had lived apart for a continuous period of at least two years and the respondent consented to divorce. Even if there was no agreement, the fact that the parties had lived apart for a continuous period of at least five years allowed the judge to conclude that the marriage had broken down irretrievably. For the first time the 'guilty' spouse could openly seek divorce against the 'innocent' spouse who had not committed a matrimonial wrong and who did not consent to dissolution. This, the cornerstone of the reform, was the statutory response to the new family morality embodied in the Law Commission's philosophy of decent burial for dead marriages. The reformers' case was felicitously put by the *New Law Journal* who reasoned in utilitarian terms that:

> There must come a point – whether after five years or some other period is a detail – where (conscientious objection apart and conscientious objection is not concerned with grounds) unwillingness to accept the dissolution of a relationship that has been non-existent for so long a period must be seen as a protest not against divorce, but against some aspect of the situation that led to divorce. In such circumstances the formal termination of marriage can have little bearing on the distress the marital relationship has caused, and will inevitably continue to cause, as long as it lasts. The recollection of it will continue to cause distress, even after it has ended, and though the continuing distress may be greater for one party than for the other (because, for example, one finds happiness and other does not) it is surely better than one should have that benefit than neither should have it. Happiness is not a matter of equity. All that the law can do is ensure that where some good is attainable it is attained – even if it is only financial security.
>
> (*New Law Journal*, 1 February 1968: 99)

But this latter 'good' was to prove unachievable.

The government had promised to withhold introduction of the 1969 Act until comprehensive legislation had been introduced to deal with the financial consequences of divorce. As the Lord Chancellor explained, these latter provisions were 'necessarily a matter for the Government'. The proposals were largely based on the Law Commission's recommendations on financial provision contained in their 1969 report. The imminent dissolution of Parliament meant that the Bill received scant Parliamentary attention through lack of time. The normally comprehensive Standing Committee scrutiny was limited to only ten hours' examination, and consequently many important amendments were not debated. The resultant Matrimonial Proceedings and Property Act 1970 codified maintenance and property matters, rationalized and extended judicial powers, and generally aimed to provide more secure financial protection to wives and children (see below pp.191–2). This Act, together with the Divorce Reform Act came into force on 1 January 1971. The two Acts were subsequently brought together and consolidated in the Matrimonial Causes Act 1973.

The new law and its philosophy was quickly accepted by both the judiciary and the public. The second couple to divorce under the new Act were told by Mr Justice Ormrod, 'there is going to be a marked difference in the way in which we deal with these matters' (*Guardian*, 13 January 1971). Time has shown this to be an accurate prediction of judicial propensity to accept the spirit of the reformed divorce law.

Three years after the Act's introduction, the Departmental Committee on One-Parent Families could firmly declare that it 'was one of those measures which commended itself to the general conscience long before it succeeded in gaining the statute book' (Report 1974: 81). Yet public opinion had never been quite so readily convinced. Shortly after the Bill was published in early 1968 separate opinion polls were undertaken by National Opinion Polls (NOP) and Gallop Poll (GP). NOP reported 44 per cent were for and 39 per cent against change. The Gallop survey indicated an opinion swing of 6 per cent over the previous ten years favoured easier divorce, though this was counterbalanced by a similar percentage towards more difficult divorce. However, the findings made it clear a smaller proportion (39 per cent compared to 51 per cent in 1958) now remained content with existing divorce law (Lee 1974: 95–6). Almost half (48 per cent) of the public approved of breakdown as the only ground for divorce, with clear endorsement of the proposed five 'facts' ranging from adultery (78 per cent), unreasonable behaviour (76 per cent), two years' consensual agreement (70 per cent) down to five years' unilateral divorce (56 per cent) and desertion (56 per cent) (Wybrow 1989: 85–6). The compromise statute reflected the diversity of Parliamentary, Establishment and public opinion upon the meaning of marriage and the role of divorce in society. The 1969 Act officially confirmed the enlarged ideological boundary surrounding marital permanancy as a core concept within family life. The state's divorce orthodoxy had formally retracted before individualism's pressure.

Introduction of the new law on 1 January 1971 led to an immediate surge of 43 per cent in annual petitions between 1970 and 1971. But the 1960s had already experienced an annual rise of 9.5 per cent, from 28,542 divorce petitions in 1960 to 70,575 petitions in 1970. The 1969 legislation was partly an acknowledgment of this steadily increasing resort to divorce. What the new Act did was to allow petitioners legally chained by unremitting dead relationships to release themselves by the five-year separation provision. Over a fifth (27 per cent) of all 1971 petitions relied on this fact to show irretrievable breakdown. Petitioners using the five-year provision were much older than the average; in 1972 two-thirds of these male petitioners and almost half of female petitioners were aged fifty or more. Such petitioners' earlier 'fault' had restrained them within the empty legal shells of long decayed marriages. These men and women were the main beneficiaries of the new breakdown approach and its philosophy of decent interment for expired relationships.

SUMMARY DEBATE

Parliament had fundamentally restructured the principles operating for divorce court clientele, but left untouched the needs of the summary courts' penurious customers. The historical juridical distinction remained; successful maintenance applications in the summary courts still depended upon the wife proving her husband's committal of a matrimonial offence. The main grounds were those largely established in the nineteenth century: wilful neglect to maintain (1886), desertion (1895), persistent cruelty (1895) and adultery (1937). It was the grievance of an unchanged and secondary system of family law lodging in a criminal court which drew the most trenchant criticism from the Departmental

Committee on One-Parent Families. The Committee, under the probing chairmanship of Sir Morris Finer, a judge of the Family Division of the High Court, produced a report in 1974 that remains essential reading for understanding the symbiotic relationship between family habits, social trends, legal options and political response. The Finer Report, and its supporting appendices of evidence, offered a cogent analysis of the matrimonial jurisdiction of magistrates courts in contraposition with that of divorce courts. They found 'two sets of laws dealing with matrimonial breakdown, operating concurrently, but in different courts, and standing, both in the spirit and the letter, in the most remarkable contrast to each other' (Report 1974: par. 4.63). Their distaste at the antinomy between the two branches of matrimonial justice led the Committee to recommend abolition of the summary jurisdiction, and the radical restructuring of law and administration within a unified family court structure.

Neither the plea for abolition, nor the Committee's other major recommendations were acceptable to the Labour government who regarded them as too costly. The Finer Report was a victim of political infanticide by a government displaying scant recognition of paternity. Rejection indicated the low political weighting of lone-parent claims to a more generous slice of the earmarked public expenditure. Time has shown the Conservative government no more able or willing than its Labour predecessor to undertake substantive reform.

The embarrassing anomalies between the two jurisdictions led to the Domestic Proceeedings and Magistrates' Courts Act 1978. The opportunity for radical reform was ignored, the matrimonial offence kept its paramountcy within the new legislation. Professor Freeman, writing in 1978, believed the Act 'could only be seen as a stop-gap, a half-measure, a clumsy attempt to assimilate that which is not assimilable, the strait-jacketing of new substance within old form' (Freeman 1978: x). This 'half-measure' legislation remains the backbone of the magistrates courts' matrimonial jurisdiction. The Act did not revive the declining resort to the magistrates courts for new maintenance orders; broken marriages increasingly turned directly to the divorce court.

TOWARDS ADMINISTRATIVE DIVORCE

Since 1977 all undefended divorces are dealt with by what is called special procedure. This, in fact, is the common procedure, for less than 1 per cent of all petitions are actually defended by the other spouse. Obtaining a divorce is now an administrative process in which both parties accept the irretrievable breakdown of the marriage. The procedure is administered by a district judge in the privacy of a court office rather than the public arena of a courtroom. His stamp of approval upon the petition and accompanying affidavit becomes formal authority for the divorce judge to award a decree. (Measures proposed by the Lord Chancellor's Department in 1990 would allow court administrative staff to grant these applications.) The daily tray of petitions are examined and certified as fulfilling legal requirements without either spouse being present for questioning. An empty courtroom stages the brusque last rights intoned upon their marriage as the judge ritually pronounces the words of divorce simultaneously upon the fifty or so named couples. The most fundamental change of policy since the introduction of civil divorce in 1857 has been the silent transformation of divorce in the 1970s and maintenance in the 1990s from judicial procedures to administrative processes.

Part III
Marriage patterns in the twentieth century

8 Changing family patterns

The family remains the pivotal institution in modern industrial society. Nevertheless, the last hundred years have witnessed powerful demographic and social changes which have altered the form and nature of the British family. This transformation largely concerns the changing position of women in both the private and public spheres of life and this chapter highlights some of the main strands of these changes. For instance, chapel tablets, church gravestones and cathedral memorials provide witness to the high infant mortality rates experienced by the Victorian family. Another facet of the changing face of mortality is seen in the age distribution of deaths occurring then and now. In the period 1901–2 one-third of all female deaths (322,000) in the United Kingdom were for girls under five and only 14 per cent were formed by those reaching seventy-five years or more. Family stability was not a feature of either Victorian or Edwardian life. Returning to today, just 1 per cent of all female deaths in 1989 were for children under five and two-thirds (66 per cent) related to women aged seventy-five or more. Such evolving patterns provide a base against which the issue of family stability past and present can be more sensibly discussed, while dispelling the beliefs of mythologers who hold that admired family values and habits are observed only in times past.

All too often research findings provide a momentary picture of the aggregated experiences of individuals at a particular time. Greater reliability and insight is provided by studying their likely life-cycle from birth, through childhood, to single adulthood, marriage and parenthood in a new household; their children grow up and depart to form their own families, the parents are alone again in middle age to face retirement, old age, widowhood and death. Each family has its own unique experience of this course of formation and disintegration which can incorporate three or more generations. A significant minority will veer from this stereotype highroad along such paths as extra-marital cohabitation, non-marital births, divorce, remarriage and a new family. The social scientist can set down some broad background patterns affecting family life and practice, though one has to confess that preparation of similar evidence some twenty years ago for the Finer Committee on One-Parent-Families produced a clearer vision of family trends in the 1960s than the more misty and obscure ones of today.

One feature still remains the common element in a person's life experience. The propensity to marry has been a demographic characteristic of those born in the first half of this century: 96 per cent of all women aged fifty in 1985 will have been married compared with 85 per cent for similar-aged women in 1950. As there will always be a number of both sexes either not wanting to marry or preferring partnerships of the same sex, the former proportion must be seen as about the highest that can be expected. The nuclear family of husband, wife and children remains the common family pattern and this chapter concentrates on changes within such a family for two reasons. First, this is still the typical experience of family life for the majority of children from birth to adulthood. Second, English family law focuses its attention on the formation and termination of marriage, for by contracting marriage the partners forthwith acquire legal rights and obligations to each other and to their children.

The nuclear conjugal family is the traditional but not the only form of raising children. There are three other important patterns of family life. These are partnerships formed by unmarried couples who live together, families with one parent present, and households formed by parent and step-parent families. Such groups will be discussed more fully later in this chapter and in Chapter 10.

MARRIAGE MOVEMENTS

The earlier popularity of marriage was linked with the overall movement towards younger age at marriage; this resulted in three out of ten spinster brides in 1970 marrying under twenty. The early 1970s saw a stop to the falling age at marriage; since then the trend has reversed to produce a clear momentum to later entry. It is too early to say with confidence whether this pattern incorporates a minority's readiness to reject marriage completely or simply a delaying action by the majority. But recent evidence gives credence to the former belief; calculations by the Office of Population Censuses and Surveys (OPCS) show that 5 per cent of sixteen-year-old-girls in 1974 who reached fifty would at that age have remained unmarried, a similar-aged 1990 cohort projects 24 per cent (OPCS 1977; 1992b: 32). This fourfold increase in less than two decades indicates rapidly changing social attitudes towards the appropriateness of traditional marriage. Today's spinster bride is now marrying at an older average age (1985: 23.8; 1990: 25.2 years) than at any time since 1939. Similar trends have occurred in mainland Europe, with the mid-1980s recording an average age at first marriage (24.2 years) very similar to our experience.

The most useful explanatory factor in the study of family life is social class. Calculations by Haskey (1983) upon a sample survey of brides marrying in 1979 in England and Wales indicate the continuing relevance of social class upon age at marriage. Male and female spouses in social class 4 (semi-skilled occupations) are at least five times more likely to marry in their teens than those in social class 2 (managers, executive officers) (Haskey 1983).

EXTRA-MARITAL COHABITATION

Arm in arm with the evidence of delay – or possibly abandonment – in entering marriage is the increasing popularity of extra-marital cohabitation. This crude term is impossible to define satisfactorily. The General Household Survey settles for an unmarried couple living together as a man and wife, although the cohabitation findings emerging from this annual investigation are likely to be below the true figure as there is a tendency for women in long-running consensual unions to describe themselves as married. But the Survey's overall pattern for the 1970s and 1980s is of the rapid increase in premarital cohabitation as a precursor to marriage.

Premarital cohabitation in the supposedly liberal sixties was a very uncommon practice. Only 1 per cent of women marrying before the age of twenty-five (both bride and groom being single) in the period 1960–4 had lived with their husbands before marriage. Twenty years on (1980–4) the proportion had become almost a quarter (24 per cent), and figures for 1987 show an increase to almost half of all spinster brides. This pattern displays little appreciable variation between the social classes. The mothers of Cheltenham and Hackney, Sevenoaks and Bolton, diplomatically accept and openly acknowledge their daughters' and sons' new life patterns. Memories of earlier unhappy marital times have cautioned the divorced from re-entering the institution without first testing their suitability; premarital cohabitation has become the standard habit (70 per cent) for marriages occurring in 1980–4 where one or both spouses had been previously married (OPCS 1987: 28). These trends appear set to continue during the 1990s and unmarried cohabitation is now an institutionalized part of premarriage selection patterns. This increasing tendency to live together before marriage should theoretically brush apart some couples whose unsuitability for life membership of the marriage club would have emerged after enrolment. In practice, pre-maritally cohabiting couples show greater vunerability to marital breakdown (Haskey 1992).

The existing problems of measuring marital and family stability are exacerbated when the socio-legal researcher attempts to incorporate knowledge concerning the new-style partnerships. For instance, the 1979 General Household Survey reports that women in longer-lasting informal unions see, and describe, themselves as married women. The date of marriage is no longer a satisfactory boundary mark to record such matters as length of cohabitation or child-spacing patterns, though it remains the most practical starting line we have, allowing comparison with already published data.

We are witnessing important demographic and social changes in long-held habits, and it is as yet uncertain where they will lead to. What is clear is that couples are increasingly living together in stable relationships and raising children out of wedlock. One in seven of all new children born in 1990 will have parents living in consensual unions (OPCS 1990d: 58). Past experience suggests most will eventually marry. But pregnancy does not propel the couple towards matrimony any more, and their parents no longer coerce them towards a proper wedding. Traditional familial attitudes and expectations have eased over the last quarter century: the social and legal stigma associated with bastardy has been rightly curtailed. This is occurring throughout all classes, as demonstrated by the editorial policy for Debrett's *Peerage and Baronetage*, 1990 edition, which for the first time allows acknowledgement of illegitimate and adopted children (though neither can inherit titles).

Changing values in Sweden have resulted in unmarried cohabitation and marriage becoming almost indistinguishable. The liberal Scandinavian stance may be heralding a new European attitude to the meaning and perception of family life. In the early 1960s most young Swedish women followed the conventional European pattern and married at a relatively early age. Then Swedish women began to cohabit before marrying and the time of this partnership increased during the 1970s; by 1980 young couples were bearing more children outside marriage than within it though it appears the majority will eventually marry.

CHILD-BEARING TRENDS

The last hundred years has transformed the married woman's lot from repetitive pregnancy to one of controlled fertility and small family size. This, and some other features of the changing life-cycle that wives have experienced since mid-Victorian times is quantified in Table 8.1. This table takes as a starting point, the 'average' spinster bride marrying her bachelor groom in the year 1886. The average age at marriage for such a couple has been recorded, and their respective life-spans *from marriage* constructed from the life tables of the period. It is assumed that five years after marriage a daughter is born who will later marry and the table records her life-cycle. It has to be remembered that it is based on raw averages and therefore concertinas the full breadth of changing patterns formed by individual experiences, but it does record the flow of some of the important changes that have occurred to the family over these last one hundred years.

Family size has declined from that experienced by the typical girl born in 1860, who would marry at twenty-six and have some five children, though 15 per cent of these wives would bear ten or more children. The reduction in the generality of large families occurred very largely in the period between 1880 and the outbreak of the First World War (Glass and Grebenik 1954: table 2). So far, no entirely satisfactory explanation has yet emerged for what the Finer Committee on One-Parent Families termed 'a climacteric in social history' (Report 1974: 31).

Our average mother, as represented in Table 8.1, who married in 1945 at the age of twenty-four, would have raised two children by the end of her child-bearing life at fifty. Only 5 per cent of these wives would have experienced the fecundity of their great-grandmothers and given birth to five or more children, and it is this fall in the propensity to large family size across all social classes that is a particularly noticeable characteristic of post-First World War marriages. None the less, low-income households still have larger families to support.

Table 8.1 The changing family life-cycle for women

Event and year	Great-grandmother		Grandmother		Mother		Daughter	
	W	H	W	H	W	H	W	H
	(wife:husband)							
Born	1860	1858	1891	1889	1921	1919	1950	1948
Marry	1886		1916		1945		1972	
at age	26	28	25	27	24	26	22	24
Husband's death	1919		1954		1989		2019	
at age	59	61	63	65	68	70	69	71
Wife's death	1924		1959		1995		2027	
at age	64		68		74		77	
Duration of (years)								
Marriage	33		38		44		47	
Widowhood	5		5		6		8	

Earlier-begun families and larger completed ones are also strongly associated with younger age at marriage. Evidence from the OPCS shows that half of the wives under twenty, who had registered their child's birth in 1983, had conceived before marriage; a percentage that had hardly changed from a decade earlier (1973: 54 per cent) (Werner 1985: table 9 recalculated). The husbands were predominantly employed (four-fifths in both years) in manual occupations and few had satisfactory accommodation in which to begin a family.

But to focus only on legitimate births to young mothers is to omit the input of extra-marital stable unions to the social and demographic patterns of the 1980s. This is reflected among the young mothers registering births in 1983 who were living with the father in either marital or extra-marital stable unions; the latter family type now accounted for 42 per cent of all births – a fourfold increase compared with a decade earlier. Unmarried pregnancy no longer creates the pressures towards marriage that still existed in the early 1970s.

Linked with all this is the high rate of divorce experienced by the young (aged under twenty) bride (Report 1967). It has been predicted half of these young wives will experience divorce compared with a third of brides aged twenty to twenty-four (Haskey 1983: tables 9 and 11). But other findings suggest early child-bearing experienced by young wives is the most important activity factor towards divorce (Kiernan 1983: 28).

Differing educational patterns is one possible factor helping to explain why women who marry and enter motherhood at an early age are associated with the lower-income groups. We know from the longitudinal investigation of girls born in 1946 that twice the proportion of those leaving school without any formal qualification had married by twenty compared with those who obtained an '0' level or equivalent grade (Kiernan and Eldridge 1987: table II). Many boys and girls from working-class homes leave school at the earliest possible age. School streaming from primary classroom days has marked such children as failures. Unsuccessful in a society which applauds the virtue of higher education and the ethic of acquisitiveness, it is not surprising that some of these girls graduate to the one role that is acclaimed by the community around them, by the magazines they read, and the television they view. For such teenagers motherhood provides a purpose to life, as well as being a clear expression of success in a role and function which is still seen by most young women as their ultimate goal. In these communities, the wedding ring, double-bed and pram are the young mother's primary marks of achievement over their similar-aged middle-class sisters. But the wedding ring is not so symbolic as it was twenty years ago.

PARENTHOOD

The procreation and rearing of children remains a general feature of married life. An attitude study by Abrams (1973) has shown that family life for many British men and women is one of the most satisfying (second only to marriage) areas of their life. Part of this satisfaction is provided by the role of parent, with its ascribed status and presumption of family solidarity. Parenthood changes the habits and needs of the couple and means that in most cases the wife is economically dependent on the husband, while care of the home and upbringing of children is still seen as the mother's task.

Delaying the start of a family allows development of a financial base to support parenthood costs, while providing opportunity for the couple to adapt to the concessionary approach required from a successful partnership of personalities. Most married couples now wait longer than their parents did to start a family – twenty-seven months being the median interval between marriage and their first child in 1990. (Though, for reasons already provided, a caveat needs to be added concerning the unknown period of premarital cohabitation that occurred for half the couples.) Wives of semi-skilled and unskilled manual workers record a shorter average time (twenty-one months) (*Social Trends* 1989: 46). Correlated with both lower social class and earlier start to family-raising (with the associated factor of premaritally conceived pregnancies) is the younger age of entering parenthood.

It is not only that family size is now smaller, but that women reach their desired completed family size more quickly than did Victorian mothers. Today, nine out of ten couples will complete their family size within ten years of marriage. Women have obtained greater social and economic freedom from the decline in large families and the associated increasing employment levels. Parental desire to control the spacing and size of their families, linked with the promotion of acceptable and efficient methods of family planning, have resulted in couples generally having wanted children. Development of oral contraceptives and IUDs allow women to be mistresses of their own fertility and time of mothering and this reformation in demographic pattern and familial habit has modified motherhood to the extent that it now occupies only a small part of their lives.

FAMILY ACCOMMODATION

The young married mother is likely to experience several forms of financial disadvantage compared with those who delay parenthood to an older age. Birth of the first child stops the wife contributing financially to the marriage and causes additional expenditure upon the new baby's needs. Parenthood also enforces the couple's need to have independent self-contained accommodation.

The nuclear family in Britain usually lives as a separate household, and it is the housing structure and condition that provide the physical framework within which a great deal of the family interaction occurs. The home is seen as an ongoing and stable base, and this characteristic of continuity is associated with the loyalty and commitment of family relationships. Personal fulfilment and satisfaction has become centred in the privacy of the home. Young Bethnal Green mothers interviewed by Anthea Holme (1985) desired a place of their own, away from the noise of neighbours destroying the privacy of their council flat. Disappointment is the probable outcome, for after two years of marriage, the young wife is twice as likely to be without a home of her own as the wife who married at twenty or over (Holmans 1981: table 1). The strains placed upon a couple by the pressures of inadequate accommodation space and amenities are far more likely to be the experience of earlier-marrying low-income couples than those from the higher social classes. This factor, linked with the earlier start to family life experienced by the younger wife, means that in many cases the couple will not have their own accommodation when the first child is born. Little wonder a national survey of family attitudes found double the proportion of those in the two lower social classes believed housing to be a factor 'thought very important to a successful marriage' compared with the less concerned response from the top two classes (Ashford 1987: 125). Poor and overcrowded housing conditions found among a sample of married women with children living in the London suburb of Camberwell, was a major precipitating factor of depression. Another characteristic of the Camberwell women was the high level of marriage breakdown (Brown and Harris 1978).

If one is going to focus on a single factor that can help to explain the association between young marriages, social class and divorce, then the financial condition of the marriage appears to be a strong contender. Available money allows suitable housing, household and family needs to be purchased. For those less fortunate, the problems of overcrowding and tight budgeting can lead to marital disharmony. The young working-class couples' accommodation problem is of course a reflection of their financial position. Newly married middle-class couples will often benefit from parental assistance towards the necessary deposit on the all-important first house purchase. We know that in marriages where the bride is twenty or more the couple are more likely to delay a family, and so have the continuing financial benefit of two incomes rather than one wage to maintain two adults and newborn baby. The former couples are usually in a more advantageous position to acquire independent accommodation at an earlier stage of their marriage than are their younger marrying counterparts.

Home ownership has become the standard family housing pattern with two-thirds of British housing stock now owner occupied compared to one-tenth of all housing in 1914 and one-quarter in 1945. The desire to acquire one's own home has been doubly fuelled by government encouragement and the lack of rented accommodation which is either affordable in the private sector or available in the public sector. Demand had driven up house prices until mid-1989 and at the same time made it harder for the first-time buyer to enter the market. The first-time buyer in mid-1988 paid an average of £43,000 (mid-1992, £42,000) throughout the United Kingdom, and required a mortgage advance of £36,000. In London the average first-time loan was over £60,000. These figures, which come from the admirable *Housing Statistics Bulletin* (January 1989) of the Nationwide Building Society, show the related gross annual income (including second incomes) to meet these new mortgages was £15,710. By June 1990 the typical mortgage interest rate was 15.4 per cent, which meant that a mortgagor with a £36,000 loan on a twenty-five-year repayment would be then paying some £475 monthly. This calculation does not allow for income tax relief, but neither does it include such additional outgoings as house maintenance, insurance, heating and lighting and Council tax costs. It is not surprising that many young couples without children, and even more so with children, simply cannot contemplate buying their own home, and those that do have a mortgaged property face the risk of repossession and consequent homelessness if unable to continue repayment. Stability was shattered for the family occupants of the 75,000 properties repossessed in 1991.

For many failed marriages the impact of large mortgage loans and high interest rates continues beyond separation and divorce. The divorce court might use its adjustive powers to make a property transfer order to the wife with the intention of providing family security, but the wife may not be able to continue the repayments out of the restraining budget of a one-parent family, and the house is either sold or repossessed. If the court makes an order for immediate sale the resulting spousal division of the equity seldom gives the wife enough capital to allow purchase of a new home. Another court option is to allow the wife to remain in the marital home until the youngest child has left school, while ordering the husband to make the mortgage repayments. The danger of this well-intentioned approach is that, in a period of rapidly rising prices, the delay only exacerbates the wife's financial problem of insufficient capital and income to a later time and age. One consequence of this combination of marriage breakdown and high-cost housing, family needs, female dependency and low wage-earning potential is that half of all separated and divorced women find themselves in public sector (local authority and new-town) housing. Such women are two and a half times more likely to have this form of housing than are still married or cohabiting couples (*Social Trends* 1990: table 8.23). Marital dissolution itself creates additional need for both public and private rented accommodation, and current breakdown rates are generating demand for some 55,000 additional tenant households every year (Holmans *et al.* 1987: 23). There is no sign of this family necessity being either met or even recognized.

Public sector housing provides over four-fifths of all rented accommodation. By the end of 1989 over a fifth of all council properties in existence in 1978 had been sold to tenants under the government's 1980 statutory 'right to buy' provisions. The desire to purchase was disproportionately higher from council tenants living in houses compared with those in flat accommodation. One consequence of the government's policy of promoting council house sales has been the severe reduction of public sector family-type accommodation and this has not been replaced. The number of public sector dwellings with three or more bedrooms annually completed in England and Wales has plunged from 52,000 in 1976, down through the 1980s (1981: 19,000) to some 4,000 in 1988 (*Social Trends* 1990: table 8.4). This depletion of council house stock has created lengthening waiting lists, especially in the expensive south. For instance, Elmbridge Council (covering the prosperous Weybridge, Esher, Cobham and Walton on Thames areas of Surrey), had sold some 1,600 homes (mostly three-bedroomed houses) over the 1980s. In 1988 the council had 5,500 properties remaining and 92 units under construction. But the surge in prices and the cuts in council house building had left 1,600 needy families waiting to be rehoused (*Daily Telegraph*, 9 August 1988).

The points system that largely dominates the system of local authority housing allocation gives priority to large family size, existing unsatisfactory accommodation, and length of time on the waiting list. Homelessness has increasingly become a characteristic of new tenancies, with 28 per cent of all new tenants in 1989–90 being previously homeless. A growing proportion (one in ten) of disadvantaged homeless families are in this situation because of mortgage default. Local authorities' legal obligation to house the homeless correspondingly reduces the housing opportunity for other families lodged on the waiting list. As public sector housing becomes increasingly scarce, the self-supporting low-income prudent couple with only a small family, living with relatives and complaining of family friction and desperate to find a place of their own, can expect little help from local authorities.

The search for independent accommodation in the private sector is equally unrewarding. Many landlords will not let to couples with young children, and those who do often charge a rent (though it may be no more than the market rate) that reduces by half the young couple's take-home wage. The combination of inflationary house prices and rent controls have largely culled the supply of private rented accommodation. Many a small landlord is discouraged by the equity of a rent-control system that sets the 1990 protected tenancy rent for a three-bedroomed terraced house in south-east London at £14 per week, which is then halved after deducting insurance, collection fees and tax. This anecdote helps to explain why the private sector has declined from a half of all owner and rental tenures in 1951 to less than a tenth today. There is little affordable private accommodation for the despairing family with an ordinary wage seeking a home.

Families rightly expect higher standards of housing than that experienced by their parents and grandparents. An elderly neighbour recollects how she and twelve other siblings grew up in my two-bedroomed home; now couples move on when their second child is contemplated. But they have a home to sell and normally profit by the price spiral (if bought before 1988). It is not to existing home-owners that the argument of this section has been directed. The family-housing quagmire impacts on young low and standard wage earners who cannot afford to buy their first home, who cannot find accommodation to rent, and can no longer look to councils for help. Nationwide Building Society figures for their first-time buyers in Surrey for the tax year ended March 1988, hammers home the dilemma. The average first-time purchaser was aged thirty-four, putting down a deposit of £11,000 and receiving an advance of £45,000. The mortgagor's annual income of £19,608 was more than a university tutor received at the top of the lecturers pay scale in October 1987. These figures complement a report prepared in 1988 by Dr Glen Bramley of the School for Advanced Urban Studies at Bristol University, for the Association of District Councils, showing over half of all working families in prosperous Surrey do not even earn enough to buy a starter flat. This unacceptable face of housing deprivation and hardship has created depression and anxiety within too many lives. If nothing is done to provide accommodation for those families, we must not be surprised if a minority do not succeed.

WOMEN AND EMPLOYMENT

A later start to maternity means that the school-leaving girl of the 1990s will experience a much longer potential employment period between ceasing education and commencing motherhood than the gap of only a few years for many schoolgirls of the early 1970s. This trend disguises likely social class variations. Full-time motherhood at home breaks employment activity, but only for a relatively short part of the women's life-cycle. But nature's reproductive prejudice creates further injustice and disadvantage for the wife intending to return to the labour market. This employment gap is often at the crucial time when men, relieved of domestic and parental involvement by their wives undertaking the household and caring tasks, establish themselves and gain promotion at the workplace.

With the youngest child reaching school age, the married mother is likely to re-enter paid employment. The General Household Survey for 1990 (table 9.11) records half (51 per cent) of all such women whose youngest dependent child was aged between five and nine were engaged in part-time employment, a further 19 per cent were in full-time employment and 3 per cent were unemployed but seeking work. The remaining 27 per cent were obtusely recorded as 'economically inactive'.

In past times, the traditional carer of the employed mother's children was the grandmother, now it is less certain that this unpaid help will be so readily available. Over half (1990: 53 per cent) of all married women aged fifty-five to fifty-nine are now active in the paid labour market, and increasing geographical mobility has separated kin. The necessity for better child-care facilities and more flexible working conditions is evident if the modern family, and especially the mother, is to cope effectively with these new life patterns.

Changing patterns of female employment over the twentieth century have helped reduce the dominance of the traditional housewife role. In 1900, only a tenth of married women worked outside the home; today, the 1990 General Household Survey indicates seven out of ten wives aged below sixty are employed. The typical British family can no longer be stereotyped breadwinner father, a home-maker mother and their two dependent children. Figures for 1981 show that among married couples *with children* 44 per cent had joint incomes and 47 per cent depended solely on the husband (Joshi 1990, table 10.2). The remaining households had either the wife as sole earner (3 per cent) or were both non-earners (6 per cent).

Married women's rising employment rates are partially explained by the interrelationship between the increasing availability of part-time jobs, declining birth rates, hankering for liberation from domestic incarceration, and economic pressures upon wives to contribute directly to the family income. Additional money allows the expanded household budget to contemplate a larger mortgage, further home improvements, overseas holidays and time-saving household appliances. Improving family choice has been the main reason attracting working-class women back to employment, while further up the social class scale the desire for career fulfilment becomes a more dominant attraction. Information from the Family Expenditure Survey for 1985 shows the significant contribution that an earning wife makes to the family finances: 25 per cent of the joint income if there were dependent children, and 37 per cent if there were not. The number of families in poverty (that is, below the old supplementary benefit level) would have increased threefold without the benefit of wives' earnings.

Social factors influencing the employment rates of wives are first, the social class grouping of the household; wives of husbands in unskilled occupations are the least likely to be in employment. The second, and more crucial determinant of whether a wife works or not, and whether it is part-time or full-time employment, is the presence, and age, of children. The likelihood of the mother being an income earner decreases with the infancy of the youngest child, so family income is thus reduced at the very time when maximum financial demands are made upon the household budget. A combination of a low wage and young family are likely characteristics of financially stretched couples. Playing the disposable income game with ineffective free-market dice means these vulnerable couples find themselves sliding further down the snake of relative poverty. The resultant stress and tension readily corrodes disheartened relationships contained in deficient accommodation to disintegration and divorce.

Greater employment participation by married women has provided them with more economic freedom and choice, as availability of paid work offers the opportunity to move away from dependency on the husband's earnings, and the means to separate if the marriage fails. Women have gained a level of financial independence and social confidence from the competition and companionship of the workplace. Within this occupational setting the observation, association and conversation of women provides social intercourse, broadens horizons and presents more opportunities than the postman ever brought. In short, new employment patterns present greater freedom and power than ever before for wives to examine the quality and worth of their marriage, and to respond if the relationship is judged intolerable. As the family expenditure broadens to incorporate two incomes, the greater is the relative decline in the accepted and expected standard of living if the partnership dissolves.

Though marital symmetry may have been enhanced, it is still the woman who invariably has the major responsibility for the constant and repetitive household chores such as preparation of the evening meal, household cleaning and washing and ironing. Caring is seen as part of the household labour in which the majority of domestic and attendant tasks all too often fall upon women. It is the mother who deals with a crying baby at night and who takes time off from employment if the child is ill. The caring role has no fixed hours, there is no contract, it is undertaken out of public view, it is seen as a task predominantly for women. An egalitarian division of domestic tasks has been the reward for only a minority of employed women. All this has produced a potential conflict of claims between the traditional expectation that wives undertake the unpaid caring and servicing of their family's needs, and the role of paid worker. The new joint-income partnership has created a more stressful and demanding day for some wives and mothers. The mental health casualty rate is highest among married women; for men the single state provides the greatest risk. And longer life is now increasing the importance of another female role, that of carer for the very elderly.

Half of all married women aged between fifty-five and fifty-nine are engaged in some form of paid work. Having reached the statutory retirement age of sixty, the wife should traditionally be seen as entering a period of tranquillity. But in many cases there will be an aged mother or mother-in-law, and of course in some cases a lone father, who may be in need of some form of care and attention. Already as many as one-fifth of women aged between forty and fifty-nine are having caring responsibilities for parents and parents-in-law (Martin and Roberts 1984).

AGEING PATTERNS

The harsh social and work environment, poor medical knowledge and public ignorance of 150 years ago all helped to create the mortality patterns whereby less than a fifth (17 per cent) of girls born in 1840 would live to seventy-five. This age mark will be passed by 54 per cent of the daughters of the 1950s, and 67 per cent of those born in the 1980s. Earlier marriage and greater longevity have meant that the girl born in 1950, when compared with her great-grandmother, would marry some four years younger and experience a further forty-seven years of marriage (the divorce possibility is discounted). This is fourteen years more than her great-grandmother. Table 8.1 records some major events in the life-cycle that draws to an end with some eight years of widowhood.

It is not that the maximum life-span is being extended, but that a larger proportion of men and women than ever before will experience longevity. Widowhood is the likely circumstance of the older woman, mainly as a consequence of the sexual variation in age at marriage whereby spinster brides still remain younger than grooms, and the longer life-span of women. The reverse side of this demographic coin shows ever-married husbands aged seventy-five or more are more than twice as likely to be living with their partners (66 per cent) than are wives of similar age (25 per cent).

The General Household Survey (1985) gives some indication of the likely future care requirements among older (seventy-five and over) women. For instance, the proportion of such women who reported that illness or disability had restricted activity in the preceding two weeks before being interviewed by the Survey doubled from 11 per cent in 1976 to 23 per cent in 1985. This rise is explained by the increasing numbers of very elderly women aged eighty-five or more. Their numbers doubled between 1961 and 1981, and are projected to double again between 1981 and 2021. The propensity to be ill or disabled rises exponentially with advancing age. This means that the very elderly are far more likely to incur some need of care and attention than those aged between sixty and eighty-five. Another characteristic of the very elderly is that they are predominantly (77 per cent) women. Their dominant source of caring continues to be the family, and it remains the case that daughters are expected to provide the major attention and services necessary to help the very elderly carry on within the community.

Daughters may be willing to take on the additional task of caring for their elderly widowed mother or mother-in-law. They may well see it as a responsibility they wish to undertake, indeed an obligation of love. This caring does reduce the daughter's independence in the same way that child-rearing had curtailed the mother's. And in the case of the elderly widowed mother aged eighty or more, her own daughter is now likely to be approaching or has arrived at retirement age and what should be a more pastoral period after parenthood and the employment years. It is time to consider the introduction of a new 'elderly care' benefit that would be payable to those who provide voluntary care service to the very old (see Gibson 1990: 94). There needs to be greater recognition by the government of the carer's role in providing company and help, thereby allowing the elderly to remain out of institutional care.

Contemporary demographic patterns and changing female attitudes impact upon this traditional network of family support which remains so important for the well-being of those elderly who need carers. Increased rates of divorce, gender differentials in remarriage opportunity, reconstituted kin obligations, reduced family size and uneven mortality patterns which cause women of eighty-five or more to outnumber men by three to one all entwine to create inescapable implications for future caring policy in general and women in particular.

FAMILY STABILITY THEN AND NOW

In the first year of this century, the Divorce Court granted some 500 divorces; in 1990 the numbers had become some 153,000: the current total, when standardized against the marriage population, is a 140-fold increase on that of 1900. But in 1900, as argued in Chapter 5, the severity of the law and restricted opportunity to the court resulted in divorce petitions making up less than a tenth of all matrimonial proceedings. The rate of divorce is a partial resultant of its availability as well as changing individual attitudes and expectations towards marriage.

The rate of divorce is only one indicator by which the stability of the nuclear family can be examined. The excessive child-bearing patterns of Victorian times, poor ante-natal care, ignorance and prolonged work in factory and home before childbirth led to some 5 mothers in a 1,000 dying in pregnancy and childbirth. Today, the risk to a mother is less than 1 in 10,000 births, a sixty-eight-fold improvement (the 'true' rate is even higher, if one allows for the then more frequent pregnancy occurrence). The end of Queen Victoria's reign still witnessed one in seven of all parents burying their newborn within a year of birth. The reality of working-class conditions at this time is made clear by Lady Bell, in her sensitive dissection of life and labour in the iron town of Middlesborough. Her account of the harsh nature of working-class family life at the beginning of this century is essential reading by which to judge the merits of Victorian standards and the resultant social structure: of the mother who 'had never got over the successive shocks' of losing nine of her twelve children in infancy (1907: 191); and the mothers who had experienced repeated stillborn labours.

> Women among the well-to-do hardly ever have this terrible experience of having one stillborn child after another. To be going to bring a child into the world; to be constantly ill before its birth, as must be the case if it dies during this time; to have either the awful suspicion that the hope is over, or else to go on to the end; to go through all the necessary agony, to bear a dead child, to have the shock of realising what has happened; then in a few months begin over again facing the terrible possibility, which in course of time comes to pass, and live through the whole dread story once more. And even when the children are born alive, what must that other woman have gone through who lost twelve out of her seventeen children?
>
> (Bell 1907: 199)

Small squalid tenement rooms denied privacy and quiet to confined mother and newborn infant; the open window offered the noise, smell and pollution of nearby smelters. All this was part of the fecund poverty drawn from the countryside and made manifest through the concentrated harshness of family conditions within the new factory landscape.

The childhood risks of Victorian times have an even more murky tinge that has yet to be properly exposed. Set against this social and demographic backcloth was the disturbing evidence gathered by the Select Committee on Child Insurance (1891) and the Northcote Commission on Friendly Societies (1874). The evidence of the Registrar General to the Commission recorded that in certain districts of northern England the infant death rate bounded up directly after the first birthday, as the child's death now brought full benefit to the insuring parents or guardians. Other government inquiries revealed the existence of large-scale baby-farming whereby infants were handed over to an unknown woman who promised to rear the child for a relatively small single payment. In reality, the child's early death allowed the supposedly caring woman to obtain maximum profit from the business. The bodies of sixteen young babies were found in Brixton and Peckham at the beginning of May 1870; in the same year some 276 babies were found dead in the streets of London. This evidence, underlined by the sensational trial and subsequent execution of a notorious baby farmer, Margaret Waters, in October 1870, subsequently caused a public outcry which led to the first of the Infant Life Protection Acts in 1872. For all the publicized horrors of modern-day child assault and murder trials it is clear that infanticide has declined over the last hundred years. Today's society expects higher parental standards of rearing, caring and protection than ever before.

The improved mortality rates of this century have also made their impact on adult life-chances. For instance, the married man in the age group thirty-five to forty-four had six times greater risk of death in 1900 than his counterpart in 1985. The improvements experienced in housing and sanitation, progress in medical knowledge, better environment, fewer wars, rising standards of living and education and the development of social services have helped to reduce significantly the mortality risks that buried the chances of a couple reaching old age together. The experience of 'great-grandmother' in Table 8.1 was thirty-three years of marriage cut short by her husband's death when she was fifty-nine. Today, almost three-quarters (73 per cent) of all ever-married women aged sixty to sixty-four in 1990 are still married, a fifth (20 per cent) are widowed and 7 per cent are divorced. Adult mortality and its impact on widowhood are reflected in the 1901 Census figures in which six out of ten widows (60 per cent) and widowers (58 per cent) were under sixty-five years. Similar calculations for 1985 show only two out of ten widows (22 per cent) and widowers (23 per cent) were under sixty-five years. The contemporary married woman has a greater chance than ever her great-grandmother had of both celebrating her sixty-fifth birthday and having her husband (though not necessarily the original) and all her children (and possibly stepchildren) beside her.

Some aspects of the changing patterns of widowhood and divorce experienced by married women this century are reflected in Table 8.2. The proportion of ever-married women who are widows has remained remarkably constant over the

Table 8.2 Age distribution of ever-married women by marital status for 1901, 1961 and 1990, England and Wales (per cent)

Year Status	15–44	Age 45–64	65+	Total	Numbers (100%) (millions)
1901					
Married	54.6	23.7	3.8	82.1	
Widowed	2.7	8.1	7.1	17.9	7.0
1961					
Married	42.2	31.2	8.0	81.4	
Widowed	0.6	5.2	11.6	17.4	
Divorced	0.5	0.6	0.1	1.2	14.6
1990					
Married	36.0	26.0	11.3	73.3	
Widowed	0.2	3.1	14.6	17.9	
Divorced	4.7	3.1	1.0	8.8	16.2

Source: Calculations based on 1961 Census of England and Wales, *Age, Marital Condition and General Tables*, table 12; OPCS 1992b: table 1.1(a).

three recorded years but, as already argued, it is the transference of widowhood to a predominantly 'older' age risk which has improved this facet of marriage stability. Set against this evidence is the steadily increasing impact of divorce, especially in the 1970s and 1980s, whereby 9 per cent of all ever-married women were recorded as divorced (and not remarried) in 1990. Professor M. Anderson (1983: figure 2) has looked at this question of breakdown and cause and calculated that there was very little difference in the marriage termination rate (death and divorce combined) after twenty years of marriage (the child-bearing period) for those marrying in 1896 compared with the probable similar marital disruption experience of a 1980 marriage cohort. The larger family size of a hundred years ago makes it likely that a higher proportion of children aged under sixteen then would have been affected by marriage breakdowns than would be the case today when one remembers the relatively high proportion (1990: 45 per cent) of current divorces without dependent children. Family breakdown is not a new phenomenom though the causal circumstances have altered.

ONE-PARENT FAMILIES

Family life for younger parents is primarily the loving, nurturing and protection of dependent children (officially defined as aged under sixteen, or between

Table 8.3 Lone-parent families in Great Britain, 1971 and 1989

| Lone parents | Numbers | | Children | Lone parents increase |
| | *1971* | *1989* | *1989* | *1971–89* |
		(,000)	*(,000)*	*%*
Mothers				
Single	90	360	504	300
Separated	170	210	399	24
Divorced	120	380	646	217
Widowed	120	70	112	–42
Sub-total	500	1020	1661	104
Fathers	70	130	195	86
Total	570	1150	1856	102

Source: Haskey 1991: table 2; and recalculation from *General Household Survey* for 1990: table 2.30).

sixteen and eighteen and in full-time education). The last two decades have witnessed a rapid increase of single parenthood within the family. The number of one-parent families has doubled over the eighteen years between 1971 and 1989; in the latter year over one million lone parents were responsible for raising 1.9 million dependent children. These 1989 figures mean that one in seven of all dependent children are being raised by a lone mother, though this may not be a permanent setting. Both the daily caring and rearing and the associated longer-term problems of heading a one-parent family largely fall upon women, for only a tenth of such households are headed by a man.

The evidence of Table 8.3 shows that the advancing count of lone mothers in 1989 largely results from the growing ranks of single and divorced mothers. Lone single mothers (that is, with non-marital children and not cohabiting) were responsible for some 500,000 dependent children. This increase is associated with changing attitudes towards family life, motherhood and independence. More women from all classes feel they have the right to choose motherhood without necessitating the father's household presence.

Non-marital births have risen from 5 per cent of all births in 1961 to 28 per cent in 1990. In some inner-city areas such as Lambeth (1986: 46 per cent) the likelihood of a birth being non-marital has become par. But it would be a mistake to assume that all these mothers are alone; study of national birth certificates shows half of all non-marital births are jointly registered by the mother and father who live together (as shown by the same address) and form a dual-parent family unit. This facet excludes them from one-parent family surveys. Only a small proportion of the remaining 'lone' single mothers place their children for adoption. Non-marital birth can no longer be seen as a sensible indicator of the incidence of unsought motherhood. Greater awareness and use of contraception backed by the safety net of the Abortion Act elevates motherhood to an increasingly deliberate and positive choice.

The surging divorced rate is the demographic feature which explains why the lone divorce mother group accounts for half of the increase in all lone-mother families between 1971 and 1989 reported in Table 8.3. Evidence from the 1990 General Household Survey suggests one in ten of all dependent children in Britain are being brought up alone by separated or divorced mothers (OPCS, 1992b; table 2.30).

The divorce rate of England and Wales in 1987 predicts almost four in every ten newly formed marriages will end in divorce (Haskey 1989a). This pattern indicates half the newly-weds will not celebrate their silver wedding; a quarter of the absentees will be recorded by certificates of human mortality and three-quarters by decrees of judicial dissolution. When insuring his life the solicitous younger husband misjudges the real family threat. One in four of all children will witness their parents' divorce before reaching the school-leaving age of sixteen.

An additional unknown number of children experience the separation of parents who do not divorce. Details of some of these broken marriages will be contained in the domestic files of magistrates courts. Even less is known about the numbers and life experiences of children affected by the broken partnerships of their cohabitating unwed parents. It is likely that there are in Britain over 400,000 dependent children living with their unmarried parents. There is no reason to suppose that such unions are any more stable than marriages. All the evidence combines to suggest that at least a third of all children will experience a one-parent household before their sixteenth birthday.

The one-parent families that mass to form the cold statistics of numbers and trends are, when observed as individuals, constantly changing in their social pattern and status. A momentary one-off snapshot of the family does not allow the detail of changing experience and realignment provided by the focus of a longitudinal study. As new lone parents increase the total at a particular time, so extra-marital cohabitation, marriage, remarriage and youngest child becoming dependent are significant life events that reduce overall numbers. A follow-up study of couples divorcing in 1973 showed half the women had married again within four and a half years (Leete and Anthony 1979). The reality of being a one-parent family may be only a fairly short period within the adult's overall life. The fact that the majority of single-parent families become reconstituted into differing new family forms has important social and legal implications which will be examined in Chapter 10.

The evidence of this chapter indicates various alternative forms of family life have become more commonplace over the last twenty years. Nevertheless, the fact that four out of five children in 1990 were living with their married parents confirms that the most popular form of parenthood remains that which regularises the relationship between family members, and formalizes bonds between family and society. The traditional family continues, yet today's evident and accepted non-conventional patterns will be more prevalent in tomorrow's family.

9 The resort to divorce: the social evidence

Divorce has become the established remedy for estranged spouses; every year in England and Wales some 300,000 husbands and wives and 150,000 dependent children witness the withered union's formal dissolution. Analysis of the available social evidence from both official data and research findings must, of necessity, freeze into cold statistical aggregates the individual experiences of unhappy families. None the less, this evidence does provide a picture of the major demographic and social associates of divorce, and they are examined in this chapter.

The Office of Population Censuses and Surveys (OPCS) collection of the yearly number of spouses judicially severing their fetid marriage bonds results in a very accurate official statistic of divorce. The annual *Marriage and Divorce Statistics* (Series FM2) provides cross-tabulations of the demographic features considered relevant and collectable by the OPCS. For instance, the reader of the 1990 edition would find the twenty-four divorce tables provided information concerning spousal age at marriage and divorce cross-tabulated by variables such as marital status at marriage, duration of the marriage to divorce, and year of marriage. Children are spotlighted to the extent that data is provided on the numbers of dependent (and independent) children of the family, family size by age of wife at marriage, and also the duration of the marriage and the ages of children by age of wife at divorce. In addition, the report provides a brief commentary on salient changes and patterns. All this provides empirical knowledge of how many men and women fall into certain demographic sets, but provides little focus on why these patterns are the way they are, or the causality between the variables. None the less, the OPCS's repeated collection and presentation of similar table formats provides the researcher with an ongoing picture of demographic trends within the *currently* divorcing population. The published statistics also provides a valuable data base against which explanations can be tested and survey material compared.

THE INCIDENCE OF DIVORCE

The total of divorces granted (the decree absolute being the final stage of the legal process, returning husband and wife to a single status, with the concomitant right to marry again) has increased each decade since the introduction of civil divorce in 1857, while their yearly number has multiplied 250 fold between 1900 and 1990. It is statistically prudent to show divorce totals as a rate for every 1,000 married women, as divorce is a partial resultant of the married population – which has doubled between 1900 and 1990 – at risk. This new baseline indicates (Table 9.1) that the divorce rate has increased twentyfold in the last fifty years. Two periods show particularly noticeable jumps. In the first example, the massive divorce surge in the period 1946–50 reflected the combined influence of the marital casualties of the war years, changing values of the post-war era and the extended grounds of the 1937 Herbert Act. This period marked a historical juncture when, for the first time, more broken marriages sought judicial termination instead of summary separation. The post-war 1947 peak of 60,000 divorces was not to be surpassed until 1971 – a pattern similar to that experienced within the United States. On the second occasion, the introduction in 1971 of a more liberal divorce legislation allowed previously restricted petitioners manacled to long-dead marriages by the clamp of 'fault' to free themselves by the new key of irretrievable breakdown underlined by five or more years' separation. Yet it has to be remembered that the 1969 Divorce Reform Act was itself as much a consequence of the legislative acknowledgement of changing social attitudes and expectations towards marriage reflected in the escalating resort to divorce as it was to the evidence of unmet needs. The 1960s had seen the annual divorce numbers continuously rising to reach 58,000 in 1970, thereby more than doubling the 1961 total. The surge following the 1969 Divorce Reform Act's introduction in 1971 led to divorces granted in 1972 exceeding 100,000 annually for the first time. Since 1980 the yearly total has fluctuated around the 150,000 mark, which means that about 13 in every 1,000 ongoing marriages will be dissolved annually. Such a rate, if it continues at the 1987 divorce level, implies that just under four in every ten (37 per cent) newly formed marriages will ultimately end in divorce (Haskey 1989b). Haskey acknowledges his calculation includes the previously divorced who had remarried, and that they both form a growing proportion of all new marriages, and experience a greater level of breakdown than do first marriages. For these reasons the true divorce risk for a couple both marrying for the first time will be lower than the calculated 37 per cent overall average.

It is clear that the rate of divorce now stands higher than at any time this century. The debate revolves around the question of whether the divorce figures are no more than a reflection of a more open democratic society changing its attitude towards divorce and lowering its legislative and procedural barriers, or whether they actually indicate a real increase in spousal breakdown. Those sympathetic to the first possibility argue that marriage breakdown has not risen in real terms, but more failed marriages are now able or willing to turn to divorce as a solution. Such a reallocation theory maintains that current divorce numbers more closely equal the real breakdown rate than occurred in past times.

In the neutral corner stand those who hold the initial question to be both delusive and unanswerable, and therefore futile. They observe there is no general

Table 9.1 Annual number and rate of divorce, 1900–90, England and Wales

Period	Average*	Rate**	Period	Average*	Rate**
1901–10	594	0.1	1961–5	31807	2.7
1911–20	1083	0.2	1966–70	47501	3.9
1921–30	3046	0.4	1971–5	106697	8.5
1931–40	5096	0.5	1976–80	137284	11.1
1941–5	10389	1.0	1981–5	148938	12.1
1946–50	39901	3.7	1987	151007	12.7
1951–5	29572	2.7	1989	150872	12.7
1956–60	24172	2.1	1990	153386	12.9

Notes: * Decrees absolute: dissolution and nullity.
** Rate: divorces to every 1,000 ongoing married women.

agreement as to what constitutes a broken marriage, and a paucity of evidence about the frequency of some forms of breakdown. These critics rightly hold that an accurate measure of marital breakdown would have to include, for instance, the number of separations recorded by court orders, voluntary maintenance agreements sealed in the privacy of solicitors' offices, and welfare benefits paid to deserted wives. Even if this information could be accurately obtained for contemporary and earlier generations, we would still have no knowledge about those whose parting left no official record, or about couples who formally remain together, even though the affective relationship has long ceased. Sympathetic analysts retreat against such a backcloth of terminological and statistical inadequacies. Yet for all such shadows and doubts it becomes increasingly hard, when examined from the observation point of 1990, to reject the second hypothesis claim that the pattern of present-day spousal separation and divorce is a meaningful and real increase from that experienced in 1900. It is known there were some 149,000 divorces and 4,000 judicial separations annually over 1981–5, evidence from the Home Office suggests some 26,000 maintenance and guardianship orders in the summary courts for 1983 (Davidoff 1984: 11). This results in a recorded indicator of some 179,000 annual marriage breakdowns. A similar calculation for 1901–5 produces an annual total of 13,000, being a combination of High Court decrees (divorce, judicial separation and restitution) and summary court orders (matrimonial and Poor Law) (McGregor *et al.* 1970: 32–3). Allowance needs to be made for the increase in married population over this century, and so the 179,000 is standardized to 83,000. A similar breakdown-rate hypothesis for the two periods would mean that the annual difference of 70,000 (83,000 less 13,000) for 1901–5 represents unrecorded breakdown at a level five times above the officially reported total. The consequent unrecorded breakdown rate of 12 per 1,000 marriages is similar to the divorce rate of 1981–5. It is hard to believe this was the reality: such unofficial separations would have rapidly accumulated to create a visible pattern of marital upheaval sufficient to create a moral panic within Edwardian society. But the Gorell Commission did not receive confirmation of large-scale unrecorded separation. Nor is there evidence of extensive extra-marital births in this pre-birth control era. The 40,000 illegitimate yearly births formed 4 per cent of all births – the lowest rate this century; the majority of the mothers were unmarried. Today, separation almost invariably leads on to divorce: some 95 per cent of separated couples will eventually divorce.[1] These figures suggest two overall conclusions. First, there has been a real rise in marriage breakdown over this century, and the current divorce rate is a realistic and reliable indicator of the growing incidence of marriage breakdown. Second, the fourfold rise in the divorce rate in the twenty years between the periods 1961–5 and 1981–5 highlights the increasing break-down trend experienced by those born after 1930.

It is not only that the resort to divorce has intensified since 1945, but that the more recently formed marriage cohorts who divorce do so within a shorter duration of marriage. This pattern is more clearly seen by studying marriage cohort trends for spinsters, thereby reducing the contaminating effect of the increased divorce risk associated with those remarrying after an earlier failure. (In 1970 three-quarters [7⁵ per cent] of all brides were spinsters aged under twenty-five: only 2 per cent of them married a divorced man.) The figures presented in Table 9.2 follow through the divorce chances for marriages occurring in post-war census years. The marked trend towards divorce intensifies with more recent marriages; for instance, brides aged between twenty and twenty-four in 1961 had, at twenty-five years' duration, double the divorce rate (1961 cohort: 19 per cent) compared to those marrying ten years earlier (1951 cohort: 9 per cent). This pattern is repeated in similar vein among brides of under twenty, but the breakdown rate is double that of their older sisters, with a third of the 1961 cohort being divorced within twenty-five years.

It is also the case that within a given shorter duration of marriage the incidence of divorce doubles for every succeeding marriage cohort. This finding applies to both age groups. For example, Table 9.2 indicates for the ten years duration point that 12 per cent of the 1971 brides aged twenty to twenty-four had divorced compared to 2 per cent for 1951 brides. The fact that a follow through of the latter cohort's divorce pattern extends to thirty-five years' duration before reaching a similar 12 per cent rate experienced by the 1971 cohort at ten years duration once more highlights the increasingly early resort to divorce of more recently formed marriages.

THE SOCIAL CHARACTERISTICS OF THOSE DIVORCING

The historical evidence has shown that the majority of matrimonial disputants were unable to seek divorce until the Second World War. In the following fifty years, society has witnessed structural modification, changing attitudes and expectations towards marriage and family life, and a dramatic switch in the legal processing of 'empty shell' marriages. Divorce has become an accessible remedy utilized by all, though evidence suggests there is disparity in resort between the social classes.

Table 9.2 Proportions of spinster marriages ending in divorce, by duration of marriage and age at marriage: 1951–81, England and Wales

Marriage: age at and date of	Duration (completed years)				
	5	10	20	25	35
	(Proportions per 1,000 married)				
Under 20					
1951	9	50	123	174	230
1961	13	96	270	325	
1971	59	226			
1981	115				
20–24					
1951	4	23	60	88	123
1961	6	44	148	187	
1971	30	120			
1981	60				

Source: Haskey (1989b: table 5).

Social class categorization is a powerful stratifying factor strongly correlated with such major life-styles and experiences as education, health, housing and income, as well as associated demographic patterns (discussed in the previous chapter) such as age at marriage and size of family. The interconnections are not always clear, but association is seldom absent. A thorough analysis of the concept of social class and its relevance within British society has led Ivan Reid to conclude 'there seems to be very little of life in our society which isn't in some ways characterised by differences between the social classes' (1981: 298). At this point a few observations should be made about the use of occupation as a means of placing married and divorcing couples into social class groups. The reason for using occupation is that it is an extremely useful tool to predict a wide range of social behaviour that coalesces to form life patterns (Kahl and Davis 1955). The Registrar General, as head of the government's Office of Population Censuses and Surveys, categorizes occupations of heads of households into five main social classes (class 3 having two sub-categories), according to character and responsibility of the work. An occupation is placed within a social class according to the prestige within the community of that work. Examples of occupational groups in each social class are provided by Table 9.3.

Social class and divorce

Examination of 1951 divorce petitions by Rowntree and Carrier (1958: 223)

Table 9.3 Rates of divorce in each social class: 1961, 1972 and 1979, England and Wales

Social class of husband at divorce	Occupational examples	Divorce rate per 10,000 marriages*		
		1961	*1972*	*1979*
1 Professional	doctors, architects	22	113	71
2 Intermediate	managers, civil service executive officers	25	106	120
3 Skilled				
Non-manual	draughtsmen, commercial travellers, clerks	43 ⎫	160 ⎫	160
Manual	coalmine face workers, engine and bus drivers	29 ⎭ 32	139 ⎭ 144	140
4 Semi-skilled	agricultural workers	25	160	150
5 Unskilled	railway porters, labourer	51	274	300
	All divorces	30	144	150

Notes: *Rate bases:
  (1) 1961 Legal Research Unit and 1972 Oxford (Gibson surveys), per 10,000 wives under 55.
  (2) 1979 OPCS (Haskey survey, 1984, table 5), per 1,000 husbands under 60. Haskey's results have been increased tenfold for comparative purposes in the above table, and thus do not entirely accurately reflect the original findings. Though there are sex/age variations in the two bases, they remain comparable when allowance is made for the wife's generally younger age.

tentatively suggested that the occupational structure of those divorcing and those remaining married was very similar, though the authors urged proper caution due to the likely bias caused by the recent introduction of legal aid. Studies that followed Rowntree and Carrier have generally reported a greater propensity to divorce among the lower social classes. A national random sample of divorce in England and Wales in 1961 undertaken by the Legal Research Unit, University of London, showed that the greatest probability of divorce occurred within those marriages in which the husband was employed in an unskilled manual occupation (social class 5) such as a labourer. Marriages within this social group had over double (2.3 times) the chance of ending in divorce compared with those marriages where the husband had a professional or managerial post (social class 1) (Gibson 1974). This study was later repeated from the Centre for Socio-Legal Studies, Oxford, when a total of 1,146 petitions filed during the first six months of 1972 formed the national random sample. The researchers found an almost similar finding of increased propensity to divorce in the lower social class grouping (social class 5) compared to social class 1 (rate of 2.4 to 1). By 1972 the proportion of divorcing husbands employed in manual occupations had risen to 68 per cent, an increase of 4 per cent on the 1961 survey result. A similar divorce rate by social class exercise was undertaken by Haskey (1984) on a sample of 2,164 divorces granted in 1979. Generally the 1972 and 1979 surveys provide a similar pattern (though the 1961 and 1979 studies report social class 1 having a lower risk than social class 2, this was reversed in the 1972 survey). The conclusion which clearly emerges from all three surveys is that marriages in which the husband is an unskilled worker have the highest risk of divorce within the Registrar General's social class groupings. A similar pattern has been reported for America (Goode 1965: ch. 4) and Finland (Anntila 1977: 29).

Even higher rates of breakdown were found by Haskey (1984: table 5) outside the social class groupings. Marriages in which the husband was a serviceman had a rate of 470 divorces for every 10,000 such marriages, providing three times the average risk. The presence of an unemployed husband also produced (rate of 340 per 10,000 marriages) a very high propensity to divorce. A range of explanations can be offered for the apparent divorce proneness of marriages within social class 5. It might be that unskilled manual workers have little or no autonomy in their work situation, which, together with low wages, leads to job dissatisfaction. The home and family become the outlet for the husband's frustration with his work (or lack of work). Within this situation marital tension arises if the wife is unable to cope with the resultant domestic stress. And, as will be shown later in this chapter, there is strong evidence that a high neuroticism score intensifies the risk. Another partial factor could be that the economic disparity between a low-wage earning husband and his wife is far less than that existing between a professional worker and his wife. The latter may well be less willing to contemplate divorce because they have far more to forfeit through loss of security and financial provision, and the curtailing of an extended social network of friends. The upper-income couple have greater economic, normative and social pressures to accommodate and compromise to the tensions and irritants of married life. Yet financial worth and social prestige do not of themselves guarantee marital security, for ten of Britain's twenty-six dukes had been divorced in 1990 – three of them twice (*Daily Telegraph*, 30 March 1990). Another explanation for the low divorce rate found in social class 1 is the direct impact of higher income, with its consequent ability to buy those items that make marriage and family life less of a potential strain upon the spouses. But these are only theories, and none are entirely satisfactory.

A useful review of the general evidence, as well as information about the characteristics of those divorcing in the early 1970s compared with that found in ongoing marriages, is provided by Thornes and Collard (1979: 40–3). Their study found higher neuroticism scores were registered by divorcing men and women than the levels found among spouses in ongoing marriages; the differences between divorcing and continuing married women were particularly marked (1979: 203–4). Divorcing women also appeared to be more neurotic than their menfolk. Those divorcing in social class 5 emerged as 'being relatively more at risk to marital stress resulting from environing disadvantage than did all the other groups' (1979: 41).

Survey findings do not provide a straight inverse association between high divorce risk and low social class. Table 9.3 indicates white-collar workers in social class 3 non-manual have a higher (1961, 1979) or equal (1972) divorce rate than that experienced in social classes 3 (manual) or 4. The divorce proneness of such white-collar marriages was particularly noticeable in the 1961 results; though the findings for 1972 and 1979 show a less marked break from the broadly inverse pattern. Two general conclusions emerge: first, the white-collar worker is the most divorce-prone within the non-manual classes; and second, their divorce rate is above that for blue-collar manual workers.

The reasons for the apparently higher breakdown risk of social class 3 white-collar marriages are not so obvious, for their life histories show many features associated with marital stability: marriage rituals like engagement and church weddings, prudent planning in both housing and timing of children, and good employment records for both spouses. Thornes and Collard (1979: 47) tentatively suggest this class has a greater propensity to internal frustration over failure to achieve expected marital roles and, at the same time, experience weaker affectional bonds with their spouses.

The overall divorce rate records a fivefold rise between 1961 and 1979. Within social classes 4 and 5 there has been a sixfold increase, suggesting divorce has increasingly become accepted as the legal remedy for low income groups' marital difficulties. It is these divorcing couples who record such debilitating social features as youngest age at marriage, earliest child-bearing, largest families, rapid job changes, lowest income and the least satisfactory housing. These material disadvantages fall upon those least able to cope with the associated tension and stress.

Occupation

It has been argued that those engaged in certain types of work are more prone to marriage breakdown (Noble 1970; Murphy 1985). Lengthy periods away from home, opportunity for extra-marital encounters, and low pay may be some of the vulnerability features working to impair relationships. The suggested association is plausible and possible, but it is unwise to base the argument on the evidence of comparing census enumeration of reported divorces to ongoing marriages (Gibson 1971b). The census figures analyse an untypical residual divorcing population of those who remain unmarried but exclude the majority of divorcees who eventually marry. But Haskey's divorce survey (1984: 427) does provide 'some credence' to Noble's original argument.

New evidence concerning the impact of unemployment on British married life emerges from a national study that interviewed some 5,000 people (ESRC, *Social Sciences*, July 1990). The findings indicate that an unemployed married person is 130 per cent more likely to suffer a separation in the following year compared with those who had never been unemployed. This expectation is confirmed by the 1984 OPCS divorce findings recording the high level of unemployment among men at the time of separation.[2] The association between low income and a high rate of divorce is once more underlined.

DEMOGRAPHIC FEATURES

Age at marriage

The association between early marriage and lower social class has important consequences for patterns of marriage breakdown. We know that couples who marry at an early age have a substantially greater likelihood of divorce. On the assumption of the 1980–1 divorce and mortality rates continuing unchanged, it seems that half of all young brides (under twenty) will not celebrate their silver wedding because of divorce (49 per cent) rather than death (3 per cent) (Haskey 1983: 11). What is more surprising is that even half of these couples will still be together.

Linked to the previous finding is the General Household Survey evidence that young marriages not only experience greater risk of divorce but they have been also significantly more prone to earlier breakdown (Table 9.2; OPCS 1989: table 4.9). The overall evidence is succinctly summed up by Kathleen Kiernan (1986: 43): 'In virtually every study of marital breakdown it has been found that marriage at young ages is the most powerful discriminant between marriages which survive and those that do not.' Kiernan's impressive study of teenage marriage resulted from the Medical Research Council's longitudinal study of people born in Britain during the first week of March 1946. The researchers found young brides were more likely to come from disadvantaged large families which had themselves experienced high breakdown rates. The brides were additionally handicapped by low educational achievement, with over three-quarters (77 per cent) lacking any school-leaving qualification (compared with 42 per cent for those marrying at twenty-two or twenty-three) that left them holding low-status and poorly paid occupations. Their husbands presented a similar associated pattern of younger age, poor education and manual occupations. The low-income dilemma of these couples is intensified by the young wife's early start to child-bearing and quicker pace of reproduction. Poor educational achievement, as well as being associated with earlier marriage (and now cohabitation), is also – according to American findings – a significant predictor of spousal distress in early married life (Kurdek 1991: 633). It is probable that early school-leaving is related to poorly developed communication skills which make marital problems and conflict more difficult.

The issue that Kiernan attempted to resolve was whether there were features causing some early marriages to survive and others to fail within this marital high-risk group. Comparison of possible explanatory characteristics distinguishing the still-married from the broken-marriage group showed both shared similar family backgrounds, educational records and occupational histories. The researchers then turned to the possibility of disparity in predisposing personality factors (as measured by the short version of the Maudsley Personality Inventory) when the women were aged (a) sixteen and (b) twenty-six years. Two major antecedent factors emerged which clearly separated the ongoing from the failed-marriage groups. First, a significantly higher 8.22

neuroticism score was recorded at sixteen for teenage brides whose marriages had broken down by the age of thirty-two, compared with the 7.30 score of those with intact marriages. The association between neuroticism and the enhanced risk of a broken marriage also held for those who married at later ages. The overall evidence was summarized by Kiernan:

> Teenage brides tend to have more unstable personalities than those who marry later. But the most striking and substantial finding was that teenage brides whose marriages broke down were, on average, significantly more unstable, even before they married, than teenage brides whose marriages remained intact.

(Kiernan 1986: 49)

The second relevant antecedent factor – though of less importance than neuroticism – was the greater likelihood that wives in failed marriages would, as children, have experienced their own parents' breakdown. Both USA evidence and this British study suggest a child's awareness and observation of parental tension and breakdown provides a role model of appropriate behaviour and response patterns for later adult pressures and problems. The learning and socialization habits acquired as a child in the home environment enforces sex-stereotyped responses for dealing with emotive situations. The woman, who as a girl felt her mother's parental frustration exploding into brutality, or who witnessed her father's desertion, is partially conditioned into accepting such behaviour as a 'normal' reaction. If the propensity to readily separate and divorce is indeed transmitted to the next generation, then the post-1960 divorce explosion can be partly explained by childhood experience. On this count divorce rates will continue to advance.

It has already been seen in the previous chapter how the habit of early marriage has rapidly declined over the last twenty years. National marriage-rate figures for young women record a sixfold fall between 1970 and 1990. As a precipitating divorce factor young bridal age at marriage is declining in terms of its numerical output. But early child-bearing remains linked with increased risk of breakdown (Murphy 1985: 460). And a speedy family start is itself associated with younger age at marriage. This is reflected in the Oxford 1972 study finding that four out of five divorcing wives who married before eighteen and with husbands in social class 5 at divorce had experienced early parenthood (defined as a child born either before or within a year of marriage). For all divorcing wives regardless of age at marriage, those with husbands in unskilled occupations were twice as likely to be mothers within a year of marriage as were wives with non-manually employed husbands.

Children

Incompatible couples are ultimately returned to a single status by the rapid stroke of a decree absolute. Behind this legal event lies the social reality of a protracted marital drama which incorporates children as both audience and cast within the unfolding chronology of discord, unhappiness, separation and divorce. Official statistics show almost three million children under sixteen experienced parental divorce in the twenty years 1971 to 1990. An additional unknown minority were witnesses to parental separation. Our current divorce trend suggests that one in four of all children will have first-hand knowledge of parental divorce before their sixteenth birthday. The United States pattern is even more depressing; their marital breakdown rates for 1970–3 indicate one in three (33 per cent) white children and three out of five (59 per cent) black children would have experienced parental disruption before sixteen (Bumpass and Rindfuss 1979: table 1).

Research concerning the impact of parental breakdown on the psychological development and life-chances of their children is limited in both range and methodological precision. Most beliefs and prejudices will find confirming evidence in the research annals. For instance, a generally acclaimed study by Wallerstein and Kelly (1980) found many children would have preferred their warring parents to have remained together rather than separating, with consequent loss of a parent and inevitable reduction in the standard of living. A third of the study's children were still experiencing moderate to severe depression five years after their parents divorced. Yet confidence in the external validity of the findings is tampered by knowledge that the sample of children, who had been initially sent for counselling help, came from white middle-class homes of Marin County, California. These findings can be set against earlier American studies which had suggested parental friction and anger were more detrimental to the children than divorce (Burchinal 1964).

Few doubt the process of separation and divorce disturb childrens' psychological and material well-being, though it is unclear what, if any, are the harmful long-lasting consequences (though see NCDS findings, p. 217 below). And are these consequences more detrimental than the daily experience of ongoing parental tension, humiliation and deception displayed in unhappy marriages? This is an obvious area needing well-designed research into household life patterns before and after separation. Such a programme would, in Allan's words (1985: 115) allow the long-term 'differential impact of material, social, psychological and organizational factors' upon children to be distinguished and assessed.

What can be assessed with more certainty are the numbers of children under sixteen (defined as dependent) directly caught up in the divorce process. Table 9.4 records that the proportion of divorcing couples with dependent children has fallen from 62 per cent in 1970 to 55 per cent in 1990, but increasing divorce in this same period has caused the numbers of involved children (at the time of divorce) to have doubled to 153,000 in 1990. A third of these children (51,000) were under five, this relatively large proportion being due to the increased tendency now for couples to separate and divorce within a shorter period of marriage.

Less than a tenth (9 per cent) of all 1990 divorcing couples had three or more dependent children. It is known that larger family size within a divorcing population is associated with lower social class. For instance, the Oxford 1972

Table 9.4 Family patterns in divorce, 1970–90, England and Wales

Year/Period*	Divorcing couples with children(%)			Numbers of children –16
	Childless	All 16+	One or more –16	(,000)
1970	26	12	62	71
1971–5	26	15	59	124
1976–80	29	11	60	156
1981–5	30	12	58	156
1990	31	14	55	153

Notes: Calculations based on OPCS, FM2 series, table 4.4.
   * Yearly average.

study found that divorces in which the husband was an unskilled labourer had three times the proportion of couples with three or more dependent children than occurred in social classes 1 and 2.

It is necessary to recognize that official statistics fail to record those children who become sixteen between the time of their parents separation and eventual petitioning. The evidence of the Oxford survey suggests a further three or four years will often pass between these two stages. The study found 70 per cent of all divorcing couples had a least one child under sixteen when they separated, this proportion falling to 59 per cent, at the time the petition was filed. A more realistic calculation showing the proportion of 1990 divorcing couples whose breakdown and separation affected one or more dependent children in their household produces a significantly higher proportion of 65 per cent, compared with the 55 per cent recorded in Table 9.4, for the time of petitioning. Divorcing households have more dependent children affected by parental breakdown than official figures suggest. Though social and legal concern is properly focused on the dependent child, the 1990 divorce web additionally involved some 68,000 teenage and adult offspring. Continuing education, unemployment or disability causes many older children to remain dependent on their parents. Adolescent youngsters especially feel the emotional upheavals, while few older offspring escape the shock waves resulting from the disintegration of a long-lasting parental marriage. Adult sibling relationships can be pulled apart in their reaction to a parent's decision to divorce. In some instances inter-family affection and loyalty will be permanently destroyed. Contamination of sibling and kin bonds are part of the corroding input of parental breakdown.

Childless marriage

Today, some three out of ten divorcing couples are childless (Table 9.4). Such marriages have increased slightly over the last twenty years. This trend partly reflects: (a) a greater propensity for women born since 1945 to be childless and,

(b) the general pattern of delayed parenthood with the consequence that an increasing number of currently divorcing couples who separate in the early years of a marriage will be childless. The proportion of couples without any children of their own will be slightly higher. Some 3 per cent of all divorcing couples in the Oxford survey only had children who were not of the marriage. Since then there has been a decline in non-family adoptions but an increase in the number of wives who bring into the marriage a premarital child by another man. This suggests that infertile (either intentionally or by misfortune) marriages currently form about 35 per cent of all divorces. Some researchers have queried the belief that divorcing couples had a higher rate of childlessness than that found in unbroken marriages. Findings from Chester (1972) and Gibson (1980) show the level of infertility recorded in official divorce statistics drops significantly once the standardized duration of time used for comparison against continuing marriages becomes that of *de facto* cohabitation rather than *de jure* marriage length. When this is done the level of infertility among broken marriages coming before the courts does not appear to be any higher than that found within the still married population. Analysis of data from the 1980 General Household Survey has led Murphy (1984) to query this conclusion and argue that childlessness and early child-bearing are both major risk factors associated with marital breakdown.

Divorcing couples who are childless have shorter periods of cohabitation. The Oxford study found six out of ten childless divorcing couples had separated within five years compared with one out of ten couples who had delayed parenthood for two or more years from marriage. This finding is partly an artefact resulting from wives who experience shorter periods of cohabitation also having less opportunity to conceive. It may be that couples who find their relationship is unsatisfactory early in the marriage, purposely refrain from having children. Also, unhappily married parents may well try to remain together and present an image of social unity for the benefit of the children, or at least continue cohabitation until the children are more of an age to cope and adjust to a legal severance of the family unit. It also has to be recognized that the very presence of children may be a source of marital conflict and disruption. These remain unproved possibilities. But what does seem clear is that childless couples are freer than those with dependent children to decide whether their marriage is best dissolved.

Duration of marriage

Marriages of divorcing couples are lasting for shorter durations than previously. For instance, the proportion of marriages lasting under ten years has increased from 41 per cent in 1972 to 51 per cent in 1990. Such calculations are based upon the formal (*de jure*) length of time the union has existed as a legal entity: that is, from marriage until the decree absolute. Marriage breakdown is best recorded by separation. This point more accurately records when the withering marital fabric of affection and compatibility metamorphosed into the reality of a one-parent household, lower living standards, bruised ego and resentment. Yet in many divorce situations such public legal markers as the date of either petitioning, decree nisi or decree absolute provide the only available indicators of earlier marital disintegration. From a social perspective it is more relevant to have knowledge about the actual (*de facto*) time the spouses lived together before parting. A divorcing population experiencing shorter-lasting marriages (say, under five years) records a significant variation between the proportion who actually obtain divorce and the larger percentage who have separated. The Oxford survey of 1972 divorces showed that five years after marriage, though only 14 per cent of the sample had proceeded to a decree absolute, there were 35 per cent who had separated. There is confirming evidence from this country that around one-third of divorcing couples have separated within five years of marrying (Chester 1971; Thornes and Collard 1979: 124; OPCS, 1990b: 11).

Early parenthood within a divorcing population is linked with short-lasting marriages. The Oxford study found 45 per cent of marriages in which a child was born either before or within a year of marriage lasted under five years before separation compared with 11 per cent when birth of the first child was delayed for at least two years. Those cases where a child already existed at marriage – usually as a result of the couple's premarital cohabitation or via the wife as a sole unmarried mother or a divorcee – were specially vulnerable to short durations. Two-thirds (67 per cent) of such 'existing family' marriages had a *de facto* duration time of under five years compared with 46 per cent for marital births conceived within wedlock. Age at marriage did not greatly affect this finding for there was little variation in this situation between wives marrying before twenty and those aged between twenty and twenty-four. What did emerge from the overall findings was the strong association between early parenthood and short-lasting marriages. This evidence provides some support to those who believe that early parenthood is more important than young age as a predisposing variable towards marriage breakdown. Newly-marrieds need time to adjust to the demands of their own relationship. Such domestic socialization is curtailed by early parenthood. The speedy arrival of a noisy and demanding baby into seldom satisfactory accommodation is a far cry from the romantic and soft imagery of a gurgling, responsive infant projected from the television screen. Parental frustration soon turns to disillusionment.

The national divorce pattern for *de jure* duration in 1972 reflected the expected young age at marriage impact, recording 14 per cent of brides aged under twenty who divorced did so within five years compared with 12 per cent for those aged twenty to twenty-four when marrying. The latest figures (from 1986 to 1990) show an unexpected change of pattern, with 1990 divorcing brides aged twenty to twenty-four having greater propensity to short marriages (24 per cent under five years) than occurred for those marrying before twenty (16 per cent). This is confirmed by the median duration being higher for young brides (12.4 years) than for those marrying between twenty and twenty-four (9.8 years) (OPCS 1992b: table 4.3). The probable explanation for this surprising new pattern is the increasing presence in current divorces where the bride was aged twenty or more of either one or both spouses being previously divorced.

Associated with a previously divorced spouse is the greater risk of further divorce and an even shorter marriage duration than that experienced by 'first marriage' divorcing couples. National divorce statistics for 1990 allow calculation within each bridal age group of the proportion of marriages containing an already divorced spouse. The results were – by wife's age: under twenty years 4 per cent, twenty to twenty-four years 14 per cent, and all ages 25 per cent (OPCS 1992b: 80). It will be interesting to see whether this new inverted age/*de jure* duration trend of the mid-1980s will continue into the 1990s, and whether a more reasonable explanation arises.

Survey findings and official figures indicate the majority of couples do not rush from marriage to divorce. The Oxford study found two-thirds of divorcing couples had maritally cohabited for a least five years. Within the 1990 divorcing population, half had marriages of ten years or more *de jure* duration while almost a fifth had continued twenty years or more.

Age at divorce

Four-fifths of all divorces occur to spouses aged under forty-five years, with a slightly higher proportion of wives due to their younger age at marriage. Among 1990 divorcing couples 83 per cent of the wives and 77 per cent of husbands were younger than forty-five. This age pattern has remained fairly constant over the last twenty years, with wives' median age at divorce rising very slightly from 32.4 years in 1970 to 32.9 years in 1980 and 34.0 years in 1990. Spouses between twenty-five and twenty-nine experienced the highest risk of dissolution; 3 per cent of both married men and women in this age group divorced in 1990. Those who divorce at a relatively younger age have a greater chance of remarriage. Evidence from both the 1961 and 1972 divorce surveys showed social class differences in age at divorce, with middle-class husbands and wives divorcing at an older age. A third of the 1972 divorcing wives in social classes 1 and 2 were aged forty-five or more compared with 17 per cent for wives married to unskilled manual workers in social class 5. The social class difference is a resultant of the former group's older age at marriage and longer marriage duration compared with social class 5. One consequence of this variation is that because the manual classes divorce at a younger age their chances of establishing a second marriage are higher than for couples in social classes 1 and 2. This means maintenance and property provisions decided at divorce are of greater importance in affecting middle-class wives' long-term financial security than is generally the case for working-class wives

The wife aged forty-five or more is especially vulnerable to the financially debilitating consequences of marriage breakdown and divorce. Over the ten-year period 1976 to 1985 the courts dissolved the marriages of some quarter of a million (245,310) women aged forty-five or more: they formed 17 per cent of all divorces in England and Wales during this period. Evidence indicates that the probability of marrying again quickly falls with age (Table 10.2). The remarriage rate also falls more rapidly for the ex-wives of non-manually employed husbands compared to those who had been married to manual workers, whatever the age of the wife at divorce.

The older divorcing wife, often having given up earnings and work pension potential by undertaking a home-care role, may well now face the loss of financial protection and safeguard in widowhood that comes from the husband's occupational pension and life insurance schemes. The judiciary in such cases have the discretionary power to try to compensate the wife. But in many cases the husband's ordinary wage and low savings, together with the utilization of his right to marry again, effectively blocks judicial power. The quagmire increases with knowledge that almost a quarter (23 per cent) of the husbands of divorcing wives of forty-five or more in 1990 were experiencing their second (or more) dissolution. Realism often prevents the court ordering either a proper level of maintenance or the direction that the husband should take out a new life insurance policy that is payable to the ex-wife. Proper compensation can seldom be provided to the divorced wife except in cases where the husband's earnings fall into the upper-income level. In demographic terms this issue will grow: the proportion of women in the sixty-five or more age group who are divorced and not remarried is likely to increase fivefold (2.5 per cent to 13.3 per cent) between 1985 and 2025.

THE SOCIAL CONSEQUENCES

According to a recent survey of British attitudes successful marriages are sustained above all by compatibility and a friendly relationship between the spouses (Ashford 1987: 124, 140). Increasing disharmony and incompatibility has brought divorce to one and a half million husbands and wives in the five years 1985–9. Democracy has allowed greater freedom and self-determination. Alongside these ideals citizens have come to expect happiness and personal fulfilment. Hedonism has become a legitimate pursuit within a free-enterprise society. Institutional displays of divorce disapproval have largely disappeared. The Establishment barometer of social mores is indicated by the rules and practices surrounding our Royal Family and the Church of England. The traditional rules of Ascot's Royal Enclosure may still refuse entry to women displaying unacceptable hats and hemlines, or men unsuitably attired, but divorcees are no longer pariahs. Sovereign acceptability has replaced fears of courtly contamination. It could hardly be otherwise, for today's Royal Family are no more immune than their subjects from the risks of conjugal breakdown. Princess Margaret, who had been dissuaded in the 1950s from marrying a divorced man, has had her marriage dissolved; the Princess Royal and Captain Phillips felt it best to separate in 1989 and divorce in 1992. Neither Princess experienced public fuss or comment on the news. In contrast, the separation of the Duke and Duchess of York in March 1992 after five years of marriage caused public criticism of one Royal breakdown too many. The Royal Family as public symbols of traditional family values suffered a further blow in a year the Queen had described as her *annus horribilis* when Buckingham Palace on 9 December

1992 announced the separation of the Prince and Princess of Wales. The heir to the throne and future Supreme Governor of the Church of England, and his wife, have taken the probable opening steps towards consensual divorce.[3] Four days later, the first Royal remarriage after divorce was celebrated at Crathie Church, Balmoral, when Princess Anne married Commander Laurence within the more tolerant atmosphere of the Church of Scotland. In England the Synod of the Church of England had finally conceded in 1981 that there were circumstances in which it could be proper for a divorced person to marry again by church ceremony during the lifetime of the former partner. The Archbishop of Canterbury, Dr Runcie, sympathetically argued that rejection of a similar proposal in 1978 had contributed to the stigmatization of those whose marriages had broken down.

Prejudice should have diminished as more people, either directly or by association, become acquainted with the world of divorce. Yet Nicky Hart's study of the divorced and separated shows many such people felt they were still looked down upon, distrusted and discriminated against; as one middle-aged man observed 'it's as though you have a disease' (Hart 1976: 153). But the very increase in divorce numbers adds weight to its acceptability and suggests both the experience and the resultant status are bearable. Spouses are now less willing to tolerate the troubles and stresses of a discordant relationship, or to see lengthy separation as an acceptable remedy. As more and more children witness parental dissolution, so this increasingly common childhood experience instils divorce as a proper and normal solution for the tribulations of domestic disharmony. In another family context one observes young children weaned from their parents and boarded out to preparatory and private schools are thereby socialized into viewing this practice as a regular part of family life which subsequently will be repeated for their own children. In a similar manner, children who experience divorce come to view it as part of life's normal pattern. The impact of marital breakdown has consequences for both the personal realm of the nuclear family and the public domain of society. Within the family it is women and children who are especially vulnerable to the consequential problems of income reduction, housing, child-caring, employment, social contacts and stress. Not surprisingly more younger women informants (aged eighteen to thirty-four) to the 1987 British attitudes survey favoured tougher divorce than did men of a similar age (Ashford 1987: table 6.1).

With most separations children experience a break of affectional ties; there is no longer an accessible father to play with or accompany them. Paternal contact may cease. The all too probable drop in the mother's household income means these children now experience further inequality in their everyday life. A child's right to expect suitable care, protection and provision has been confronted with parental inability to live together. For some mothers and children the move to lone-parent status will bring improvement over past conditions. It might be relief from fear of violence or the mother's awareness that income support will give her assured money for the household budget compared with the husband's uncertain provision. Such social accounting reflects diverse beliefs as to what practices and habits the good family should display.

Many divorced men and women will form new relationships and eventually marry again. This means the disruption and possible ending of existing non-custodial parents' kin networks, while step-relationships come to play a more important role. The husband who marries anew a mother with children implicitly accepts responsibility for their day-to-day welfare and support, though few men have sufficient income to maintain adequately both old and new families. Appended to the second union comes step-grandparents, uncles, cousins and siblings. At the same time old relationships can die or be destroyed. For instance, children and paternal grandparents may no longer have opportunity or encouragement to meet, though patterns vary a great deal. New children of the marriage join their older step-siblings. This constellation of old and new kin is extended even further if this second union fails and a new partnership is formed.

It could be that divorce disrupts the bonds between children and parents so that the former are no longer available or willing to provide care in old age. We have no firm evidence on this question, though the older divorcing husband who remains unattached might be especially vulnerable to lack of a supporting kin network. Similar questions can be asked about the family consequences if one of the parents' children experience divorce. Such a break may especially cause the loss of a daughter-in-law from the family and the rupture of previously close supportive contact between the in-laws and the ex-wife (Finch and Mason 1990: 232). One social consequence of kin disruption can be seen in the ageing population that is projected to contain two and a half million women aged seventy-five or more in 2021. Both community and government have seen daughters and daughters-in-law as the traditional carers of their ageing mothers and mothers-in-law. A high rate of divorce has impact for both the nuclear and the extended family.

Within the public domain high rates of cohabitation and remarriage after divorce together with standard wage packets has meant the level of maintenance ordered is neither sufficient for effective support, nor is it regularly paid. The ex-wife and children experience a fall from the family's previous standard of living. Some 400,000 separated and divorced wives heading lone-parent households were in receipt of income support in 1990. Further non-contributory expenditure entitlement include lone-parent benefit, housing benefit, council tax rebate, and the net cost of social fund loans and family credit to women on low earnings. To this list can be added the expense to local authorities of taking children into care, and health service costs resulting from illness and the emotional toll of breakdown. The doctor's surgery has become a marital stress service post prescribing relief, contributing therapy and offering referrals to marriage counsellors. Child-care provision at both public and private levels is generally inadequate in availability, setting and facilities for the needs of employed lone mothers. A national matrimonial ledger will also debit Treasury costs for legally aided matrimonial disputants. State pension contributions can be credited without payment from the divorced woman who has not remarried and is not earning. The public and voluntary bodies providing community and client services include the judicial system and its administrators, the advisory professional groups like the probation service, counselling bodies such as Relate (formerly the Marriage Guidance Council), court conciliation services, Citizens' Advice Bureaux, the Salvation Army's Missing Persons Bureaux, the National Council for One-Parent Families and Gingerbread. This provision has to be paid for. Whatever way the matrimonial account is audited the personal and public costs of disharmony and breakdown are enormous.

10 The reconstituted family

Lord Devlin, in a public lecture upon morals and the law of marriage, raised the question: 'What then is the divorce court really doing when it pronounces a decree of divorce?' The judge answered his own query: 'The State is . . . saying that it will recognize any other marriage that either party chooses to make. That is the practical effect – indeed it is the only effect, unless it is supposed that the court has spiritual powers – of the decree' (1965: 66). This remains the divorce decree's only important legal consequence in the regulation of private habit.

Unsuccessful marriages are provided with the remedy of divorce which returns both husband and wife to the status of single persons. But the law cannot dissolve away the couple's children nor their existing kin relationships. For the majority of the 153,000 dependent children whose parents divorced in 1990 the family continues in a form similar to that experienced since parental separation. The decree absolute legally confirms for these children and the caring parent the reality of lone parenthood. Divorce does not record the end of family life and structure, but rather marks one point in a particular family's life course which will continue in an amended form. For many couples contact and communication is maintained because of the presence of children and family kin.

Remarriage in the first half of this century never formed much more than a tenth of all new marriages and generally concerned those who were widowed. Divorce played little or no part in this pattern, as Table 10.1 indicates. From 1947 this was no longer the case and the earlier divorce of one or other spouse became the increasingly common feature within second marriage. It was not so much that mortality risks slowly declined but that the likelihood of divorce escalated, thereby projecting increasing numbers of divorced couples back into the non-married population. This trend intensified with the divorce explosion of the 1970s.

In 1961 it still remained demographically correct to observe that married women aged between twenty and forty-nine as a group faced similar risks of divorce and widowhood. By 1990 the possibility of dissolution had become eleven times a greater threat than the death of the husband (calculations based on OPCS 1992b: tables 1.1a, 4.1 and 5.1; and earlier editions). Wives aged forty to forty-four provide a fairly similar pattern; their divorce rate experience is six times higher than that of widowhood. This current evidence concerning marriage

Table 10.1 Remarriages of divorced persons as a proportion of all marriages: 1900–90, England and Wales

Period/ year	Annual number of marriages	Both single	Widowed	Divorced (Marrying)		One or both divorced
			Widowed or single	Widowed* or single	Divorced	
	(,000)			(a)	(b)	(a)+(b)
1901–05	260	88	12	(0.2)		(0.2)
1921–2	301	86	13	1		1
1931–5	326	89	9	2		2
1951–5	351	82	7	9	2	11
1961–5	355	84	6	8	2	10
1966–70	398	83	5	10	2	12
1971–5	399	73	4	16	7	23
1981	352	65	3	20	12	32
1988	348	63	2	21	13	35
1990	331	63	2	22	13	35

Notes: *In this classification the divorced spouse marrying a widowed spouse has been counted as 'divorced' (column (a)). Such marriages formed 2.3 per cent of all 1990 marriages.
Calculations based on OPCS, (1992b: 24); and earlier numbers.

breakdown risks shows that a far larger number of divorced compared with widowed wives find themselves free to marry again at an age when the probability of remarriage remains high.

The majority of divorced men and women will utilize their right to marry afresh. Secular marriage provisions have supported institutional morality by solemnizing in 1990 three-quarters of the 115,000 marriages that embraced a divorced person, so avoiding probable refusal by religious authorities. Over a third of current weddings in England and Wales (Table 10.1) unite a spouse who has been divorced. This feature of modern marriage is both a consequence of the high divorce rate and a reflection of many divorcees' desire to seek happiness with a new spouse. Marriages involving a previously divorced spouse now dominate the world of remarriage; they formed 94 per cent of all second marriages in 1990 (and even if those 'divorced' marrying 'widowed' marriages were transferred from 'divorce' to the 'widow' count, the latter group would only rise from 6 to 13 per cent of all second marriages). Remarriage now follows divorce rather than death.

The question of maintenance and parental support never lies very far from the world of the remarried. A new marriage reconstitutes the lone-parent family into a fresh structure which creates important legal and social consequences. Divorce law tells the wife that her maintenance claims upon the ex-husband cease when she marries again; for the obligation to maintain is now transferred to the new husband. The latter relieves the state of its liability to the claimant and her children receiving income support. And if the new husband is also divorced, then realism also ensures the current household takes priority over his former family within a society where male wage packets are designed to support only one household. Not surprisingly the first wife, who may have been left to raise their children as best she could, resents the visual signs confirming the much higher living standard often experienced by the ex-husband and his new family. So the carousel of support and obligation permeates the world of divorce and remarriage. Through marriage (or cohabitation) the lone divorced wife gains a strengthened economic base and a more assured financial future. Survey findings (see pp. 182 and 210) show the most generally effective way for divorced wives to regain their pre-divorce financial situation was by marrying again.

Evidence indicates remarriage can also be a major means of improving the standard of living experienced in the first marriage by women who were then 'in relatively less advantaged circumstances – those married to a spouse in a manual occupation, those in private tenancy, and those living in households without access to a car or a van' (Bhrolcháin 1988: 33). The same OPCS longitudinal study findings also show those men and women who, by the same indicators, were initially in better circumstances before divorce appeared more likely to undergo a deterioration in their socio-economic circumstances following a second marriage.

RATES OF REMARRIAGE

The demographic evidence of twenty years ago suggested some three-quarters of all divorcing couples married again (Gibson 1974). It still remains the case that the majority of spouses passing through the divorce courts will marry again, but not to the same degree as in the 1960s. The remarriage patterns of the 1980s indicates around 70 per cent of all divorced people will remarry, though age, sex, social class, employment and attitude towards marriage are all factors affecting the rate of remarriage.

Considering their earlier marital unhappiness, it is perhaps surprising to find divorced people displaying greater willingness to re-embrace the institution of marriage than shown by single people. This pattern applies to men and women of all ages. For instance the marriage figures for 1990 indicate divorced compared with single women aged twenty-five to twenty-nine had a third greater likelihood of marrying in that year. But more divorced people are now inclined to view remarriage in the worldly manner of Dr Johnson as 'the triumph of hope over experience'. Premarital cohabitation has become a more common practice, being the habit of a quarter (28 per cent) of single-status divorced women under fifty surveyed in the 1988 General Household Survey. It is the standard precursor to marriage when one or both spouses have been previously married (OPCS 1990e: tables 3.2 and 3.9; OPCS 1990c: 15). This is part of the shorter, pragmatic and domestically directed courtship pattern displayed by the more sexually aware and experienced separated and divorced compared with younger unmarried couples. The former are impelled towards cohabiter relationships by immediate practical and economic factors such as housing, money and the necessities of everyday living which provide material backbone to successful family existence. One informant provides the following practical reasons for his remarriage.

> Well, we were both of us on us own . . . well, you see, I were travelling up there three and four times a week . . . she didn't come down here, not unless I brought her down. . . . Because of travelling time and bus fares . . . we thought it were just a waste really to keep two houses on, you know, her having that up there and me down here. We were paying two rents, two lights, two 'gases', you name it, we were paying it, so . . . I said we could cut half of these expenses down.
>
> (Burgoyne and Clark 1980: 14)

Increasing popularity of unwed cohabitation, linked with the general trend to delayed marriage entry (for all marital status groups) helps to explain why remarriage rates for divorced men and women recorded in Table 10.2 have

Table 10.2 Numbers and rates of remarriage for divorced men and women, by age, for selected years 1961–90, England and Wales

Year		*Numbers*	*Remarriage rate (per 1,000) for age groups*		
		(,000)	*All*	*25–29*	*35–44*
Men	1961	19	163	474	198
	1971	42	227	509	251
	1981	79	129	261	142
	1985	81	95	173	110
	1988	85	82	144	97
	1990	80	70	122	82
Women	1961	18	97	410	112
	1971	40	134	359	140
	1981	75	91	202	96
	1985	77	71	163	76
	1988	82	63	147	70
	1990	78	55	130	62

Source: OPCS, 1992b: tables 3.2 and 3.3, and earlier editions.

declined from their 1972 peak which followed the previous year's introduction of more liberal divorce legislation. As well as changing normative patterns there has been a reduction in prejudice against divorcees, thereby reducing the appeal of remarriage as the appropriate avenue towards respectability. In the past, marriage held greater popularity as the only appropriate means by which a divorced mother could shield herself and children from the harsh realities of being a one-parent family. Today, the availability of improved welfare services, government financial provision, better employment opportunities and more equal pay have especially helped divorced mothers by allowing greater freedom of choice when considering the possible benefits and disadvantages of a new marriage.

As well as declining remarriage rates, two other noticeable patterns are recorded in Table 10.2. First, the annual numbers of divorced persons who remarry has steadily increased as a consequence of the rising divorce population. (Though in some cases divorce can be initiated by desire to marry a lover.) Second, the likelihood of remarriage falls rapidly with age. Demographic evidence strongly suggests age is the major determinant influencing remarriage chances, though gender becomes a differentiating factor of increasing relevance at older age (OPCS 1990c: 14). For instance, Table 10.2 records divorced women aged twenty-five to twenty-nine were twice as likely to marry again in 1990 than those aged thirty-five to forty-four. Within this older age group divorced men had a third greater chance of remarrying compared with similarly aged divorced women. Our experience of higher male remarriage rates is similarly found in the 1970s demographic experience of eighteen European countries examined by the writer. Remarriage rates of two-thirds or more for divorced men were recorded in ten countries. Bulgaria was the only country to produce a similar rate for women (United Nations 1976: 585–96, 640–3).

The time of separation indicates the *de facto* end of marriage. The couple's age at separation, with its association to age at divorce, is the most important factor in determining the likelihood of a further extra-marital or marriage partnership. Recent findings linking greater chance of remarriage with younger age and gender are provided by Coleman's life-table calculations upon 1981 OPCS data (1989: 99). The probability of a divorced man aged thirty-five marrying again before his sixty-fifth birthday remained remarkably high (95 per cent). Similarly aged divorced women still had a high chance (81 per cent) of remarriage. This latter rate suggests nine out of ten of the 81,603 women *under* thirty-five who divorced in 1988 will marry again. Divorce is a transitional state for most younger men and women. But increasing the age level by an additional fifteen years produces a significant drop in the remarriage rate. Now, at age fifty, only 60 per cent of previously divorced men and 31 per cent of divorced women can expect to eventually marry again. These figures underline that though remarriage rates decline with age for both sexes, it is women's chances which fall most rapidly. This gender and remarriage rate differential widens with each increasing year, so that at sixty a divorced woman records only a quarter of the rate for divorced men.

Younger age at divorce not only increases the probability of remarriage; it is also associated with shorter time between divorce and a new marriage. The work of Haskey (1987b: table 6) upon a sample of divorcing couples in 1979 shows one-third of all divorcing wives had remarried within two and a half years. The proportion increased to half (49 per cent) for those aged under twenty-five at divorce and fell to 16 per cent for those aged fifty or more.

Age at divorce is also strongly linked with the social class of the husband. The previous chapter showed that the highest rate of divorce is experienced by the lower manual classes; they also experience earlier age at marriage and shorter marriage duration which in turn leads to younger age at divorce. Conversely, middle-class divorces tend to occur at a later age, which in turn reduces the wife's chances of establishing a second marriage. These demographic patterns help to explain why it is that divorced wives of manual workers have higher rates of remarriage than found among wives of non-manually employed men (Haskey 1987b: table 2 and figure 1).

The presence of dependent children does not necessarily lessen a wife's remarriage chances. Earlier evidence from the USA reported larger family size was a positive feature of early remarriage (Goode 1956). More recent, 1980, American findings indicate 'young divorced mothers were becoming more likely than childless divorced women to remarry and to do so rather quickly, while young childless divorced women were becoming more likely to delay remarriage and to do so for a rather long period of time' (Glick and Lin 1986: 744). Findings for this country also suggests the existence of a child makes less negative impact on remarriage chances than might generally be expected (Coleman 1989: 107; Leete and Anthony 1979: 5; Ermisch 1989: 50). In 1988 the majority (60 per cent) of divorcing mothers with dependent children (under sixteen) were themselves aged under thirty-five (OPCS 1990a: 77). These patterns combine to suggest some two-thirds of all dependent children experiencing breakdown of parental marriage will find themselves in a reconstituted family unit of mother and stepfather.

The gender differential in rates of remarriage is most sensibly examined from knowledge of existing social mores and processes. In nine out of ten divorces the parent with responsibility for the daily care and control of the children is the mother. We know that in about 45 per cent of all current divorces the wife has to bring up at least one child under ten. It is these lone mothers with young children who are especially liable to find themselves confined to a domestic role which severely limits their ability to get out and meet other people, especially in evening leisure activities. Separation can force the employed wife to give up her occupation to look after the children in what is now a one-parent family. Men have greater opportunity to meet women in the workplace and in leisure activities such as membership of social clubs and sports centres. But the mother forfeits her chance of meeting people at work by her caring activity, and thereby lowers her chances of remarriage compared with those who remain employed (Ermisch 1989). Removal of a wage packet creates economic hardship, which in turn reduces the mother's ability to present an appearance that is seen as attractive both by herself and by others. The same tight budgeting and the associated problems of running a fatherless family can lead to a deterioration of the general structure and quality of the accommodation and its furniture and fittings to a level that discourages the mother from inviting friends home. Dennis Marsden in his penetrating 1969 study of fatherless families observed: 'It was not just that mothers needed to make special efforts to start up new relationships. They must work hard even to keep those friends they formerly had.'

Further male advantage in remarriage opportunity is contained within the arena of courtship. Gender differences found in cultural and social patterns of behaviour and in personal attitudes benefits the male seeking new female friendship. For all the talk of woman's liberation we still have a society in which men expect, and are expected, to make the initial approaches to women. Yet divorced men whose social life during marriage had been centred in home and family might well have lost the knack of approaching women and making their acquaintance. At the same time facilities for meeting the opposite sex are very largely orientated to the needs of youth. Such meeting places as dance and disco halls and youth clubs do not cater for the middle-aged woman (half of all divorcing women in 1988 were aged thirty-four or more) who, because of family responsibilities, do not even have the opportunity of meeting people provided by employment.

Many divorced women do not wish to marry again and risk lacerating existing marital scars (Mitchell 1985: 150). For others, a fresh marriage to a low wage earner encumbered with maintenance commitments might cause a reduction in the standard of living experienced by those with a large family maintained by income support and ancillary state benefits. As one mother told Marsden (1969: 159): 'It would be no good me marrying an ordinary working man . . . I want somebody to pull me out of this rut.' A Bristol University survey records a third of wives with care of children reported being financially better off since separating, because for the first time they controlled the family income. One wife reported, 'I never had so much money in my life. I know how much is coming in every week which I didn't know when I was married. . . . I don't mind living on a reduced income because it's secure' (Davis *et al.* 1983b: 222). For those who receive maintenance a new marriage causes the wife's order to be revoked. For some divorced wives the single status is preferable to once more risking the hazards of wedlock.

The reality of cohabitation with a new partner effectively removes some of the problems facing the lone divorcee. Such a relationship can begin before a divorce has occurred. Mitchell's study of family disruption in Scotland, for instance, reports one-third of the departing spouses almost immediately commenced a new partnership (1985: 149). In some cases a formal dissolution of the dead marriage is never sought. Cohabitation may operate as a substitute for, or as a preceding stage to, marriage; or as an event occurring before an eventual marriage with another person. A significant minority of divorced cohabitants see and refer to their relationship as a marriage (OPCS 1979: 39). Half of the wives in Dunnell's study who separated in 1970–1 had within four years formed a new relationship by marriage (28 per cent) or cohabitation (20 per cent) (Dunnell 1979: 38). More recently, the OPCS *Consequences of Divorce* study reports a new partnership had been formed within twelve weeks of the decree absolute by 36 per cent of interviewed men (remarried: 11 per cent; cohabiting: 25 per cent) and 25 per cent of women (remarried: 7 per cent; cohabiting: 18 per cent) (OPCS 1990c: 13).

These rates of remarriage and extra-marital cohabitation indicate divorce is a transitional event for the majority of disunited couples and their children. Our couple-orientated culture has created a social landscape which discriminates against the single adult and the lone-parent family. The alternatives can appear decidedly less attractive than the companionship and acceptability secured by the return to a conventional two-adult household. There are also practical and financial advantages, and it is therefore to be expected that the majority of divorced persons will form new relationships. Within this variegated family web can be seen the breakdown of old commitments and the formation of new associations and bonds of attachment and obligation.

THE NEW MARRIAGE

Marriage registers chronicle the increasing presence of previously divorced persons. One in four of all spouses in England and Wales entering wedlock in 1990 had been previously divorced. Similar nuptuality status rate calculations for European countries in the years 1980 or 1981 indicates the English experience (1981: one in five) provided one of the highest rates, exceeded only by Denmark (one in four). The demographic and social impact of divorced persons in new marriages can be observed in all European countries allowing divorce. For example: Sweden (one in five), Scotland and West Germany (one in seven) and France (one in ten). As would be expected, there is a direct association between these remarriage rates and national divorce rates (United Nations 1984: 670–7). In most industrialized countries divorce and remarriage have become life events which the majority of married couples will encounter either directly or through involvement of kin.

Family patterns are altering as a consequence of the accumulating number of remarriages that embrace younger brides. A quarter of the brides under thirty-five in 1990 were wed in remarriage nuptials; they were either single women marrying divorced men (29,000), divorced women marrying single men (21,000) or divorced women marrying divorced men (16,000). Regardless of the bride's previous status, it is natural and reasonable to conceive children. Most of these marriages will be fertile, though only a few remarrying husbands will be wealthy enough to maintain two families.

Previously divorced women now bear one in ten of all marital births. This rate has doubled over the last twenty years, being a further consequence of rising divorce numbers (CSO 1989: 47). Socially, the formation of new families once more extends the kin network within both the nuclear and the extended family. This is especially the case when there are already children of an earlier marriage to magnify the complexity of kin arrangements within second marriages.

The presence of children from a previous relationship means many remarried couples begin life together with an existing family already around them. Such remarriage structures do not differ from those of earlier centuries except that today's absent natural parent remains alive. The likely range of family structures are summarized in Table 10.3, though some other possibilities have had to be excluded. But the table does provide an indication of the ongoing social movements whereby remarried adults can become step-parents, parents, or both, and some children acquire step-parents and half-siblings. Such realignments confound some of the basic expectations of Western family life; we can no longer suppose a couple's children are their progeny.

The consequences of divorce and remarriage spread out in all directions and they clearly affect children. Marriage breakdown means most children lose regular contact, and a minority (possibly even a half) relinquish all contact, with their father. American evidence shows the father's remarriage is a major factor reducing paternal involvement.One mother explained to Arendell: 'He used to have them come visit him, but he just has no room for them anymore now that he's remarried. It's like the kids don't belong in his life anymore.' Another interviewed mother in the same study observed: 'My children refuse to accept his new wife. It's because of the way it was done: he started living with her immediately, as soon as he left here' (Arendell 1986: 116–7). Severance may well be extended to paternal grandparents, uncles and aunts. Over time old networks and links are fractured or destroyed and replaced by new and more complex relationships involving step-parents and their new extended family. The judiciary have no means of foreseeing the nature, quality and durability of these associations. Yet Parliament creates the myth that the courts have a welfare calculus which forecasts the child's best interests.

The mother's new spouse might welcome the chance of having replacement stepchildren as surrogates for his lost earlier family. Brenda Maddox, in her study *The Half Parent* reports: 'Many stepfathers, unlike stepmothers, told me how much they loved their stepchildren. "It was far, far easier than being a parent – all of the satisfactions and none of the guilt."' The next of Maddox's informants displays a more doubtful attitude: 'I love some of my wife's children; my wife feels guilty because she doesn't love mine' (Maddox 1975: 155). A resentment of the children's presence can create tension between adults attempting to mould new marital relationships in delicate and testing circumstances. The ambiguity of emotions facing step-parents is described by Allan:

> At the head of the problem lies the different significance of children to parents and step-parents. Whereas children are taken, ideally, to bind their parents together and symbolize their unity, step-children in effect do the opposite. Rather than being a joint 'creation', socially as well as biologically, step-children represent an unshared past and a somewhat divided present.
>
> (Allan 1985: 123)

Many remarried couples see the begetting of their own children as underlining the normality of their partnership (Burgoyne and Clark 1986: 193).

Society is puzzled and uncertain as to the correct and proper manner to handle these step-family relationships. This rapid development of new family patterns has failed to provide either a cultural framework to handle, or a suitable vocabulary to describe, such alliances. For instance, where does the stepfather stand at his wife's daughter's wedding reception; or what name does the child call his stepfather, and if it is 'Dad', might not the latter's own children in the same household see this as a threat to their paternal claim?

An American study of 30,000 households has shown that the presence of children from a previous marriage increases the probability of the remarried wife experiencing further breakdown, while the presence of children from the new marriage reduced the probability of divorce (quoted in Cherlin 1978; see also, for a critique, Furstenberg and Spanier 1984: 186–91). A whole range of conflict situations can arise in the step-family household, such as the problem facing the mother when tension arises between her children and the stepfather. Should she support the children or the new spouse? Or it may be that each parent's children wish to celebrate Christmas in their own past way. In another situation, stepchildren who do not live with the stepmother can also, by their visits, be a regular source of intense difficulty and tension. A recent English study of the consequences of divorce reported objections to access were more likely to come from new partners than from either the custodial or the visiting parent. One father reported his experience as: 'Her new husband [new partner of custodial mother] didn't approve of me seeing them, and didn't like me going up to the house or anything' (OPCS 1990c: 156). These role ambiguities, uncertainties and issues combine to increase the relationship problems contained within step-families.

THE PROTRACTED FIRST MARRIAGE

The reassuring presence of a new partner rekindles social links of affection and attachment within survivors swimming from the wreckage of a collapsed marriage. Those who remain alone see divorce as the symbolic burial of an unhappy association. Nevertheless, in many instances and situations the former marital relationship and kin networks are not so readily dissolved. This is especially so when there are dependent children. Divorced parents, and particularly the mother, simply cannot make a new beginning completely severed from past familial affiliation.

We know the majority of those who divorce will marry again. The marital distribution pattern for the 167,000 (100 per cent) previously divorced persons who re-entered matrimony in 1988 shows 'both divorced' (55 per cent) formed the largest group, followed by divorced men and spinsters (21 per cent), divorced women and bachelors (19 per cent) and divorced and widowed spouses (5 per cent). It has already been seen that remarriages containing step-parents and children have potential for far greater points of stress, conflict and ambivalence than that found within a first marriage. Manners, habits and expectations attached to Western culture's traditional lifelong marriage have lagged behind the aftermath of the divorce explosion. All this helps to create a web of undefined parts for the cast of the reconstituted family. Their private stage displays the personal stresses and problems associated with past ties and present ambiguity of parental behaviour. It is this backdrop which encumbers the remarried as they learn new and uncertain roles. As Mrs Graham informed Burgoyne and Clark (1984: 187): 'When I got married to Martin . . . I was going to imagine that I had never been married before and I was going to start afresh, and it hasn't been like that. It would appear that our marriage, on both sides, has taken over from where our last one ended and it's very frightening.'

An earlier American study found that remarried mothers, in contrast to those who had not remarried, wished the father would visit the children less frequently or not at all (Goode 1965: 324). The remarried mother may believe the absent father's access contact with his children restricts the development of binding links within her new relationship. Exuberant children returning after an exciting day with their father may be seen by the mother and her new husband as confirmation that these visits are an unnecessary brake to their development of traditional family bonds. Limited weekend time when mother and stepfather are both free for family trips has been curtailed by parental contact, and irritation grows as they lack the means to compete with the father's gifts and outings. The children develop divided loyalties, they are uncertain about the stepfather and his claims to their mother, and resent his discipline in the home. The new husband's presence alongside the children's mother emphasizes the acquired responsibility of social parenthood, and he naturally wishes to incorporate the identity and role of father both with his stepchildren and with the community. Yet the step-parent role is really one of being an added parent rather than a substitute father for an orphaned child. The children retain the name of their natural father. The Children Act 1975 restricted adoption of children following remarriage of the natural parent (normally the divorced mother) and the new step-parent. As a result the annual number of legitimate children who were adopted fell by 60 per cent between 1976 (9,100) and 1986 (3,800) (CSO 1988: 46). The law of 1975 returned to an emphasis on genetic or 'blood' relationships and ignored the social day-to-day environment of the child. But it remains the case that the child's future best interests now reside in the success of the newly formed household relationship.

Court intervention may ensure a father's continuation of contact with his children (and vice versa) and simultaneously stop the mother's freedom of choice and movement. This is reflected in *Tyler v. Tyler* ([1990] FLR 22), when the divorced mother of two young boys brought up on a Lincolnshire farm had her application to take them to join her parents in Australia turned down by the Court of Appeal. Lord Justice Kerr observed the boys needed a father. The mother had not formed a new stable relationship since divorcing three years earlier. The judgment, decided on the boys' best interests, ensured the mother's self-determination was seriously curtailed by the continuing family bonds of a severed marriage.

Family law is also in a quandary as how to deal with the step-parent and stepchild relationship. This predicament stems from the already explained historical background whereby in times past the new association inevitably resulted from the biological parent's death. Now the latter lives on as a paternal shadow desiring levels of parental involvement ranging from forceful commitment to minimal or non-existent contact. The first marriage's established boundary of parental rights and obligations have been jolted by divorce. The second marriage creates a hazier map of the step-parent's claims and duties. For instance, the step-parent does not have authority to act *in loco parentis*, and accordingly has no right to make decisions affecting the child such as giving consent for an operation. If this is the case then one may well ask under what circumstances does the stepfather have a duty to maintain the child? The Child Support Act of 1991 appears to place full responsibility on the natural parents.

If the new marriage should break down the court can make an order against the stepfather for his stepchild's support, but only if satisfied the latter has been treated as a child of the family. The more inclusive the stepfather's acceptance of his new family the greater the likelihood of being judged liable for their financial support. What will the newly established Child Support Agency do in such a double-bind situation? Some other legal areas clouded by uncertainty towards claims recognizing the presence of stepchildren and their relationship with the step-parent are those of workmen's compensation, social security benefits and inheritance. They indicate some of the new legal problems that might arise for 10 per cent of all children who are brought up in step-parent households. New family patterns have rushed ahead of legal acknowledgement.

Children are witnesses to developments, events and new relationships occurring in both parental households. The innocent comment of such a go-between can readily inflame the embers of bitter resentment in the other parent. The effects and consequences of parental antagonism are all too often seen by domestic panel magistrates. An arrears hearing where the ex-husband excuses his non-payment by saying the children were so shoddy and ill-dressed at contact time that he bought them new clothing rather than pay the court order. The employed mother who resents Sunday's access departure on her one free leisure day, and the children's joyful return with presents and pocket money from their father while the carer's mortgage arrears, household debts and maintenance arrears mount up. On the next Sunday's visitation the children are not waiting to be collected but have been taken to their maternal grandparents, and another access dispute is born. And while the father vents annoyance, his new companion resents this domestic intrusion into their courtship. Or the newly married wife complaining of the irked ex-wife's telephone harassment of the non-paying father. Such verbal action can be part of the weaponry of the divorced wife who resents her replacement experiencing better living standards. All this, of necessity, reduces to stereotyped situations the uniqueness of personal life patterns acted out on each family's stage by the main players' interaction that links past and present.

CHANGING SOCIAL NETWORKS

The traditional nuclear family has a network of reciprocal social links with a

Table 10.3 Family sets following remarriage

current marriage of wife and husband	*Children from:* Wife	*previous marriage of:* No	Husband Husband (*number of sets*)	1st wife
No	No	–	1 H	1 E
	Yes: with Wife	1 W	2 HW	2 WE
	1st Husband	1 E	2 HE	2 EE
Yes	No	1 C	2 HC	2 CE
	Yes: with Wife	2 WC	3 WHC	3 WCE
	1st Husband	2 CE	3 HCE	3 CEE

Notes: Children in the family household may result from: (W) previous marriage of the wife; (H) previous marriage of the husband; or from (C) their current marriage. The couple's children (especially the husband's) from an earlier marriage (or relationship) may be external to the current household (E).

constellation of spousal kin. Grandparents obtain satisfaction and pleasure from contact with their grandchildren, their caring provision benefits both parents and children. Friendships develop between the spouses and their respective uncles, aunts and cousins. The reality of separation lessens commitment, support obligations and goodwill to, and from, the other spouse's relations. Divorce creates acrimony, residential moves reduce contact, and time further weakens earlier familial ties (Finch and Mason 1990: 230). Nevertheless, established links are not always broken by divorce; a study of family life in north London reports the person one divorced woman was closest to was her first husband's sisters's daughter (Firth *et al.* 1970: 288).

It is fairly common for men and women who experience accommodation needs following marriage breakdown to return to the parental home for at least a while (Finch 1989: 25–6). This kin group support can be seen as a form of the extended family, and often continues to the grandparents providing child-care for the mother. As fresh friendships develop into marriage, so new webs are once more woven between previously unknown families. The complex new kin networks affect both personal relationships and the interests of children.

In Britain today, a tenth of all couples are raising children from a previous marriage (OPCS 1990c: 10). The remarrying husband may have three sets of children at home: those of the first marriage, stepchildren from the wife's previous marriage, and children of the new marriage (Table 10.3). Siblings from their respective parents' first marriages are stepbrothers and stepsisters to the other group; they all become half brothers and sisters to children of the second marriage. In the realm of adults the marriage of divorced spouses creates an affinal relationship between the ex-spouse and the new groom or bride. If a second marriage causes an entanglement of old and new kin associations, then a further divorce and third marriage creates a labyrinth of extended relationships.

INSTABILITY IN SECOND MARRIAGES

The emotional inheritance of the first marriage adds to the complexities and problems facing those divorcees who marry again. This is only one feature which helps to explain why it is that second marriages have a greater risk of divorce; the probability is double that of a first marriage (Haskey 1983; OPCS 1990a: 88). A somewhat similar conclusion has been reached by Coleman (1989) from age-specific divorce rates produced from 1981 Census data. The much higher divorce propensity found within remarriage is also confirmed by studying the subsequent marital experiences of single and previously divorced men aged twenty to twenty-four who married in 1966. Comparing these two cohorts fifteen years after their weddings shows the bachelor grooms (19 per cent) had half the divorce rate experienced by those previously divorced (35 per cent). Half the latter group will live through a further divorce. The experience of women also aged twenty to twenty-four is very similar to the men; previously divorced brides (31 per cent) had double the divorce risk of spinster brides (15 per cent) (Haskey 1989b: table 5). A similar variation is recorded for divorcing women of all ages in 1990 (Table 10.4). The American experience is like ours (Cherlin 1978: 638, table 5). Marriages embracing a divorced person are particularly prone to breakdown.

Those who divorce again also experience shorter durations of marriage compared with those who divorce for the first time; for instance, 50 per cent of previously divorced brides who divorced once more in 1990 had marriage durations of under eight years compared with 36 per cent for spinster brides who also divorced in 1990. The pattern for men coincided with that for women (OPCS 1992b: 83, 87). Second marriages' propensity to early breakdown is confirmed for this country by marriage cohort data from Haskey (1989b), while Furstenberg and Spanier (1984: 183) provide supporting evidence for America. Such trends, linked with the increasing number of non-marital household relationships, affect the stability and continuity of parental socialization. One in twenty of the 1980s newborn are likely to share the confusing childhood experience of at least two more partners taking up residence with the custodial parent.

Serial divorces are having increasing influence upon the overall divorce pattern of England and Wales. A quarter of all divorces in 1990 contained a previously divorced spouse. In almost a tenth (8 per cent) of all cases dissolution for the second (or further) time was the lot of both spouses. At the level of individual divorce experience, 17 per cent of the spouses were undergoing their second (or further) divorce; this was double the proportion recorded ten years earlier. The impact of sequential divorce upon overall divorce rates is under-emphasized in demographic, sociological and legal discussion. The increasing numbers experiencing sequential divorce means it has become too simplistic to equate reconstituted families with a second marriage (or cohabitation). We now have several parallel stuctures of family life-cycles (first, second, third or more) with their own demographic (age, fertility), social (kinship, multiple parentage) and legal (support obligations, custody) characteristics.

Why is it that remarriages display this vunerability to further breakdown? Explanation most sensibly focuses on the interaction between the structural, institutional and behavioural features which affect family life. At the structural level, the new family can experience financial hardship through the husband's ongoing maintenance liability and this creates pressure on the second wife to earn, which in turn causes her irritation at having to contribute to past marital obligations. Resentment may also be created by the divorced spouse's continuing contact with the ex-partner; in Sanctuary and Whitehead's experience (1972: 151) 'the children of a former marriage are usually acceptable, but not the parent whose place the new partner has taken'. These two situations are further examples of the protracted first marriage detrimentally affecting the quality and binding of the new relationship. Many reconstituted families will begin their new life in unsatisfactory accommodation because they are too poor to obtain a mortgage, while having little chance of being rehoused by the local authority unless classified as homeless. The study of step-families in Sheffield by Burgoyne and Clark (1980) brings out how the economic, social and emotional inheritance from the earlier family are carried into the new marriage.

It has been seen that divorced persons who marry again face special family problems and strains unknown in first marriages. Reconstituted relationships produce more opportunity for disagreement and division through the absence of effective institutional and cultural guidelines, controls and solutions found in the management of first marriages. For instance, there are no socially prescribed roles and models of behaviour for stepmothers to present to their stepchildren. Study of newly married couples shows the factor most associated with stress and unhappiness among wives was having to cope with stepchildren (Kurdeck 1991: 634). Earlier similar American evidence had led Cherlin (1978) to describe remarriage as an 'incomplete institution', and to argue that it is this normative uncertainty which helps makes the preservation of family unity more difficult. Though Cherlin's argument has appeal, it does not entirely explain why there should be a sixfold greater propensity for further divorce found in 1990 divorce rates (Table 10.4) among younger (aged twenty-five to thirty-four) previously divorced brides – an age group that avoids the special factors associated with 'older' widows – compared with similarly aged widowed brides.

A more individualistic explanation contends that the divorce-prone display a personality and disposition for the marriage stakes which more readily gives up or veers away from the challenging threat than resolves it. In addition, such people may be less adept at choosing the right partner. The divorce experience

Table 10.4 Comparison of bride's marital status by divorce rates experienced in 1990, England and Wales

Period of marriage	Bride's marital status	Age at marriage		
		25–29	30–34	All ages
		(Rate per 1,000 related marriages)		
1985–9	Single	15.2	11.9	24.5
	Widowed	20.9	15.9	11.0
	Divorced	26.1	21.4	21.8
All years	Single	3.8	2.6	6.3
	Widowed	2.4	2.1	1.3
	Divorced	16.1	13.2	12.6

Source: OPCS (1992b: 88).

acclimatizes a segment of its population who are already temperamentally predisposed to form incompatible relationships. Those remarrying line up again at the institutional tape innoculated with the techniques and experiences of post-breakdown survival and knowing there is life after divorce. This cognitive awareness ensures less hesitancy next time around if once again the new spouse fails to provide personal happiness. There is American data from Thornton (1985: 868) to support this argument, while their interviews led Furstenberg and Spanier (1984: 192) to be 'continually struck by the admissions of many of our informants that they were prepared to dissolve their second marriage if it did not work out'. A more rapid conjugal assessment and pronouncement is particularly true of those remarrying at a younger (under thirty-five) age. This tendency is shown within the short-lived recent 1985–9 marriages recorded in Table 10.4 whereby the younger previously divorced and widowed brides displayed a greater readiness to come out of unsatisfactory marriages more quickly than did similarly aged spinster brides.

If the arguments of personality and temperament, poor selection ability and knowledge for surviving breakdown can be validly related to individuals, then new partnerships bringing together two divorced persons appear especially vulnerable. This expectation of incompatibility is confirmed by both Monahan's American results (1958: table 5) and by the 1972 Oxford divorce data which allowed precise marital status pairing to be made. Calculating the percentage of divorces lasting under ten years from marriage to decree absolute in each marital group within the Oxford study showed: any single or widowed combination – 41 per cent, divorced and either single or widowed combination – 63 per cent, both divorced – 84 per cent.

Lord Devlin's authoritative analysis of the practical effect of divorce has proved to be a timely caution. A combination of changing social attitudes and the divorce courts' authority to issue liberally licences for new marriages have together produced the conditions for sequential divorce. It is impossible to imagine Parliament legislating to debar divorce second time around – what if the other spouse was initially single? – and ineluctably enforcing its new rule by declaring adultery and desertion to be criminal offences. Such an unworkable authoritarian code would not be tolerated by a democratic electorate. We are left with our existing divorce structure within which the statutory concepts of the paramount welfare of the child and the husband's obligation to maintain are in many cases legal fictions.

Part IV
Marriage breakdown today

11 Divorce: the legal evidence

English divorce law has always insisted a certified cause be shown to dissolve the marriage partnership; a mutual agreement to divorce is not accepted as sufficient reason for immediate termination. When the last Royal Commission on Marriage and Divorce began in 1951 to inquire into the law affecting marriage breakdown, it was examining a legal process designed to ensure an adversarial contest between the petitioner and the respondent. The rules of engagement required the wronged spouse to come to court with 'clean hands' and prove the respondent's voluntary committal of a matrimonial offence judged so heinous as to cut at the heart of marriage. In practice the vast majority of respondents offered little resistance at the court confrontation: the licence to marry again was a prize bestowed on both parties.

THE GROUNDS AND FACTS OF DIVORCE

1950–70

The three fault grounds of either adultery, desertion or cruelty accounted for 99 per cent of all divorces. Adultery remained the most commonly presented ground; it was easy to prove against a respondent equally desiring divorce. Resort to this ground increased between 1955 (43 per cent) and 1970 (55 per cent), though the rise was largely due to increasing usage by wife petitioners. In the same period use of desertion halved, its decline equally spread between men and women. Wives began to petition more readily on cruelty, encouraged by the easing of judicial interpretation. The latter trend also reflected women's changing normative expectations of what was acceptable within married life. By the 1960s wives were no longer so forbearing of behaviour their mothers had accepted because there had been no other choice, or so willing to continue in relationships offering no satisfaction or happiness. As the number of divorce petitioners advanced through the 1960s, so the proportion formed by wives steadily increased to form 63 per cent of all petitions in 1970 – the last year of the 'offence' law. This trend partly reflected the rules of legal aid which specifically benefited wives, as well as the changing mores and declining stigma attached to divorce.

Table 11.1 Facts supporting breakdown by petitioning husband or wife, for selected periods 1972–90, England and Wales

Spouse granted divorce: period

Breakdown facts	1972			1975–9			1980–4			1990		
	H	W	T	H	W	T	H	W	T	H	W	T
		%			%			%			%	
Fault												
Adultery	15	17	32	13	17	30	12	18	30	12	17	29
Behaviour	1	17	18	2	27	29	3	32	35	6	39	45
Desertion	4	6	10	1	3	4	1	1	2	0.2	1	1
Sub-total	20	40	60	16	47	63	16	51	67	18	57	75
Separation												
2 years	7	11	18	10	17	27	9	16	25	7	12	19
5 years	12	10	22	5	5	10	4	4	8	3	3	6
Sub-total	19	21	40	15	22	37	11	20	33	10	15	25
Total	39	61	100	31	69	100	29	71	100	28	72	100
Numbers (Decree nisi)		118,253			130,825			145,672			152,120	

Note: Calculations based on Law Commission (1988: 47–9); OPCS (1992b: table 4.6); *Civil Judicial Statistics* table 5.3

Failure to prove fault against a spouse unwilling to be divorced meant the marriage formally continued its dead legal existence though its social form had dissolved long ago. The following extract from a letter to a national newspaper in 1951 tells its own tale:

> She will not divorce me, and we have been parted 26 years. I have been living with a lady for the past 17 years and have two fine boys 16 years and 13 years and an adopted daughter aged 6 years. I would clearly love to get married before I die, but I cannot see how I can do it so would you please advise me.

Post-1970

The doctrine of fault held firm until the beginning of 1971, when introduction of the 1969 Divorce Reform Act brought in irretrievable breakdown of the marriage substantiated by one or more of five 'facts'. Three of the five supporting facts are simply the old fault offences shaped to new outlooks. The act of adultery remains what it has always been, though petitioners now have to now certify additionally that they find 'it intolerable to live with the respondent'. Generally the provision allows divorce without delay. Since 1971 the usage of adultery as a 'fact' has remained a fairly constant proportion of some 30 per cent of all petitions, though husband petitioners have been more likely to utilize adultery than wife petitioners.

The 1969 legislation reduced from three to two years as the minimum period before desertion could be used as a 'fact'. This easing did not stop the continuing dramatic fall in the use of desertion to a level where it has now almost disappeared in practical relevance to form 1 per cent of all petitions.

Since 1971 'unreasonable behaviour' has gained in acceptance to become in the 1980s the most commonly used 'fact' supporting breakdown; it is the most noticeable trend recorded in Table 11.1. This rise in resort to behaviour is associated with increased usage by women. In 1990 behaviour represented 45 per cent of all divorce 'facts'; for every one such husband petitioner there were six wife petitioners. An already tense and unhappy domestic situation is further corroded when the respondent reads the petition's list of alleged behaviour failings. The Matrimonial Causes Committee under Mrs Justice Booth report: 'The practice . . . can exacerbate and prolong bitter feelings [and] lead to a defended suit and to disputed issues as to custody and finance' (Report 1985: par. 4.25).

The pre-1971 era required cruelty as a fault to be supported by full supporting evidence which became subject to judicial scrutiny. Now the 'fact' of unreasonable behaviour has been reduced to the petitioner's bald statement that the complained behaviour makes it unjustifiable to expect this petitioner to live with that respondent. Though legal text books properly record the courts have to apply an objective test to the evidence (Cretney and Masson 1990: 108), in causal terms it is the spouse's subjective response and attitude to this behaviour that creates the breakdown. A wife in the 1970s successfully petitioned that the marriage had irretrievably broken down through the husband's constant demands to have his feet tickled! In earlier times this would have judicially seemed an irritating tiresome desire but not sufficiently grave and weighty to satisfy proof of cruelty. The spouse who now complains the marriage consortium has ended due to the behaviour's detrimental impact upon the petitioner is assured of a divorce as long as the other spouse equally wishes for dissolution and therefore does not defend the complaint. The processing of undefended petitions is undertaken within the format of special procedure whereby the district judge examines and normally approves the petition without the parties being present and available for examination. The introduction of special procedure has led to this fact becoming, in the words of Davis and Murch (1988: 87) 'the catch-all basis for divorce'. As a respondent informed the researchers: 'if you can't find anything really solid, then have a go at unreasonable behaviour'. Judges have accepted the breakdown approach, and virtually every undefended petition recording behaviour as a supporting 'fact' is allowed even though the allegation may appear trivial to everyday folk (Law Commission, 1990: 179). This judicial approach is a contemporary culmination of the growing recognition since 1900 that lifeless partnerships embalmed in the rigidity of a restrictive fault-based divorce law regulated within inaccessible courts were inducements to non-marital unions and thereby threats to the institution of marriage.

The two remaining facts focus directly on breakdown, and do not require evidence of a matrimonial offence. Confirmation of the couple's living apart is the most meaningful indicator of the irretrievable breakdown of their marriage. The couple are required to have lived apart for a minimum period of either: (a) two years, if the respondent has agreed to the separation; or (b) five years if there has been no agreement. Table 11.1 reports a steady decline in the use of the very facts which were believed to more properly reflect divorce law's new breakdown approach. One practical reason that helps to explain this surprising trend is it is generally easier for husbands to leave home and find other accommodation. Social needs have created practical barriers which discriminate against four-fifths of wife petitioners in 1990 being able or willing to utilize either of the separation facts.

Two years' separation brought divorce by agreement into the statute book. This way was intended to be the conciliatory civil approach to divorce for couples who recognized their relationship had irretrievably come apart. Yet the mutual consent 'fact' has for most of the time since 1971 been used by no more than a quarter of all petitioners. Couples are not prepared to wait two years when the facts of either adultery or behaviour provide an alternative and much quicker route to the court.

Separation without either offence or consent was introduced as the radical solvent to be unilaterally applied to long-dead unions. A minimum period of five years' separation was evidence of irretrievable breakdown, even though the respondent had neither breached the old fault framework of expected conduct, nor consented to divorce. This was the cornerstone of the 1969 reforms. The first year of the new legislation saw some 30,000 previously debarred petitioners seeking divorce through the five-year fact; they formed 27 per cent of all 1971 petitions. Evidence from the Oxford 1972 divorce survey confirms most of the petitioners using this fact, in the very early period of the new liberal provision, were seeking legal internment of relationships effectively ceasing long before 1971. The length of time from separation to petitioning averaged fifteen years compared with three years for the combined four other 'facts'; a quarter of the former petitioners reported separations of twenty years or more. The wave of five-year fact petitioners experienced in 1971 quickly subsided into a steady stream as the backlog of previously debarred petitioners were cleared. By 1975 the numbers had fallen to some 14,000 petitions, a tenth of all petitions filed. Since then, resort to five years, as Table 11.1 indicates, has decreased further to form 6 per cent of all divorce facts in 1990.

Early critics of the Divorce Reform Act, such as Lady Summerskill, feared provision of non-consensual divorce would be a Casanova's charter, licensing lustful husbands with younger and more exciting replacements for fading matronal wives. The needs of wives denied opportunity to remarry by both husband and offence-based law were never discussed or recognized. In practice non-consensual divorce has never been the monopoly of husbands; even in the first year of usage (1971) 45 per cent of petitioners were wives. Since 1973 there has been equal spousal resort to this fact. Changing mores have blown the earlier forecast inside out. Calculations focusing on those who were under forty-five and using five years' separation in 1990 reveal wife petitioners (2,652) outnumber husbands (1,695) by one and a half times (OPCS 1992b: 91). Presumably these husbands were both free of matrimonial fault that would have allowed their wives more rapid freedom and aversion to being divorced. Many wife petitioners using this fact wish to marry a new partner; Haskey (1986: 145) has shown 42 per cent of these wives remarried within two and a half years of divorce compared with less than a fifth (17 per cent) among the discarded ex-husbands. The evidence of this paragraph is a clear indicator of one of the most dominant forces creating change within marriage form and habit. Women in the latter half of this century have rising expectations of the quality of life coming from marriage. Traditional female attitudes have reshaped during a period experiencing a reduction in divorce stigma. Structural modifications in the form of government family policy, increasing female employment opportunity and better wages have created improved financial support for lone wives and mothers. All this has allowed wives greater (but not equal) freedom and ability to choose whether they wish to continue an unhapppy marriage or seek divorce. It has been these social transformations that have helped create the patterns and numbers of divorce rather than reform of divorce grounds.

Lawyers soon realized the statutory defences inserted to neutralize criticism of non-consensual separation were falling on deaf judicial ears. The courts' rejection of such pleading was not sexist bias against women respondents but, rather, a consequence of the judiciary's wholesale acceptance of the new philosophy obligating the formal ending of long shattered marriages. Five years living apart must be conclusive evidence of a marriage's irrevocable death. A determined respondent's bitter court defence acrimoniously denying the partnership's irretrievable breakdown only parades the propriety of the petitioner's claim.

Threat of a defence is an effective tool for respondents to negotiate better financial terms. Bargaining and adjustment over these terms often removes the respondent's initial opposition and the petitioner's need to wait for five years. The spouses broad economic agreement allows their lawyers to more readily settle on use of a quicker acting fact. This is why the five-year 'fact' is resorted to less than might have been expected.

NEEDS, FACTS AND TIME

The necessary two-year delay has proved a deterrent for consensual spouses seeking speedy release. This is especially so for poorer wives with children who have difficulty in arranging to live apart from the husband and one or other obtain the separate accommodation usually necessary to satisfy the condition of separation. In some courts a decree absolute is withheld if the couple are still living at the same address, and at the same time local authorities will not rehouse individuals until they have obtained the decree (Law Commission 1990: 173, 175). Information obtained by the Law Commission's courts record study shows, first, petitioners with children used two years separation far less (15 per cent) than those without children (34 per cent) and, second, that this pattern is especially true for the divorcing working-class population (Law Commission: 1990: tables (i)3, (ii)2 and 4 recalculated). All these factors help to explain why two years' separation was used in less than a fifth of all 1990 divorces.

The two quickest divorce access grounds of either adultery or unreasonable behaviour are more commonly used by petitioners with larger families (Haskey 1986: table 1). Couples without children displayed far greater readiness to utilize two years' separation, regardless of who actually petitioned. This pattern is confirmed by Gregory and Foster (OPCS 1990c: 12–17). Their study reports almost three-quarters (72 per cent) of wife petitioners using behaviour had been separated under six months when the petition was presented. Wives resort to this fact because they feel it important to obtain a quick divorce (Davis and Murch 1988: 81). Yet the pressure is not so much towards formal dissolution as the practical necessity of resolving the problems pressing down on the family following breakdown of marriage (Elston *et al.* 1975: 637). Mothers with young children can be faced with such urgent matters as the violent husband's continued presence in the home, the need for maintenance support, and assurance upon the children's future care and control. The truth is these so-called ancillary matters are the pressing and important family issues within the framework of special procedure and assured divorce. But it is necessary to bring such disputes to the court's notice before adjudication can proceed, and solicitors have a duty to direct their client's attention to the most direct and practical manner to attract judicial attention. Filing the divorce petition starts the cogs of the formal divorce machinery, which in turn activates the court's settlement role towards property, financial support and custody concerns.

Practical urgency causes many petitioners to turn to a fact which neither demands delay before use nor seeks positive acknowledgement of fault (as adultery does) from the respondent. But the price can be high, for evidence shows unreasonable behaviour as a ground fuels far greater resentment and ill-will to an already inflamed marital situation than the other four facts do (Davis and Murch 1988: 83). The respondent reads the allegations of behavioural wrongs put against him (or her) which itself creates a feeling of injustice. It is one factor which makes this ground the most likely to generate defensive responses. Consequently, negotiations on the ancillary issues of financial settlement and occupational rights display greater acrimony. This is why behaviour petitions produce the longest time gap between filing and the decree nisi: 36 per cent of such petitions record an interval of six months or more compared with 24 per cent for the combined other facts (OPCS 1990c: 18, table 2.37 recalculated). The paradox to this is revealed by the same survey's data (table 2.40) upon the crucial socially relevant time interval between separation and decree nisi. Two-thirds (68 per cent) of behaviour petitions obtain a decree nisi within a year of separation compared with 55 per cent of adultery petitions. The other three facts cannot enter this time-ranking exercise until a period of at least two years have formally passed. The evidence suggests pressing domestic problems generated by matrimonial breakdown have greater influence than legal veracity on the choice of presented fact.

Behaviour is the most commonly used fact because it allows the home-maker quick progress to court. The association between resort to behaviour and the requirements of property and accommodation is seen in the needs of low-income mothers; Haskey's study found 62 per cent of all divorcing wives with husbands either in social class 5 or unemployed petitioned through behaviour (1986: table 3 recalculated). Yet this same fact creates most bitterness and ill-will, and this can continue long after the divorce in situations where spousal association is maintained through paternal contact with the children. It is incongruous and absurd that the pathway to quick divorce is by the 'fact' known to promote the greatest spousal hostility.

PROCEDURE AND FORM

The most important consequence of the 1969 legislation was an unplanned and indirect sequence of events that transformed the divorce process into an administrative affair. The bureaucraticization of our divorce procedure is a strange and not entirely clear tale, though this section attempts to lay some markers. The one certainty is the absence of any meaningful Parliamentary or public discussion. Over some twenty years the legislature had fully debated the principles and issues surrounding the substantive grounds for divorce before half heartedly agreeing to extend them in 1969. Now Whitehall's regulatory powers were to side-step Parliamentary consent on the primary question of how the divorce process should be properly and considerately conducted.

The civil formalities of the marriage ceremony and the requirements of registration have long been entrusted to either clergymen or superintendent registrars. The act of divorce until recent times required the presence and authority of a senior judge. This status distinction in conducting the making and breaking of the marriage contract was usually explained by reference to the public interest. As Mr Justice (now Lord) Scarman observed in 1965: the public 'over-riding interest is that the institution of marriage should not be undermined by an unworthy and disreputable market in its dissolution' (*Nash v. Nash* [1965] P.266). The actual processing of undefended divorces in the High Court, London, in the late 1960s is observed and recorded by Norman Shrapnel: 'There were 73 undefended cases the day I went, mostly going on in this pair of starkly unadorned rooms which could almost be termed cells, pumping out divorces like a two-stroke engine. The law makes no pretence of majesty here. Productivity is the thing' (Shrapnel 1969: 11–12).

Lawyers, as much as any other interested pressure group, are liable to create myths which mask reality. In 1946 the Denning Committee on Procedure in Matrimonial Causes had affirmed divorce should be handled by the highest courts available. Their report went on to explain:

> In our opinion the attitude of the community towards the status of marriage is much influenced by the way in which divorce is effected. If there is a careful and dignified proceeding such as obtains in the High Court for the undoing of a marriage, then quite unconsciously the people will have a much more respectful view of the marriage tie and of the marriage status than they would if divorce were effected informally in an inferior court.
>
> (Report 1946: 7)

It is not known whether the guardianship of High Court divorce judges made couples more decorous within their marital relationships. But it is clear that the vast majority of divorces were undefended petitions which were speedily processed by Special Divorce Commissioners masquerading as High Court judges. Undefended cases, as Mr Harvey QC explained in a caustic exposition of the post-war divorce procedure, 'works almost on the slot machine principle' (Harvey 1953: 133). Sir Hartley Shawcross, the Attorney-General, recalled to the House of Commons in 1951: 'One used to handle these undefended cases at the rate of about one in two minutes . . . it did not impress me at the time that there was any real principle operating in practice in the administration of our divorce laws' (McGregor 1957: 141).

The courts, the lawyers and the public were increasingly seeing the administration of divorce as a charade serving little purpose yet costing a great deal to undertake. During the 1960s divorce numbers rose steadily as did the cost to the legal aid fund. Law Society figures for 1963/64 show over 80 per cent of the annual civil legal aid bill was due to divorce actions. This led the Lord Chancellor's Advisory Committee to express concern that 'the taxpayer was left to pay the lion's share' of legally aided matrimonial costs (LCD 1965: 56–7). A consequence was the demotion of undefended divorce hearings from High Court to County Court status in 1968, thereby giving solicitors similar rights of advocacy as barristers; the move was expected to save £400,000 a year.

County court judges already sat in London and at selected provincial towns as

Special Divorce Commissioners with the dignity, rank and pay of a High Court judge. All the 1967 legislation ritualistically achieved was to allow lawyers to address the judge in the recognized term of 'your Honour' rather than 'my Lord'. Little else changed in the procedure; it was the same courtroom, and the same judge wearing the familiar purple robes of a County court judge rather than the black robes of a High Court judge. This was the first of many lost battles the Bar experienced when defending their monopoly rights. Treasury power was beginning to dominate the barrister-manned citadal surrounding the Lord Chancellor's Department.

Widening the statutory framework in 1969 helped to accelerate the already increasing resort to divorce, consequently the 110,000 petitions of 1972 were threefold the number ten years earlier. Increasing consumer demand became a major (though not the only) contributory element causing civil servants and judges to instigate a complete change in the labelling of divorce processing and control procedures. This was still presented in 1972 as a judicial public process. The Court of Appeal felt it proper to emphasize in *Santos v. Santos* ([1972] Fam. 263–4) that even two-year consensual separation petitions required proper judicial scrutiny to ensure the breakdown test was applicable. In Lord Justice Sach's opinion the divorce should be allowed only after a hearing involving 'judicial care as opposed to rubber stamping'.

The legislation of 1969 had not altered the public procedure by which divorce was judicially granted; every petitioner appeared in a divorce court, testified to the judge's examination, and witnessed pronouncement of the decree nisi. By 1977 the divorce process had been changed into a private arrangement validated within an administrative setting. This most radical transformation in the approach to, and meaning of, divorce took place without serious Parliamentary debate. The new process was essentially the outcome of a cost-saving exercise rather than a purposeful Parliamentary rethinking of what the legislative, administrative and social needs of a modern divorce policy should be.

When introduced in 1973 the new arrangements were properly termed 'special procedure', for availability was restricted to petitioners without dependent children who sought divorce on the fact of two years' consensual separation. Two further extensions have meant that since April 1977 all undefended divorces are dealt with by special procedure. And this, in fact, is the general everyday procedure used by 99.9 per cent of all petitioners. The parties are not required to appear before a judge unless there are dependent children or if there are ancillary matters to be resolved. The district judge examines the papers in his office for both conformity to administrative requirements and assurance that the petition and its supporting affidavit evidence meets the substantive requirements for divorce. When satisfied on these two counts the district judge certifies his approval. This is the crucial decision, for with this certificate to hand the divorce judge must pronounce the decree nisi.

The national newspapers reported the working of special procedure one May day in 1978 when Judge Willis dealt with a batch of twenty-eight registrar (now termed district judge) certified petitions. A common feature for twenty-seven of the petitioners (which included a chambermaid, a housing officer, an office cleaner and an ex-guardsman) was that all had brought their own cases and were not legally represented in court. The remaining petitioner, Princess Margaret, had benefit of professional preparation for her petition of irretrievable breakdown after two years' separation, with the consent of Lord Snowdon to the ending of their eighteen year marriage. The Royal couple were not in court to hear the judge formally pronounce a divorce for all twenty-eight petitioners. Some judges were dissatisfied with their automaton role in special procedure. Earlier in the same May, Judge Grant 'under considerable protest' granted twenty-nine decrees simultaneously, complaining that he was being used 'as a rubber stamp' (*Daily Telegraph*, 9 May 1978).

The universalization of the special procedure records a fundamental change in our approach to the administration and regulation of divorce. A special exception brought in for a minority of petitioners had rapidly become the standard divorce procedure. The Bishop of Durham could write to *The Times* (4 April 1977):

> I am disturbed at the implications of divorce by post, and even more disturbed by the apparently casual manner in which such a fundamental change has been made. . . . To avoid public action tilts the concept of marriage breakdown dangerously in the direction of divorce by consent, and in so doing widens the gulf between Christian and purely contractual understandings of marriage. I believe it would be an immeasurable loss if those who, from both sides, wish to widen this gulf were given encouragement to do so by a piece of administrative convenience.

But executive endorsement of special procedure was not governed by a radical belief that divorce should now be seen as an essentially administrative process that no longer required a court hearing. Rather, at a time of economic crisis, causing the Treasury to insist on major cuts in public spending and the government to announce that there was to be little or no increase in expenditure on legal aid for the next five years, the Lord Chancellor concluded that there was only one area within civil legal aid where sizeable savings could justifiably be made. This was the field of divorce where calculations show (see p.89 Table 6.1) that 82,000 petitioners in 1976 had obtained legal aid, a figure that exceeded all petitions filed in 1970. All the evidence indicated that both the yearly net cost resulting from the availability of legal aid for petitioning and the proportion that this sum formed of the overall civil legal aid bill were increasing annually. The result was the removal of legal aid from undefended divorce petitions.

Under the rules governing eligibility for legal aid the separated wife is treated as a single claimant rather than being aggregated with her husband's income. Consequently, marriage breakdown has functioned to allow separated wives to more readily clear the means test access barrier to legal aid. The overall increase between 1970 and 1975 of 73 per cent in the yearly number of legal aid certificates issued to petitioners had largely been created by legally aided wives (89 per cent increase compared with 14 per cent increase for husbands). Wife petitioners were the major claimants to the civil legal aid funds in a situation where there was in reality no legal litigation or contest. It became increasingly hard to justify public expenditure upon lawyers' presence at proceedings where both spouses agreed their marriage had irretrievably broken down.

When Lord Chancellor Elwyn-Jones announced in 1976 the extension of special procedure to all undefended divorces he also declared that legal aid would no longer be available in such proceedings. The rationale behind this change was that as determination of the undefended petition would not now require a court hearing there was no longer need for a lawyer's attendance at court. However, legal aid would still be available where the need for a hearing arose for which legal representation was necessary. This covered contested petitions and such matters as disputes over ancillary questions involving maintenance, property or arrangements for the children. Ancillary proceedings were, in the words of the Lord Chancellor, 'the areas of real contest between the parties to divorce proceedings today, not the question whether the petitioner should get a decree' (*Hansard*, HL, vol. 371, cols 1218–19).

The procedural changes had been helped by findings from a 1973 survey undertaken before special procedure was introduced. The field work of Elston, Fuller and Murch (1975) gathered petitioners' reactions to their court experiences. The researchers found that in most undefended hearings only the petitioner and accompanying lawyer were in court. In three-quarters of the hearings the judge did not ask a question about the marriage, and 85 per cent of the hearings lasted less than ten minutes. A divorce was always granted. The authors concluded: 'At present the community is paying a high price for preserving an inefficient system which exemplifies the adversary system under maximum strain' (Elston *et al.* 1975: 640).

Special procedure has guillotined the outmoded 'inefficient system'. Today only the defended divorce petition goes to trial before a judge. The burden of proof is now upon the respondent to show the marriage has not irretrievably broken down but, as already argued, this final courtroom declaration of affection underlines the futility of the pleading. Contested hearings have become almost extinct because they are normally doomed to fail; in 1988 only 67 respondents (4 in every 10,000 processed petitions) persuaded the judge to reject the petition (LCD 1989: tables 5.5. and 5.6). Defended actions are discouraged by the courts, the lawyers and the Legal Aid Committees who all recognize the low chances of success must be set against the formidable legal fees and the debilitating emotional costs.

Divorce trials do not take up much judicial time; in 1988, a total of 367 defended petitions were dealt with in the High and County courts. Even this figure overstates the true number of full trials because of the legal pressure towards conciliation that leads on to an agreement before entering the court. The expert view of Sir John Arnold, President of the Family Division of the High Court in 1987, was that annually all divorces excepting '100 or less . . . are made without being opposed in the full rigour of litigation'.[1] Sir George Baker, a former President, could report in 1972 after twenty weeks of trying defended cases that there was 'not one single fight. They all settled.'[2] The divorce process has been radically transformed from a public judicial inquest titularly undertaken by High Court judges to a private administrative ratification of the spouses' decision to divorce. The legal setting for the vast majority of divorces is the County court; a structure designated and formulated for the quick, cheap settlement of debt disputes, minor accidents, breaches of contract and, since 1968, undefended divorce cases.

LEGAL AID AND ASSISTANCE

The motivating force towards a cost-effective functional divorce procedure came from the Treasury's necessity to reduce public expenditure upon an escalating divorcing population rather than from external pressure groups or official committees of inquiry. The reformation in administrative policy does not appear to have harmed or inconvenienced the clientele of this family welfare law service. Nor has there been any evidence that the removal of legal aid from *undefended petitions* has brought hardship or undue inconvenience to petitioners.

Successful applicants for legal aid have to clear the twin tests of legal merit and financial eligibility. Full legal aid remains available for the contentious and important practical matters of injunctions, custody, maintenance and property resolution. As compensation for the removal of legal aid from undefended petitions the Legal Advice and Assistance Scheme (often referred to as the Green Form Scheme) covers preliminary advice and assistance in divorce cases. Solicitors can normally undertake three hours of written work or oral advice. The third form of available legal aid is the Advice by Way of Representation (ABWOR) Scheme, which is mainly used for representation in summary court domestic proceedings. The latter Scheme assisted 36,000 people in the tax year 1986/87.

In the tax year 1986/87 some 116,000 new full legal aid certificates were issued for matrimonial work in the High and County courts, of which 86 per cent were related to divorce matters of ancillary relief or custody and access (LCD 1988: 53).[3] Wives continue to be the main beneficiaries of matrimonial legal aid: 70 per cent of all new certificates (116,000) went to wives (62 per cent as petitioners and 8 per cent as respondents). This is a consequence of, firstly, the means test rules benefiting those who are either not employed or are on low income (see above, p.178); and second, the certificated disputes of financial support and custody especially concerning women. But the low qualifying levels means that as more women earn a wage so they increasingly need to find either a considerable proportion, or all, of their legal expenses.

The Green Form Scheme provides a primary advisory function in the majority of divorces, helping some 63 per cent of all those who benefited from legally aided matrimonial assistance in 1986/87 (the remaining 37 per cent consisted of full legal aid certificates (27 per cent) and ABWOR (10 per cent)) (LCD 1988: xiii). Its existence means that wives especially are able to seek professional advice and guidance from solicitors in the Scheme. The dilemma remains that some poorer people perceive lawyers as an alien body having little relevance to their needs and problems. Solicitors' offices remain under-represented in working-class areas, and there is evidence that some firms are now pulling out of matrimonial legal aid. Citizens in times of personal crisis need ready access to available and willing specialist consultation and representation. There is little purpose in enacting legal rights if a victim of domestic violence has to approach twenty solicitors before finding one willing to take her case (*The Magistrate*, February 1991).

The study undertaken in 1984 by Gregory and Foster throws important light on public resort to both solicitors and legal aid. Their findings show that among divorcing wives, virtually all petitioners (97 per cent) consult a solicitor; but a quarter (23 per cent) of respondents omit such professional advice (OPCS 1990c: 144). Most wives (80 per cent) who sought professional advice benefited from legal aid (OPCS 1990c: table 9.15). Consultation of a solicitor and the presence of legal aid were both strongly linked to whether the petition was based on fault or separation facts (OPCS 1990c: 145, and 150). Among women petitioners, 87 per cent of the 'fault' compared with 72 per cent of the 'separation' petitioners obtained legal aid. This pattern of usage reflects the correlation between the lower income groups and their resort to fault-based facts and especially behaviour. The results also underline the affirmative role that accessible legal aid and assistance continues to offer divorcing women. The latter's ongoing demand for this service explains why the 1976 changes in availability have not reduced matrimonial legal aid expenditure to the degree its supporters expected. The £80 million net cost in 1986/87 was an increase of 50 per cent in four years. And matrimonial matters continue to take over half of civil legal aid and 30 per cent of all civil and criminal legal aid (OPCS 1990c: xiii). The most recent figures show an escalating trend: by 1991–2 the government were spending £192 million on legal aid in matrimonial and family proceedings (*Independent*, 2 November 1992). Legal aid will continue to remain a major feature influencing changes in divorce procedure.

CONCLUSION

The absence of a full trial hearing has removed the stigmatizing and useless experience of a court appearance from all but a few cases. In times past the trial functioned to reflect institutionally the community's distaste of divorce and its solidarity with the concept of lifelong marriage. The legal processing of divorce has become little more than a mail order transaction except that the petition with covering cheque of £40 is posted to the Divorce Registry. But the untoward individual rupturing of marriage as a social institution is still publicly marked by the decree nisi being pronounced by a judge.

The court's application of special procedure has, in Judge Latey's words, the objective of 'simplicity, speed and economy'.[4] District judges have no means to undertake their statutory duty (Matrimonial Causes Act 1973, s. 1(3)) and verify the petition's content; indeed they are realistically advised by Judge Latey not to be too meticulous or over technical in approaching their task. This realism is supported by the Law Commission's study of divorce files which concluded that intervention by the divorce courts did not make 'a noticeable impact' upon eventual outcome of the cases (1990: 179). In most situations it is hard to see how current divorce law is procedurally little (if anything) more than judicial ratification of the petitioner's claim for divorce.

The practical relevance of special procedure is to bring within the legal orbit of negotiation the relevant practical issues affecting the family future which needs to be speedily considered and equitably resolved. These issues and problems are more fully discussed in the next chapter. Howbeit to say that once the marriage has broken down it is the ancillary concerns that are the essential matters for legal attention and resolution. Divorce is an assured formality.

12 Family breakdown, protection and the law

A society proclaiming concern about the well-being of family life has to study legislative success in guarding the more exposed members of the collapsed two-parent family. This chapter examines how effectively the interests and needs of wives and children have been protected by the law. The greater vulnerability of children is given predominance within the court's protective function, and this aspect will be examined first before turning to the matter of maintenance.

RESPONSIBILITY TOWARDS CHILDREN

Some 153,000 children aged under sixteen in 1990 saw their parents divorce. The yearly numbers of these principal witnesses of parental dissolution had risen from some 82,000 in 1971 to 163,000 in 1978 and 1980. The doubling of numbers in the 1970s was a direct consequence of the divorce surge. As a result one in five of all fifteen-year-old children in 1980 had already experienced the divorce of their parents.

Legislative policy

Family law reasonably and realistically directs its concern at children dependent on parental care and maintenance. The law's difficulty is deciding what are the best interests of children and how they should be promoted and enforced. The Royal Commission on Marriage and Divorce had recommended in 1956 (par. 372) that divorce procedure should be amended to ensure parents gave proper consideration to their childrens future welfare and upbringing. The Report's proposals led to the Matrimonial Proceedings (Children) Act of 1958. The petitioner now had to file with the petition an accompanying statement setting down the proposed parenting arrangements. This requirement was incorporated within the Matrimonial Causes Act 1973 (section 41); these statements are accordingly commonly referred to as section 41 affidavits. The 1958 legislation said that a final divorce (decree absolute) was only to be granted after the judge certified the parental arrangements for their children were either satisfactory or the best that could be devised in the circumstances, or declare that it was impracticable for such arrangements to be made. The same legislative intent continued to operate until October 1991 when the new non-interventionist policy of the Children Act 1989 came into effect to amend (but not remove) this section.

Parliamentary intention in 1958 was to encourage divorcing couples to fulfil their parental responsibilities, and to ensure that spousal interests would not override those of the children. Such worthy legislative dictates are unnecessary for the reasonably minded, but troublesome and virtually impossible to implement against those who remain vengeful and warring. Family law may express hope and provide restraints, but enforcement of parental obligations by rigid coercion is an inappropriate court tool. Legal intervention at the divorce stage can seldom be more than conciliatory; the family's dissolution occurred in times past.

Judicial policy in mid-Victorian times reflected the patriarchal view that a child's needs were subsumed within the father's right to have control of his children. By the beginning of this century the judges had become more sensitive to these needs. The Court of Appeal in 1910 could declare 'It is always to be borne in mind that the benefit and interest of the infant is the paramount consideration, and not the punishment of the guilty spouse'(*Stark v. Stark and Hitchins* ([1910] P.190). The welfare approach to decisions affecting children became statutory in 1925; the Guardianship of Infants Act requiring the court to 'regard the welfare of the infant as the first and paramount consideration'. Judges were given an unfettered discretion in interpreting Parliamentary intent. The welfare approach was reinforced by the Matrimonial and Family Proceedings Act 1984 instructing the court, when exercising its powers over financial and property matters, to 'have regard to all circumstances of the case, first consideration being given to (the child's) welfare'. The Children Act 1989 now requires the child's welfare to be treated as 'the paramount consideration'. This principle is the tenet guiding judicial adjudication upon any question relating to the custody or upbringing of a child. The legislators have dutifully expressed their concern but failed to provide any significantly new indication as to how the judges should go about reaching a decision. Is it intended that the court, giving first consideration to the welfare and financial well-being of the petitioner's children, should ignore the presence of the father's second family? No guide exists as to the worth or weight to be set against the multitudinal facets forming children's welfare needs and parental duties. This latter hesitation is understandable, as experts in the fields of child-care, psychology, psychiatry and law differ in concluding what are a child's best interests. Judicial decision making in these matters of necessity continues to operate under the umbrella of wide discretionary powers.

Since October 1991 district judges have authority to deal with section 41 affidavits. Before this change child welfare and custody matters were the significant tasks reserved for the divorce judges. They undertook two functions. First, to superintend and protect the interests of children of divorcing parents; and second, in care and custody disputes, to adjudicate where the child should live and to define conditions of access by the absent parent. Research findings indicate most parents reach custody agreement, thereby making the court's work mainly the former one of protection (Maidment 1984: 61–2).

Court practice

Section 41 statements normally provide information about where, and with whom, the children will live; their proposed education; who will maintain them; and what arrangements have been agreed for the other parent to have access. Assertion of the child's orderly future contrasts with the problematic life patterns facing many parents. Their optimistic viewing of a misty crystal ball provides no certainty to the central question of what will actually happen to these children as the family changes over time.

Between 1977 and 1991 the judge was expected to hold a 'Children's Appointment' at which the petitioner might be questioned about future plans for the children. This was the set standard interview for parents who were in basic agreement over their children's care and upbringing. An extensive investigation of the working of section 41 requirements found that normally only one parent attended the hearing, which on average lasted less than five minutes – one-fifth of the observed hearings took two minutes or less. In a system of perfunctory examination, the Bristol researchers forcefully declare: 'judges have to conduct as many as 50 appointments in a day, their capacity to assimilate a great deal of information in a short time is severely tested . . . . The "conveyor belt" feel of the system encourages, and indeed almost demands, a routine, mechanical approach' (Davis *et al.* 1983a: 133).

There does not appear to be any recorded case of a divorce being consistently denied because of judicial concern over the parental arrangements. This is not surprising, for refusal of a decree absolute would not in itself change the child's situation, though the possibility of delay may act as a lever towards improvement. But judges have no power to see that declared arrangements are actually undertaken in the future. As Lord Chancellor Elwyn-Jones informed the House of Lords in 1976: it was 'very difficult for the judge to do more than approve whatever arrangements the petitioner proposes' (*Hansard*, HL, vol. 371, col. 1216).

Judicial policy is to leave the children where they currently reside. In the vast majority of divorce cases parents voluntarily present sensible arrangements for their children and the courts accept them. The introduction of judicial scrutiny of parental plans in 1958 was the token response to society's embarrassment at its powerlessness to provide any meaningful prescription to neutralize the corrosion of broken homes.

Checks and reports

The judge may order a court welfare officer to prepare a report on the children's case if either more information or an independent check would be helpful. This judicial power has been used sparingly. A report was sought in 5 per cent of all appointments observed by the Bristol researchers, though it rose to a quarter (28 per cent) of the adjourned cases. The officer has the sensitive task of intruding into the privacy of an unhappy family.

The Committee on One-Parent Families was divided on the suggestion that all divorce cases involving dependent children should have welfare reports attached. Pragmatic reasoning prevailed. More recently, the Booth Committee on Matrimonial Causes Procedure (Report 1985: 63) was similarly opposed to mandatory independent investigation for all children. There are insufficient welfare officers to cope adequately with existing work. It is by no means clear why, if society should demand a thorough investigation of divorcing parents' fitness and habit, that only this particular group is singled out as causing special concern compared with, say, separated or indeed married and unwed parents. Problems that faced the Cleveland Inquiry (Report 1988) into allegations of child abuse (mostly within marriage) underline the Pandora's box that awaits the implementation and consequences of such a proposal. Too great a level of intervention is seen as a threat to family autonomy and individual freedom; too little, and criticism comes from those seeking greater protection for vulnerable and dependant children.

Intervention and best interests

The issue of intervention raises the whole nature and administration of decision making, the acceptable level of risk taking, and the choices open to the court. These matters need to be set against our social, psychological and parental knowledge of childrens' needs for security and stability. Behind this discussion lies the fundamental question of what a judge can, and should, do if all the evidence mounts up to a likely very disturbing future home situation for the child.

Overturning parental agreement by court-enforced transfer of children from one home to another generally flies against common sense. Unwilling parents cannot be forced to accept, raise and nurture their children. If the judge feels the child's future welfare is seriously threatened, he can make a care order giving the local authority a trust to protect the child. This would normally mean the Social Services Department removing the child from its home. These orders are seldom made; they formed under 1 per cent of all custody orders made in 1987. The court's protective function can also be exercised by the making of a supervision order (1.2 per cent of all 1987 custody orders), whereby the court welfare officer or social worker keep contact with child and home. Even fewer care and supervision orders should follow the new Children Act requirement (s. 31(i)) that an order will not be made unless the test of 'significant harm' to the child is proved to the Divorce Court's satisfaction.

We know survey evidence reveals judges have not called for welfare reports in as many instances as might have been expected, or seldom intervened to alter the parentally agreed children's residence. This might seem to fly against the spirit and intent of the legislature. Yet, paradoxically, children's best interests were being supported by judicial recognition of what was possible, combined with the policy of minimal disruption to the child's existing ties within home and community. Ultimately, all that the judge can do as a measure of last resort, against a backcloth of highly disturbing evidence, is to place the child in care.

The 'significant harm' test of the Children Act might discriminate against the lower-income households who fail to present the expected behavioural and structural patterns displayed by the more affluent. These matters involve the imposition of values about which there is little general consensus. The Children Act does not resolve what risk calculus Parliament expects our courts to operate. Generally, the underlying philosophy of the 1989 Act suggests judges in borderline cases will conduct an even more restricted investigatory and interventionist policy.

Summary matters

Similar policy issues occur in the summary matrimonial jurisdiction. Since 1960 magistrates have been required in all matrimonial disputes to consider the welfare of the children as a separate matter. Their powers and duties are, in general terms, similar to those operating in the divorce court, and they must treat the welfare of the child as the 'paramount consideration'.

A large proportion of magistrates' domestic court panel work involves post-divorce cases. This is partly a result of divorce court maintenance orders being transferred to the summary court for enforcement. The five-year period 1983–7 saw 56,762 such divorce court orders registered in magistrates courts; in other cases the original summary maintenance orders usually still remain enforceable after divorce. This background explains why three-quarters of recent (1990) matrimonial hearings involving children and resulting in an order, coming before the writer as a member of a domestic court panel, were post-divorce cases.

Registration of a divorce order means that the domestic panel would normally be expected to deal with access and custody disputes. Access disagreements are the most aggressive and bitter form of spousal conflict. In too many such hearings the child is used as a bargaining tool against the father by a mother understandably annoyed by non-payment of maintenance or the difference in their respective standards of living. Fathers get irritated and angry over what are seen as intentional acts of humiliation and hostility at visiting times, such as having to wait outside the garden gate rather than walk up the path and knock on the door. Or the mother who sought change of access conditions so that her ex-husband's new partner should not be with him (and barge uninvited into the flat) when the father came to collect his infant – and pram – from the mother housed on the third floor of a liftless block. Children have a right to keep in contact with the absent parent, and courts hope that a combination of parental good sense and conciliation will ensure compliance to the order defining access. But if this optimism proves false, there is nothing to be gained for the child and its future welfare by sending the recalcitrant parent (normally the mother) to prison for contempt of court.

This section has argued that in practice the courts' powers to recast the child's environment are very limited. Society also has to recognize the dispute may offer no obvious and correct judicial decision, as the ensuing custody case concedes. This summary of one family's anguish once again raises the question of how one judges a child's best interests. Upon divorce the parents had agreed that the son and his two younger sisters should stay with the mother, the father having agreed access over the weekend. The parents lived a short distance apart; the father with his own mother. The father now wished the son of fifteen to live with him. The mother opposed, saying it would break up the family. More worryingly, there was convincing evidence that the two daughters aged eleven and nine were seriously disturbed over the real possibility of their brother leaving. Both parents were unimpeachable in their behaviour and home conditions. A court welfare officer's interview with the son reported mature awareness of the distress his departure would cause to both mother and sisters, but he remained adamant in wishing to live with father. The chairman of the domestic panel was convinced that any son should be living with his father, and that was that. The lady justice fully acknowledged the son's wish, but cogently argued that his decision would be bitterly regretted in later years. The panel had to give paramount consideration to the future welfare of all the children. Therefore we should recognize on the son's behalf that it was in his best interest to stay with mother in the family home. The third member, though sympathetic to the mother's case and the appeal of his colleague's contention, believed the overriding factor was that an intelligent youth of fifteen had the right to determine his own upbringing and welfare. The father succeeded in this case of many years ago; equally the court could properly have rejected his application.

Many parental disputes adversarially fought against the setting of severed family relationships prohibit manifest judicial resolution. Courts remain powerless to settle disputes unless both parents accept the judicial decision as being in the best interest of their children. This is why availability of trained conciliators becomes a necessary adjunct to the court processing of divorce.

Minimal disruption legislated

Family law's child protection function has been exercised in a hierarchy of courts regulating a range of procedures contained in a diffusion of inconsistent Acts designed for the regulation of distinct social groups. The Children Act of 1989 has attempted to iron away some of the associated legislative complexities and anomalies. Parliamentary purpose was provision of a statutory concordance of procedure and practice – regardless of the origins and causes of concern – for the future upbringing of children coming before the courts. The 1989 Act's overtones of Conservative political philosophy emphasize individual parental responsibility to the detriment of public intervention. Lord Chancellor Mackay declares the preliminary question is, 'Need this case go to court at all?' (*Family Law*, 1991). The earlier evidence of this chapter supports the new realism towards parental breakdown. Many children face marital rupture's exactment of emotional strain and disruption, uncertainty and conflict, split loyalties and awkward parent-contact meeting places. The Children Act instructs courts to ensure disputes concerning these dependent casualties are resolved with the minimum delay. Emphasis on the needs of children is reinforced by section 1 making their welfare the paramount consideration in matters concerning the upbringing of a child. The court still has a duty to consider the practical arrangements proposed for the children – the 1989 Act substitutes a new section 41 in the Matrimonial Causes Act 1973 – but the decree will only be delayed if this is in the child's interest. In practical terms the court's regulatory role has been reduced.

Adjudication is constrained by the new policy of minimal intervention. This requires courts to predict the child's future well-being, and to intervene only if the evidence weighs heavily enough to suggest an order would be better for the child than no order at all. Such prognosticative proficiency requires forensic skill, as well as a broad band of interdisciplinary knowledge: the theory and process of child development and education, family life and practice in modern Britain, child psychology and psychiatry, the nature and habit of child abuse, and the working of the social services. Who assesses judicial ability to decide the child's future best interests? And do we know what these 'best interests' are? The new judicial style is seen in the reported views of Lord Justice Butler-Sloss: 'There's not much *law* as such in the Family Division. We're looking at how people behave. We're looking at emotions . . . and if certain facts show the risks are such that children should go home to their parents, then you're not worried about the law at all' (*The Times*, 4 October 1991).

Behind the legislation lies the belief that children's best interests are primarily served by encouraging parental co-operation, conciliation and eventual agreement for shared future responsibility despite their separation or divorce. The Act purposefully moves away from parental rights to an emphasis upon parental trust and obligation to find common ground towards the children's future. Most spouses reach agreement over their childrens' upbringing before the divorce petition reaches court (see Eekelaar 1991: 161, n.41). Consensual parents no longer have to make formal application for what we knew as custody, care and control, and access. Under the terms of the Act, both divorced parents are assumed to hold joint responsibility for their children. Yet the likely future pattern of orders will not change significantly. Professors Cretney and Masson, in their detailed analysis of the 1989 legislation, suggest: 'In most cases, confirmation of arrangements for public authorities responsible for housing or income support, and the clarification of the parties' respective roles may make an order desirable in the interests of the children' (Cretney and Masson 1990: 563).

Where family strife continues unabated, the courts can intervene to make new-styled residence orders (section 8) 'settling the arrangements to be made as to the person with whom a child is to live'. This order replaces a custody order. The parent without a residence order still retains parental authority, though as Cretney and Masson record (1990: 545), this 'is little more than symbolic, but may help reshape societal attitudes'. Access orders are similarly supplanted by contact orders, the new term emphasizing the child's entitlement to parental contact. Courts are provided with a checklist of welfare matters for consideration when deciding contested matters. But the Children Act gives no indication of judicial importance to be attached to each factor (s. 1(3)), nor by what calculus a final decision is arrived at. Embittered parents are offered professional help and advice in the form of family assistance orders. A probation officer or social worker can be assigned to assist and encourage resolution of this parental enmity.

The information-gathering function of the courts is supported by wide powers to order welfare reports. Maybe this is for the good, though Whitehall clearly has no understanding that in early 1991 domestic panel magistrates were experiencing a delay of three months for the preparation of such reports. These delays mean justice is withheld and family concerns are prolonged. The perception, practice and momentum of the conciliation movement is given impetus by the rationale of the Children Act. Nevertheless, the Act's impact on the course and consequences of matrimonial breakdown is likely to be slight. The paramountcy of the child's welfare has long been a prominent concept within family law. It is hard to see how the legislative changes of 1989 will neutralize the spousal poison recently displayed in a 1990 court hearing upon an application by a father already possessing a 'reasonable access' order and now seeking defined interim access of one day a month to his two young children. Nothing emerged in the interim hearing (following an unproductive pre-in-court conciliation meeting) to suggest the application was unreasonable or against the children's interests. The inculcated emotionally disturbed atmosphere would pervade these children's lives. The Act's aim of encouraging parental co-operation and shared responsibility for maintaining the links between parent and child will do little to remove the fearsome enmity, resentment and hatred within a minority of separated spouses. But at least solicitors are formally sanctioned to foster conciliation among such accusatorially clashing parents. Nor will the Act alter the parenting pattern whereby some half of separated and divorced fathers give up seeing their children. Parliament's worthy intentions are dissolved by the limited practical options open to the courts and the fact that existing parental attitudes, habits and relationships are not readily amended by legal intervention.

A QUESTION OF MAINTENANCE

The wife is the economically weaker marriage partner. Social conditioning, job opportunity, wage differentials, child-bearing, infant-rearing and housework are some of the features behind the unequal marital distribution of power and wealth.

Paper protection

The common law has long declared the obligation of the husband to maintain his wife and family. Matrimonial law offered the wife who properly fulfilled her side of the male-shaped marriage contract the reassurance of indissoluble marriage and, more problematically, the security of financial protection. The legislation of 1969 changed the rules significantly and allowed the 'guilty' spouse to seek divorce. It was the economic consequences of the five-year non-consensual separation 'fact' that brought most hostility from critics who held the Act contained inadequate financial protection for the 'innocent' wife divorced against her will. Parliament tried to provide a safeguard for such cases by allowing the court a discretion to refuse a decree if it was felt that divorce would 'result in grave financial or other hardship to the respondent and that it would in all the circumstances be wrong to dissolve the marriage (Divorce Reform Act 1969: s. 4(2)(b), consolidated in Matrimonial Causes Act 1973: s. 5(1)). The clause had been restrictively drafted to ensure that each of these two distinct conditions had to be satisfied. In practice this provision soon became of little value or relevance and very few wives have benefited by its statutory presence. It has been termed by Cretney as 'the defence of last resort' (1984: 162).

In the twenty years since the divorce reforms were introduced the judges have displayed a liberal affirmation of the new mandate authorizing decent burial of long-dead conjugality. The judiciary had no option, for dissolution will not exacerbate either the economic or social hardship that has befallen the wife. It was a Parliamentary delusion to believe that the new law could and would protect discarded wives, and at the same time encourage legal dissolution of irretrievably broken marriages.

Family obligation

The reality of the newly legislated 1969 Act's provisions were, according to Lady Summerskill, to provide sexual licence for the generality of men: 'Most men cannot afford to keep two wives. That, shortly, is why I said this is "a Casanova's charter". None of the arguments apply to the rich men' (*Hansard* HL, vol. 303, col. 310). To mollify such fears the government introduced the Matrimonial Proceedings and Property Bill, following a Law Commission Report (1969) on financial provision after breakdown of marriage. The Bill's proposals did not allay Lady Summerskill's fears; her concern remained 'with the first wife in the lower income groups, who, unless specifically protected and given first claim on the available resources, will be denied elementary justice. . . . The women of this country are being cheated. They are not going to have protection.' Similar outrage was expressed by practically every women's group in the country.

Lady Summerskill's analysis was only partially correct. Survey evidence from the 1968 Report of the Committee on Statutory Maintenance Limits clearly showed the existing pre-1970 law had failed miserably to provide effective levels of maintenance for the great majority of separated and divorced women and their children. Almost two-thirds of such wives on social security benefit in 1965 did not receive maintenance, mainly because husbands lacked the necessary resources. The one proven effective personal way to ensure regular payments is through secured maintenance, and only very wealthy husbands have such means.

The eventual 1970 Act gave divorce courts significantly wider discretionary powers over the division and redistribution of the husband's income, capital and matrimonial property and assets. The new property adjustment orders allowed matrimonial property – the most important example being the matrimonial home – to be transferred or settled for the benefit of the wife and children. Maintenance was to be provided through the making of financial provision orders. (The 1970 Act was consolidated with the 1969 Act to form the Matrimonial Causes Act of

1973: this latter Act provides the basis of our current divorce legislation.) However well-intentioned the legislators were in their provisions for the financial protection of wives and children, it remains the case that no Parliamentary wand can soften the harsh economic fact that only a few men have the wealth to support two households effectively, and more often than not two families. The divorced man is free to pledge himself to further lifelong financial obligation, and some 70 per cent of these men utilize this authority.

Justifying maintenance

Debate about the nature of, and justification for, maintenance following marriage breakdown centres around two conditions. The first focuses upon the mother and child application, and here there is a generally positive public approval. The second condition concerns the claim of the wife without dependent children; this situation has caused most debate, and is examined next.

The 1857 legislation recognized both the status of 'wife' and the attached support obligations of the husband had been simultaneously extinguished by divorce. Yet Parliament was forced to acknowledge the injustice of leaving the ex-wife destitute within a society that denied employment opportunity towards self-support and had upon marriage transferred her property rights to the husband. The newly created Divorce Court continued private Act practice by ordering maintenance – but only if circumstances made it appropriate – against that part of the husband's property set aside to provide secure provision. The divorced wife's future support claim was not against her ex-husband but upon his property assigned to produce the ordered income. The arrangements underlined legislative expectation that divorce would remain confined to a very small element of the wealthy property-owning population.

At common law the husband's obligation to his wife terminates with cold historical logic at divorce: this is currently reflected in the Department of Social Security having no power of prosecution against the ex-husband for non-support of the ex-wife. But liability for support of his children continues beyond divorce. The divorced husband's financial obligation towards the ex-wife rests entirely on statutory law.[1] How then in modern times is a continuing financial obligation justified after the marriage has been legally terminated and the spouses returned to a single state?

The ex-wife's right to maintenance had been attacked by those such as Deech (1977) who believe if women are to obtain true equality they must expect to be self-sufficient and not present themselves as economic dependants of men. Maintenance should become a limited duration rehabilitative provision for wives unable to earn through child-rearing, incapacity or age. Continuation of the obligation to support acted as a restraint on the movement to female liberation. Nor should divorced husbands be penalized for a social system that treats women as inferior citizens, restricts their work opportunity and pays them lower wages.

These arguments, so critics like O'Donovan (1978) respond, ignore the nature of marriage as a dual form. There are two experiences of marriage – his and hers.

The wife's marriage presents a gender-based division of strongly weighted household labour and caring tasks. Parenting means mothering and loss of earning opportunity, while crucial family decisions -- such as whether to move home -- are made in the light of the husband's career needs. The performance of this traditional home-based role allows the husband freedom to earn and advance his career within an economy offering men greater employment and promotion prospects, and higher wages. Within this discriminatory private setting and public structure, maintenance becomes compensatory payment for the wife's restriction of both income and current independence forgone by earlier domestic activity and the associated sacrifice of income potential. It is also recompense for lost opportunity to a continued share in the husband's future monetary prosperity, partly achieved through the economic value of the wife's past household commitment. The ex-wife's loss of claim in the prospective 'new property' of expected promotion, insurance coverage and pension rights provides a further justification for compensation.

Such maintenance support arguments are applicable regardless of whether there are children or not. There is less controversy when the spotlight is turned towards mothers with dependent children. We know in some 55 per cent of cases there are dependent children at the time of divorce, and in almost nine out of ten cases the essential ongoing caring role is undertaken by the ex-wife: in 89 per cent of cases in Gibson's 1972 Oxford study, in 83 per cent according to Eekelaar and Clive (1977), and 87 per cent in Gregory and Foster's study (OPCS 1990c: tables 7.4, 7.9). It is generally accepted that parents have duties towards dependent children: they are expected to protect, support and maintain them while the children are unable to care for themselves. Equity and morality requires the father to contribute towards the cost of his children's upbringing, and at the same time reimburse the mother for her ongoing sole custodianship duties. In this situation maintenance becomes a measure of recompense and equalization to the carer of the parental offspring. The courts acknowledge the lone-mother household's social and economic viability generally governs the quality of parental welfare and care. A divorce philosophy centred on irretrievable breakdown and declaring the children's welfare as the court's paramount consideration of necessity transfers attention from the past and the causes of breakdown to concentrate instead on the family's future interests and economic requirements.

These justifications of accountability within a male wage economy designed to maintain one household only become feasible when moderated by pragmatic awareness of findings reporting the support obligation's negative features. These are, first, the limiting half chance that divorced fathers will provide financial support (see p.196); second, the courts set the majority of maintenance orders way below full support level due to the economic and social circumstances of the father (OPCS 1990c: 141; Bradshaw and Millar 1991: 67); and third, there is the state's interventory economic role through income support provision. Evidence indicates that the paternal accountability promised by family law is an illusion and should be seen as such.

Judicial attitudes

Divorce court maintenance hearings are mainly adjudicated by district judges. Little was known about the unreported exercise of their discretionary jurisdiction until eighty-one were interviewed by W. Barrington Baker and the writer in the first of two Oxford Centre for Socio-Legal Studies inquiries. This pioneering 1973 survey of judicial attitudes showed that the registrars' (as they were designated until 1991) approaches to maintenance resolution could be polarized into two contrasting types. The majority felt their role to be that of an adjudicator, as expressed by the comment 'my job is to ensure the proper distribution of the available resources, both capital and income, according to the statutory provision' (Barrington Baker *et al.* 1977: 63). On the other hand, about a third of the registrars felt it was their duty to encourage conciliation between the parties.

The inquiry was repeated in 1988/89 by Barrington Baker once more seeking the opinions and preferences of registrars upon the more problematic issues surrounding dispute resolution. This valuable study records, as in 1973, the informants' considerable variation in attitude. Discretion creates variation, and this is mirrored in the registrars' views on the acceptability of post-1984 clean-break orders. A significant minority (40 per cent) strongly disliked the finality of an order which later stopped the former wife coming back to court (Eekelaar 1991: 63). The 1984 Act requires courts to have 'regard' to a wide range of circumstances including the possibility of either spouse increasing their existing 'earning capacity'. As one registrar explained 'Now even older women who have never worked may not expect to get maintenance; it's a very noticeable change in attitude' (Eekelaar 1991: 70).

In most divorce situations the clean break can only operate effectively for childless couples. In this sense the obfuscatory Matrimonial and Family Proceedings Act of 1984 only confirmed the established judicial attitude that believed childless ex-wives should normally seek self-sufficiency rather than look towards their ex-husbands for long-term support. One registrar declared: 'Assessing maintenance for women is becoming a lost art; I haven't done it for a long time. As I said, it's all a result of our property-owning democracy and escalating property values' (Eekelaar 1991: 70). But in other divorcing conditions the shuffling ghost of indissolubility cannot be exorcized so judiciously.

The problem judges and magistrates constantly face is the perennial one of trying to conjure one man's standard wage packet into maintaining two households. Similar findings indicate that less than a fifth of divorcing men come from the higher income brackets of social classes 1 and 2 (Gibson's 1972 survey: 19 per cent; Haskey's 1979 survey: 19 per cent [1984: table 3]). Husbands described as 'not economically active' formed 13 per cent of Haskey's sample; half of such men were 'unemployed' and within this latter group 25 per cent had three or more children and 15 per cent had experienced an earlier divorce (Haskey 1984: tables 3 and 7). (The depression of the early 1990s creates a higher proportion of unemployed men within the current divorcing population than the

6 per cent recorded in Haskey's survey.) These findings highlight one of the major realities within the current maintenance question: namely, that marriages in which husbands have the lowest incomes have the highest rate of marriage breakdown and the largest family size (see Chapter 9, pp. 136 and 142).

The overall requirements of the ongoing family have to be considered and especially the totality of financial support to keep both the children and their carer. Registrars confirmed that ordering child maintenance from the ex-husband's limited income resources seldom left anything for the court to award the mother (Eekelaar 1991: 69). Should the ex-wife then be expected to seek employment? Half the registrars indicated a general preference for mothers to be at home when the children were young, but this view was more qualified as the children became older. Yet the benefits of the mother aiming for self-support have to be placed in the social and economic context of the poverty trap. This is seen in the reported experience of the divorced mother with two young children, who, because she was unable to deduct the full cost of a child minder from her family support benefit, found she was £10 a week poorer when in part-time employment than on state benefit (*Daily Telegraph*, 10 March 1992). Such a mother's dilemma is recognized in the following registrar's comment:

> In this area women want to go back to work, but the difficulty is the poverty trap; they have got to earn enough to ensure a better income than they would have got from the State or their husband. I have to take into account the minimum expenses incurred with children, which could easily be £40 per week for child-minding. I have a daughter myself and I am quite aware of these things.
>
> (Eekelaar 1991: 67)

A significant proportion of divorce maintenance work is actually undertaken at summary court level. The vast majority of magistrates who undertake this work are not legally qualified, but they do have the assistance of a legally trained clerk to advise them on matters of law. Survey findings suggest the major function of the summary matrimonial jurisdiction has for some time been the enforcement or variation of divorced wives' maintenance orders rather than resort by still-married wives seeking maintenance under the 1978 Act (Gibson 1982). These trends have resulted in some 70 per cent of all maintenance orders held in the magistrates' courts being for the benefit of divorced wives or their children rather than for separated wives. Once again there is no clear statutory policy to guide magisterial discretionary powers in the manner of distributing one separated or divorced man's below average wage (Gibson 1987: 90; Report 1990, vol. 2: 21) between two households.

The remainder of this section gives special attention to maintenance arrangements for the support of separated and divorced lone mothers. Official statistics upon maintenance orders made in the divorce and magistrates courts are of dubious precision and restrictive content; no detail is provided on amounts ordered. Consequently, survey findings become the main source of information.

Parental disorder and state support

A national survey of petitions filed in 1972 and examined by the writer some two years later (to allow for delayed financial settlements) showed a maintenance order existed in almost three-quarters (72 per cent) of the cases where there were dependent children. An investigation of the financial consequences of divorce by Eekelaar and Maclean (1986: 90) found 55 per cent of the wives with dependent children had maintenance orders while a further 10 per cent benefited by voluntary arrangements. Only half of divorced lone mothers, when interviewed in a 1984 national study sponsored by the Lord Chancellor's Department, reported they received maintenance for themselves (22 per cent) or their dependent children (26 per cent) (OPCS 1990c: table 8.7). A similar finding was recorded for divorced mothers with new partners. The reliability of the mother's evidence is underlined by the very similar proportion of divorced fathers (47 per cent) who acknowledged they were not paying any maintenance (OPCS 1990c: 132, tables 8.7 and 8.8). These studies show it is by no means the general practice for divorcing mothers to have either maintenance order or voluntary agreement. Indeed it seems probable in 1990 that as many as half have not secured a claim. And mothers who are successful may establish only a relatively small claim which is all too often not paid.

The generality of low amounts is reflected in Gregory and Foster's 1984 interview data reporting the divorced mother's receipt of weekly payments averaging £10 per child; those with two children secured personal and child maintenance totalling £40 (OPCS 1990c: 132, table 8.28). At this time the National Foster Care Association calculated in 1983 that the weekly cost of maintaining one fifteen-year-old child in the provinces to be £35. The collectivity of three decades of survey data exposes the monotonous depressing and threadbare canvas of low amounts and non-payment.[2]

This backcloth creates a 1990s structure in which the family economy of 80 per cent of divorced mothers are either currently (61 per cent), or had been previously (18 per cent), reliant upon income support (Bradshaw and Millar 1991: 67, table 6.6 recalculated). Only a fifth of the mothers had never utilized this state provision. The same dismal display of inadequate paternal support largely accounts for the 412,000 ex-married mothers (separated and divorced combined) and their 808,000 dependent children in 1990 who were caught by public law's subsistence safety net of income support as a consequence of family law's unenforceable promises (DSS 1992: 35). The quagmire of responsibilty and enforcement intensifies when one examines paternal liability under public law. Government statistics allows one to calculate that a third (33 per cent) of separated and divorced husbands have no liability to maintain their wives under existing Department of Social Security rules (DSS 1992: 35, 49).

In cases where a direct liability to maintain was established, the DSS figures record ex-married mothers on income support received in 1990 support payments totalling almost £1 billion. Income support provided 89 per cent and husbands' direct payments to the mothers formed the remaining 11 per cent. The DSS recovered from the liable men 2 per cent of Departmental expenditure (DSS 1992: 51). The latter figure will drop to an even lower proportion when set against all ex-married mothers' lone-parent expenditure (though the DSS statistics do not provide this basic information) regardless of whether or not there is a parental liability. All of this is a reflection of the officially assessed inability of these men to contribute no more than a minute proportion of public expenditure on the support of their families. The pattern should be remembered when the implications of the Child Support Act are discussed in the next chapter.

CONCLUSION

The courts have been unable to offer either assured financial support for wives and mothers or protection for children.[3] This is not because the judiciary have failed in their professional duties. It is, rather, a reflection of both the average man's wage packet and the law's lack of usefully enforceable sanctions against separated recalcitrant parents linked only by continuing vexation and disharmony over their children's future. The majority of divorcing parents who sensibly and civilly resolve disagreements in the light of their childrens' needs present the law with no great problem.

The Children Act's philosophy emphasized that prime responsibility for their children still lay with the divorcing parents. The 1989 legislation reflects the desirability of parental freedom from state interference; the Child Support Act of 1991 declares executive commitment to enforcing private obligations. The escalating outflow of public expenditure on lone-parent families galvanized Parliament to relegate family law's adjudicatory authority and discretion in matters of maintenance. Instead trust had been placed in the regulatory powers of a newly formed administrative Child Support Agency.

13 Accounting for family support

The problems and concerns of single-parenthood are significantly reduced for carers with adequate financial support.[1] The evidence presented in Chapter 12 recorded the general low level of maintenance received by separated and divorced wives and mothers. One harsh consequence is that only a minimum of the 600,000 such lone mothers have a constant and adequate income from this source; a minority depend on earnings, the majority rely on public benefit. The findings of Gregory and Foster (OPCS 1990c) underline the dire financial predicament constantly facing the majority of lone mothers. The OPCS divorce survey findings have been reformulated for this chapter around a net weekly income of £80 as an indicator and measure of low income. (Less than a quarter [23 per cent] of the men and women informants interviewed in 1984, reported net weekly incomes of under £80 when they had lived as married couples with dependent children [OPCS 1990c: 55]; the *Family Expenditure Survey* records the 1984 average weekly household expenditure for all households was £152 [CSO: AB 1987: 260]). It is the immediate post-separation period that presents the low financial point within the cycle of events following breakdown. At this stage over four-fifths of the lone mothers recorded net weekly incomes of under £80. Awareness of, and resort to, state benefits and entitlements helps to raise her income level; so that by the time of the 'post-decree' interview the proportion of lone mothers below an income level of £80 had fallen to two-thirds (though it remains well above the 17 per cent level reported by those with joint income through a new partner). This former proportion is still reflecting an unacceptably high segment of impoverished female carer family life. One has only to examine Table 13.1 to see that only a third (half the mothers' percentage) of single divorced men who were raising children had incomes below £80.

The preceding chapter examined the justification for the ex-husband's ongoing duty to support his children and the lone mother, and concluded the paternal obligation was reasonable. But the father is only one of several possible financial support avenues for the family. This chapter sets the question of spousal and family support claims in the broader context of both personal obligation and governmental strategy towards family matters.

The mother providing care is already undertaking an essential role for the children of the marriage. Her care continues to relieve the father from direct

Table 13.1 Proportion of divorced persons by household type in 1984, England and Wales: (a) with net weekly income under £80; (b) receiving supplementary benefit

Household type	(a) Proportion under £80 (%)	(b) Proportion in each type on SB (%)
Single		
(1) no children:		
(a) Female	70	24
(b) Male	35	16
(2) with children:		
(a) Female	65	55
(b) Male	32	21
Couples		
(1) No children	10	6
(2) Children	17	20
All	44	30

Source: OPCS (1990c: 67–8, table 4.33, and recalculation upon table 4.35).

involvement in the time-consuming duties of child-raising; it is work with high replacement cost value. (And the costs fall on the community via the local authority if neither parent is able – or suitable – to undertake child-care). Is it reasonable to expect the carer additionally to contribute financially towards her household's support?

Apart from the parents there are three other possible financial avenues for child support. First, a permanent new male wage earner entering the family unit is a major means of lifting the household's standard of living. The evidence of Table 13.1 (column a) indicates the wide variation in low-income levels (below £80) between divorced lone mothers (65 per cent) and those mothers who had since breakdown acquired a new partner with a male-weighted wage (17 per cent). The former group had almost three times the likelihood of having to depend on welfare support (55 per cent) than did mothers in a male-supported reconstituted household (20 per cent). Such economic facts underline the nature of motherhood's dependency within both marriage and the wider social structure. Secondly, kin, relatives and the community can provide support. The abolition of the Poor Law removed the legal obligation on relatives such as grandparents to maintain needy and destitute grandchildren. Today, unforced kin ties cause grandmothers to be the most common carer of their employed daughters' pre-school children. Third, Parliament has set down a range of financial support entitlements for those with dependent children.

FAMILY POLICY

The welfare state was designed, promoted and developed with the aim of removing some of the gross inequalities and injustices restricting opportunity to equal citizenship. Yet the modern child's welfare, likely life-chances and opportunity still largely depend on the lottery of umbilical attachment.

One may talk of governmental family policy to the extent the official format recognizes in varying degrees that the rearing of children requires time, effort and money from the carer. All three main British political parties acknowledge child-rearing is no longer a private matter left entirely in the hands of parents. Tomorrow's society depends on the maintained well-being and nurture of our children, and governments affirm their obligations through provision of social services and by contributing towards the parental costs of child-rearing. Beyond this level of basic public commitment the main current of governmental policy meanders and becomes uncertain through absence of guiding principles regulating child support. The one observable characteristic is the continued focus on the husband as the expected wage earner and financial provider within the nuclear family household. Emphasis is directed towards the husband to insure the family against future contingencies by both public and private schemes. In the former case state-levied national insurance contributions upon employed persons covers such eventualities as family health care, widowhood and pensions in old age. In return the government provides more generous entitlement rates to contributory claimants than to those who have not paid into the Scheme. This is why widowed mothers with dependent children receive a higher rate of benefit than other lone mothers. The policy reflects the state's perception of the wife's economic dependence upon her husband. The National Insurance Scheme of 1948 recognized the possibility of the husband's death but ignored divorce as an agent of family vunerability.[2]

Current debate centres around the degree of, and justification for, state intervention within the varying forms of family condition. Analysis occurs against the interrelated setting of, first, contributory and non-contributory entitlement; and second, universal and income-related benefits. The one benefit specifically for children that is universally paid to all parents regardless of income or marital status is child benefit. This is paid directly to mothers and other carers, thereby providing women with some independent control over family expenditure. Child benefit also has the advantage that, being tax-free and non-means tested, it is neutral between non-employed and employed mothers. This benefit has been index-linked since April 1991. Increases in child benefit rates do not help lone parents on income support as the benefit is incorporated within the scale rates. It is a question of policy whether it would be more beneficial for the £4.5 billion child benefit paid out in the year 1988–9 to be targeted instead to families (whether married or lone-parent) seen as in need. Facile though it be, it is essential to stress there are no easy or direct answers to this or other related crucial questions of choice in family policy.

Social policy at governmental level combines commitment and pragmatic decisions as to how the social expenditure cake should be cut and distributed. Lone parents are competing against other claimant pressure groups who believe their cause is paramount. For instance, non-contributory social security expenditure in Great Britain in 1989–90 was £20 billion (CSO 1992: 94). The point being made is that it is remarkably hard to alter the rules and rates for one claimant group without equally acknowledging the hardships pressing upon other groups within the same benefit catchment net. As a pressure group lone parents do not attract wide public sympathy. Claims from interest groups like the disabled or the elderly housebound receive wider support, and this response is reflected in Parliamentary action.

It has been seen that low income is a major characteristic of lone mothers. At the same time one in ten of two-parent households contain the same low income pattern, and in sheer size they record larger numbers than lone parents. There are a significant residue of married couples bringing up children (600,000 in 1985) with levels of income on or below social security rates. More recently a report examining child welfare in Europe has estimated one in four of British children were living in poverty. This figure, based on an EC standard which defines poor families as those having less than half the national average income, is exceeded only by Ireland and Portugal (NCH 1992). Two-parent low-income households exist as a constant reminder of residual family hardship and inequality in Britain.

The policy maker confronts, as always, a range of value positions camouflaging economic and political resolution. Improving the financial lot of lone mothers cannot create a situation in which low-income married couples feel aggrieved by believing personal hardship would be lessened by separation. Policy proposals which simply present improved benefit levels for lone mothers without consideration of other competing claims in and out of the family setting have little chance of public or Parliamentary acceptance, especially in the present ideological and economic climate. And anyway women do not want reliance upon welfare benefits. Improvement lies in structural change through the provision of effective avenues towards financial independence that offer lone mothers real gains over the state's terms of support.

Lone mothers form one type of family structure and for many single parents dependency is a transitory stage towards either a reconstituted two-parent household or single independency. The question of financial provision for mother and children means, in practice, examination of support options provided by the state, the marketplace, community and kin, and the ex-husband and father.

Divorced and separated mothers experience a combination of factors causing resort to social security. The previous chapter explained that family law's expectation of the father maintaining his marital family is confronted by many mothers' experiences of irregular or non-existent maintenance payments. If the amount due is paid, it is all too often a sum below the amount necessary for adequate family support. The marketplace offers wives limited availability of well-paid local work, discriminative promotion prospects, and conditions of employment which pay little regard to the needs of mothers. Poor employment and maternity protection, linked with low pay and recessionary unemployment restrains the woman contemplating part-time employment. These obstacles especially operate against the lone parent (Joshi 1990). Women who have worked at the same firm full-time for less than two years, or part-time for under five years, are particularly vulnerable because they do not have clear protection against dismissal (CAB 1992). All of this is set against a general lack of access to obtainable and affordable child-care provision (see Cohen 1988).

The child-caring role is traditionally seen as unpaid women's work and not a state responsibility as in the rest of Europe. We continue to have the lowest level of publicly funded child-care in Europe. Less than 2 per cent of children under three receive day care, compared with 44 per cent of children in Denmark. The Danish government spends seven times more per child than we do on child-care services. The fact that lone mothers in employment are more likely to be concentrated in low-paid jobs is reflected in the 104,000 such mothers who in April 1989 received family credit benefit as a supplement to their earnings. Poor child-care facilities, low wages and limited work opportunity make it uneconomical or impossible for many mothers to seek employment (see Brown 1989).

As the proportion of joint-earning parent households increases (see p.123) so the low-paid part-time lone mother employee finds her household income falling relatively further behind the national average. Absence of a full-time wage has long-term implications for her pension entitlement over some twenty-five years of likely retirement life beyond the age of sixty. This argument applies more poignantly to the non-wage-earning lone mother. The structural barriers experienced by lone mothers has led to a one-fifth employment rate drop over the last decade, though in the same period the wage trend for married mothers with dependent children has increased. In 1990, 61 per cent of married mothers were in some form of employment compared with 40 per cent of lone mothers (OPCS 1992a: 193). When focus is placed upon employed mothers whose youngest child is under five years, the variation intensifies to double the proportion of married women (43 per cent) compared with lone mothers (20 per cent). This move away from paid work linked to the failure of absent fathers to provide maintenance has helped to cause lone mothers greater resort to the DSS.

Income support – together with the all-important additions of housing and council tax benefits, free school meals and other related support – provides regular and reliable financial help. The new (post-1988) earnings rule allows a weekly disregard of £15, but takes no account of child-care bills while in employment. Nor can these costs be set against taxable income for Revenue assessment. Such deterrents to employment help to explain why an increasing proportion of lone mothers remain on income support.

PUBLIC SUPPORT AND MAINTENANCE BREAKDOWN

Some twenty years ago the Finer Report established that the primary source of income for all lone mothers and children were the minimum rates of provision offered by the Department of Social Security (henceforth DSS) rather than maintenance payments from fathers (Report 1974: 104, 136). Currently some

Table 13.2 Numbers of lone mothers receiving income support, and as a proportion of all women in age groups 15–45: for years 1961, 1971 and 1990, Great Britain

Lone mothers receiving income support*	Year		
	1961	*1971*	*1990*
Single (,000)	21	61	347
Ratio (per 1,000)	7	20	73
Separated, divorced and prisoners' wives (,000)	55	151	415
Ratio (per 1,000)	8	21	57
All** (,000)	92	238	774
Ratio (per 1,000)	9	23	64

Notes: *Termed national assistance in 1961 and supplementary benefit in 1971.
**Including widowed mothers (hence does not total). They formed less than 2 per cent of all lone mothers on income support in 1990.

three-quarters of all lone mothers receive income support. The government's concern about the relative demands placed upon public and private support obligations takes place against the rise in both the number and percentage of families with dependent children headed by a lone mother who was either single, divorced or separated. At the time of the Finer Report such lone mother families formed 7 per cent of all British families with dependent children; by 1989 the proportion had surged to 18 per cent or one in six of all families.

Nature's discriminative treatment and society's child-care expectations creates dependency among women. It is the state which provides the financial support for the majority of lone mothers. Table 13.2 sets down the accelerating number of female one-parent households reliant upon income support, which totalled three-quarters of a million in 1990. Within three decades the proportion of lone-mother claimants, when standardized against the female population aged fifteen to forty-five, has recorded a sixfold increase – a reflection of the former group's expanding population, and their widening resort to income support. Overall, some 6 per cent of all women aged between fifteen and forty-five in Britain today are lone mothers dependent on income support to maintain their family.[3] This trend creates a political conundrum: at what point is the state entitled to say our system of non-contributory welfare benefits was simply never designed to cope with this pressure of demand? By 1988/89 social security expenditure on income-related benefits for lone-parent families (excluding widows) had reached £3.2 billion (at 1990/91 prices) (Report 1990, vol. 2: 11). Government-supported research by Bradshaw and Millar found maintenance payments form less than 10 per cent of lone parents' net income.

Even more significant has been the increasing propensity of lone-parent welfare payments to take an ever larger bite of all social security expenditure on families with children. This proportion is now more than half. It was against this backcloth of changing family habit and escalating welfare expenditure that the government's radical prospectus for reconstructing the system of financial support for lone-parent families was presented in the October 1990 White Paper *Children Come First* (Report 1990), and legislated in the Child Support Act 1991.

NEW LAMPS FOR OLD

The government's solution is in essence to make the father reimburse the Treasury for undertaking his primary duty of parental support. The Child Support Agency (henceforth CSA) has been formed as a public sector management 'Next Steps Agency' having semi-independent authority within the DSS. It is basically a device to reduce public expenditure on lone-mother families by tracking down and extracting a far larger part of the public support costs from fathers than the enforcement officers of the DSS succeeded in doing. The extensive new powers attached to the Agency make the programme this century's most radical innovation in the public approach to maintenance.

Mrs Hepplewhite, the first head of the CSA, will have opportunity to change what she reasonably analyses as the 'frustratingly inadequate' present system of assessing and collecting maintenance for mothers and children from absent fathers. The lone mother's new champion (or is it the Treasury's?) has made clear her terms of engagement with defaulters: 'We have a job of ensuring that children receive maintenance and we shall do it in whichever way is available to us' (*Daily Telegraph*, 24 January 1992).

The Agency began operating in April 1993. Eventually the CSA will have responsibilities for the assessment, review, collection and exactment of child maintenance claims. At the end of the Agency's three-year phasing-in period 'the courts will no longer have responsibility for assessing new claims for maintenance awards or for dealing with applications for a variation of awards' (Report 1990: 28). The courts will still encompass spousal maintenance as well as their continuing jurisdiction in disputes affecting property and matters concerning children's general welfare, residence and upbringing. The summary courts' maintenance jurisdiction retains its terminal enforcement role against recalcitrant defaulters. Magistrates will be authorized to make a liability order upon the CSA's application, and to commit to prison if this order fails. Similarly, the Sheriffs' courts preserve power to enforce relevant Scottish law. The method of enforcing community charge debts shows the procedural dangers that lie ahead. Will magistrates be presented with lists of a 100 or more defaulters and, upon the assurance of the CSA official to the veracity of the listed names, make liability orders against all the proscribed names in the space of ten minutes? Judicial enforcement should be seen to have more substance.

The CSA now apply a newly devised formula to assess the extent of the father's financial liability.[4] He is expected to meet the state's maintenance bill whenever possible. The bill consists of those current elements of income support allowances to which the qualified lone mother is entitled: the child and carer allowances element together with additional premium elements for (a) families and (b) lone parents.

The amount the father will actually pay is calculated by the CSA operating a further formula that claws back half of his assessable income until the liability is met. The safeguard of a protected level of income operates to ensure the employed father, and any new family, has a residual income above income support levels after all his current household's 'inescapable financial obligations' have been met. The protected figure results from the sum of all income support allowances together with housing costs that would be payable to this man as a claimant, plus an additional margin of £5. By this means the liable father is offered a minimal safety net designed to ensure his net wage after deduction of maintenance does not quite fall to income support levels.

The new formula does not directly raise the non-earning mother's entitlement provided under current regulations, but it will oblige the majority of fathers to pay a larger proportion of the state's bill. Behind this legislation is the government's desire for a policy of equalization between the parents. Those husbands with incomes allowing their former family to be supported above the basic formula level become liable to an additional 15 per cent levy upon their remaining assessable income. The previous family's standard of living is thereby commensurately linked with the father's. The earned income of the employed mother is also recognized in the formula's rules. In addition, the CSA proposes to review its orders annually, allowing adjustment for inflation and the changing economic and social circumstances of each parental household. The probity of the regulations may raise doubts and concerns, yet there is no disguising the radical attempt to build a causeway across the current maintenance quagmire.

The introduction and enforcement of standard public rules to calculate child support ought to ensure a greater degree of precision and certainty to the determination of maintenance. Claimant mothers benefit by knowledge of the probable resultant amount, liable fathers will be equally forewarned of their likely support contribution. Similar cases should get comparable treatment from the new statutory authority wherever the parties reside. A regulated administrative procedure also allows lawyers to advise clients on likely maintenance orders. Bargaining and resolution can occur in the light of a known formula producing certain regulatory outcome.

A weakness of the present system of enforcement is that it can be a slow and inefficient process. The delay may well be a consequence of the situation in which the wife has no interest in seeking enforcement because, as an income support recipient, she recognizes that regularity of maintenance payment and a reduction of arrears will only benefit the DSS. Under the new scheme the CSA should be able to take prompt and effective enforcement action against recalcitrant husbands. The government expect that up to 200,000 more lone parents will receive maintenance regularly. But at what cost to the fabric of new families headed by an ex-husband with continuing maintenance obligations? Chapter 10 discussed the special problems facing reconstituted families which made them more vulnerable to breakdown. The pressure of financial liability is one such problem. There are other worries and concerns about the practicality and morality of the scheme's implementation. These are briefly examined.

The very presence of the formula is likely to make the private resolution of maintenance and property matters conditioned and channelled by the shadow of the Agency's practice. The Oxford 1988/89 study of district judges' work and adjudication underlines this concern. The interviewed judges observed wives were increasingly consenting to forgo future maintenance claims in return for house possession (Eekelaar 1991: 72). Their belief is confirmed by official statistics showing a 6 per cent decline in decree absolutes – divorce and nullity combined – between 1985 and 1989, while lump-sum and property orders increased by 26 per cent in the same period. A judicial willingness to transfer dependency to the state can be observed in the judge who believed it was better from the wife's point of view to have the home and let the Department of Social Security pay her mortgage interest (and provide income support) (Eekelaar 1991: 69). Financial matters that in the past would have been resolved and settled by agreement will now become more contentious and acrimonious. Solicitors should be advising male clients that such transfers – with their reciprocal lower maintenance payments – could leave the husband with a heavier financial liabilty. Under the formula rules a husband will be less willing to agree to settle his share of the house equity to the wife in return for her agreement to lower maintenance.

The courts will still decide the wife's financial needs and the husband's contribution. Are agency and court to be barricaded from the other's existence? For instance, the new formula has inbuilt a 'parent as carer' allowance (at income support adult rate: currently – 1992/93 – £42.45 per week) for the mother's own support. Will the judiciary be expected to adjudicate in the knowledge of CSA practice? The restructuring of family support should have been extended to its realistic completion and incorporated wife maintenance into the Agency's programme. Instead, family law continues within the jurisdictions of divorce and summary courts and welfare law remains the administration of the DSS: three parallel but separate systems for resolving and enforcing maintenance. But the omission of such authority and power from the CSA becomes logical if the new proposals are seen as a further step onwards from the 1984 legislation (The Matrimonial and Family Proceedings Act, section 3) towards eventually removing wife maintenance – other than in exceptional circumstances – from the statute book.

The formation of the CSA as an executive agency raises basic questions concerning protection of citizens' rights by improper, defective or unjustified administrative decision making. It is established that the quality of initial claimant determination within the DSS is unacceptably low. This belief is confirmed by the monitoring audit conducted by the Chief Adjudication Officer in which he found that the quality of DSS decisions upon new and repeat income support claims warranted comments in 37 per cent of the examined cases. The Chief Adjudication Officer observed the standards on income support decisions 'overall remained disappointing'.[5]

Accountability within the administrative framework becomes an issue. A new Child Support Appeal Tribunal will handle maintenance assessment appeals, but they can only correct errors that are brought to their notice. Should legal aid be available for appellate tribunal hearings? Advocacy for a positive outcome is likely to produce a Treasury-inspired rejection. Lord Justice Woolf, in his 1989 Hamlyn lectures, declares, 'The outstanding defect of the tribunal system is the absence of virtually any legal aid' (Woolf 1990: 101). Yet a consequence of 'this substantial blot' requires the aggrieved citizen claiming abuse of administrative power to tackle and overcome both the complexity of law and the professional resources of the public body. It is known that appellants and applicants have a greater chance of success at tribunals when they are supported by specialist representation (Genn and Genn 1989). Under the new Agency regime family lawyers will require expertise in both social security and administrative law.

The legislation brings a real danger of decision making in the areas of property resolution, wife maintenance and child support being seen as separate parcels being delivered by the judiciary, the magistracy and the civil servants: each only vaguely aware of the others existence. This can already be seen in adjudicating the future of the matrimonial home. Judges will, of necessity, consider the resolution of the home as part and parcel of the court's maintenance and child welfare decision-making function. After examination of the financial evidence, the divorce court makes maintenance and property orders. Yet, if the maintenance order is eventually transferred to the summary court for enforcement, the magistrates are not provided with details of the parties' circumstances at the time the order was made, or what weight the judge gave to property division when deciding maintenance. But the magistrates are expected to reach variation, enforcement and remittance decisions against a backcloth in which consideration of changing circumstances usually plays a significant part. Present unsatisfactory practices will continue unchallenged and unreformed unless far greater case communication develops between concerned maintenance agencies and the courts.

The question of conduct once more surfaces now that the administrative formulae will make a larger number of divorced husbands far more accountable for their ex-wives' and children's financial support. Yet some of these men might argue that separation was caused by the mother's own volition, and consequently it was unjust for the state's support costs to be transferred to the father.

To many observers the 1984 legislation's clean-break principle appeared too generous towards husbands' interests. The scheme now shifts the balance too far against the 'innocent' standard wage-earning husband and father. By his wife's unilateral action the husband loses the comforts of home and family companionship, and now becomes publicly liable for both wife's and children's support. Is court discretion and flexibility to be revoked for the interests of administrative expediency and Treasury needs? Though family needs have nothing to do with morals, obligations cannot be entirely set apart from conduct. The cost of justice should fall upon the state.

SECOND FAMILIES: A REVISED ORDERING

Parliament has felt it proper to provide easy access to readily obtainable divorce. The evidence of earlier chapters highlighted the reality behind the current maintenance debate; namely, that marriages in which husbands have the lowest incomes undergo the highest rate of marriage breakdown and that second marriages are especially prone to divorce. One result is that almost one in five (17 per cent) of divorcing husbands in both the years 1989 and 1990 had been previously married. The maintenance dilemma intensifies.

Reconstitution, by cohabitation or marriage, into a two-adult household is a major avenue by which many mothers and children are lifted out of the economic dependency of lone parenthood. Cohabitant relationships are essentially trial unions that will often become marriages. The majority of divorced mothers will be marrying a groom who has also been divorced. For instance, marriage statistics for 1990 indicate 56 per cent of previously divorced brides married divorced men. One in seven of spinster brides under forty-five wed divorced grooms. Most of these marriages will be fertile, though only a few husbands will be wealthy enough to maintain two families.

Past policy of the DSS, and its predecessors, had recognized the financial capability of a standard wage earner did not extend to maintaining both past and present households. When it came to deciding between the claims of the wife and a paramour family, then practical consideration suggested, in the words of the National Assistance Board's Annual Report for 1953, 'It is easier to enforce the maintenance of those with whom the man is living than of those from whom he is parted' (NAB 1954: 19). The courts have largely accepted this approach. The Court of Appeal felt it was unrealistic to order weekly maintenance of £30 against a former husband who set up home with a new partner on his limited wage of £115 per week (*Delaney v. Delaney* [1990] 2 F.L.R. 457). They held that courts could not avoid recognizing availability of social security benefits for the former family. The appellate court substituted a nominal order, thereby implementing the clean-break policy. As Mr Justice Ward declared in this case: 'Among the realities of life is that there is a life after divorce.' Thus, the last forty years has seen develop both departmental and court acceptance that a wage structure designed for one household limited expectation of proper maintenance for the former family if a more recent ongoing family obligation existed.

The new scheme severely jolts the weight of obligation given to the current family. The former children's needs are given first consideration before the new partner and stepchildren. Allowances are made for the father's liability to support later progeny but not his stepchildren, though the latter are legally and socially children of the family. The first mother now has a parent-as-carer allowance built into the formula calculating her support, thereby adding to the father's liability; yet the fact that the second mother equally has to be supported in order to undertake her caring role is deliberately omitted from the calculation of the husband's exempt income. Does the government really desire second-grade second families? Administrative expectations and economic reality are incompatible.

The safety nets of exempt and protected incomes will safeguard men placed in the very lowest decile of national income. It is the lower and standard wage earner supporting a new family who is caught in the formula's pincers. Some fathers with new family obligations may well find that unemployment does not significantly reduce net income, and the state is left with two households to maintain. The poverty trap created by a low wage structure once again operates. The ingredients of economic reality, current commitment, legal expectation and administrative formula produce a half-baked loaf unable to sustain satisfactorily either past or present family. Effective enforcement of the formula could create unintentional consequences. Will over-crowded prisons be additionally congested with civil prisoners incarcerated for failure to meet child support commitments?

Many defaulting fathers live in depressed inner-city areas. Lone motherhood is shown by OPCS estimates for 1987–9 to occur more readily within certain ethnic minority groups (Haskey 1991); these patterns mirror the American experience (Wilson 1987; for a discussion of ethnic minority patterns in Britain see Goldthorpe, ch. 12). For instance, a lone mother headed every other 'West Indian' family and 27 per cent of 'African' families, compared with 13 per cent of 'White' and 6 per cent of 'Indian' families; though a significant number of these households will involve an 'associated' man. Where are the absent fathers living and how will they be traced? If an address is established and a liability order results, will the bailiffs be calling to take away the father's possessions? In short, some of the politically and culturally sensitive areas of greatest urban deprivation could erupt against officialdom's enforcement of the scheme. The cost might be unacceptably high.

POOR FIRST FAMILIES

The United Kingdom survey findings of Eekelaar and Maclean confirms marriage breakdown causes lone-parent families to descend rapidly into financial hardship. For instance, 56 per cent of the still-single caring parents, when interviewed, were mainly reliant on welfare support. Yet fathers without children in their current household did have some surplus income remaining in their wallets after discarding any maintenance contribution and allowing them twice their welfare entitlement. Lenore Weitzman's study of maintenance resolution in no-fault divorce California provides graphic evidence of a shift of economic resources from divorced mothers to ex-husbands. In the year following divorce, women and children underwent a 73 per cent drop in their standard of living compared with a 42 per cent improvement experienced by the ex-husband. But the United Kingdom evidence records the disappearance of this surplus income once the divorced man has a new family to support. Their wages were so low that little could be taken from the household income without the risk that the new family would consequently be brought below the average standard of living (Eekelaar and Maclean 1986: 98).

The paradox facing the government is highlighted by Eekelaar and Maclean's finding (supporting the evidence of Gregory and Foster in Table 13.1) that the most effective way of divorced wives regaining their pre-divorce financial situation was by marrying again. More than three times the number of remarried wives with dependent children (39 per cent) reported at the time of the interview that their household incomes were above the researchers' measure of poverty (140 per cent of supplementary benefit entitlement) compared with 11 per cent for similar mothers who remained unmarried (Eekelaar and Maclean 1986: 68). For the ex-husband, a further marriage means that he takes on the legal duty of supporting his new wife and any children of the new relationship. He becomes 'social' father to children the wife brings to the marriage, and often accepts financial responsibility for his stepchildren. A consequence of the new child support regime might be to cause divorced men to be less prepared or financially less able to contemplate new marriages. This result would leave a greater proportion of lone mothers dependent on income support for an even longer time.

The Child Support Act enforced by the new Agency introduces far-reaching implications for both family and public law arenas regulating family support and liability, and the broader horizon of both citizen's rights and parental morality and duties. Crystal ball gazing suggests some broad patterns are being set for future maintenance policy. Divorce will become fault-free, supported by a clean-break philosophy encouraging wives to be self-sufficient through employment. The intention to remove child support enforcement from the legal arena is for the good when set against the present ineffective court maintenance structure. A similar scheme has produced a 70 per cent compliance rate in Australia (Parker 1991). Establishment of a Child Support Agency considerably reduces court maintenance and enforcement hearings within magistrates courts. An effective executive agency reduces Treasury outgoings on lone parents, preparing the way for the Inland Revenue eventually to deduct and collect maintenance through PAYE.

The prerequisite of expenditure restraint has created a scheme designed to recoup welfare payments from absent fathers. This is the state's response to the question of who should bear the cost of a combination of fertile wedlock and repetitive marriage practised by a minority of people of modest means. Ensuring parental responsibility is a proper aim so long as the father and second family are not reduced to unacceptable income levels. The very real dilemma and dangers government policy finds itself facing is underlined by Lord McGregor's (1987: 55) observation: 'A democratic government is entitled to ask questions but it cannot regulate the marital and sexual behaviour of citizens in accordance with their incomes and ability to pay maintenance.'

Will the second wife have to seek or continue employment in order both to maintain her family and support the husband's first wife and children? The White Paper does not seriously debate the justification for the lone mother's right to remain at home until the last child is sixteen. The force of the Child Support Act will impose practical financial liabilities on fathers who until recently have been largely protected by the umbrella of the DSS's support of lone-parent households. The couple by their marriage contract and their parental status have a joint responsibility to safeguard and support their children, and this trusteeship continues though the marriage has ended. Does the caring role still warrant the mother's domestic full-time commitment, or should policy be reformulated to modern habit? The question highlights the need to find an agreed method by which the financial value to society of the mother's child-caring role might be assessed. Some may now argue that it is no longer reasonable to expect either the father or the state to be the sole financial supporter of the non-income-earning lone-mother household once the youngest child has reached eleven years. The issue is a political hornet's nest the present government is ill prepared to tackle, though it is well aware of the likely stings. On the one hand, wives have the laudable right to earn in an enterprise society, while at the same time, the child-caring role is traditionally seen as unpaid women's work. Limited work opportunity, low wages and poor child-care facilities make it uneconomical or impossible for many mothers to seek employment. The new scheme has done nothing to improve the financial lot of mothers on income support or give these women the means to be self-sufficient. Few will be significantly better off.

The scheme is essentially about reducing welfare expenditure, as underlined by the Agency's first clients being income support recipients rather than non-claimant mothers for whom maintenance payments are a positive top-up to her earnings and a contribution towards the costs of child-care. Treasury needs precede those of carers, witness 'the taxpayer has an interest in whether maintenance is paid' (Report 1990: 11). Whitehall has lost sight of the underlying fundamental problem of family hardship encapsulated by low wages and second families associated with many liable fathers. The scheme's rationale of equal distribution of the father's assessable income will only ensure impartiality of poverty between first and second families. This is an inept benchmark for constructing future maintenance and family policy towards the casualties of broken marriages.

14 Marriage breakdown in the 1990s

CHANGING ATTITUDES AND FAMILY STRUCTURE

The broadening attraction of earlier marriage witnessed in the post-war period until 1970 has almost disappeared. Arm in arm with the delay, or possible abandonment, in entering marriage is the increasing acceptance and popularity among younger couples of living together and raising children out of wedlock. There is a growing tolerance and recognition of non-traditional family arrangements,[1] and marriage has become a choice that an increasing proportion of younger men and women will deliberately refrain from.

The concluding section of Chapter 8 recorded that parenthood is normally still confined to the married couple, with four out of five children being raised in conjugal family households. Nevertheless, this projects a current picture which is too conservative an overview for likely future patterns. The demographic momentum of the 1970s and 1980s have produced fundamental amendments to the traditional nuclear family structure model of a married couple with dependent children. The 1990 figures for both the proportion of children born out of wedlock (28 per cent in the UK), and the divorce rate (12.9 per 1,000 married couples in England and Wales; a rate of 10.5 in Scotland) provide a similar twofold increase above 1970 levels; the numbers of children under sixteen annually affected by parental divorce in England and Wales has more than doubled to some 153,000 (CSO:AB, 1992). Such trends project an increasing presence of a non-traditional family form within the United Kingdom. This is a pattern that is being repeated in varying degrees in other Western industrialized countries, as both the current divorce and extra-marital birth rates and the related period increases recorded in Table 14.1 confirm for certain European Community countries. Comparison between the eight listed countries in 1988 shows the UK had the second highest divorce rate and the third highest proportion of extra-marital births.

These fundamental modifications to our marital orientation are not explained away by the suggestion that the changes, when viewed over the last fifty years, are no more than a historically normal progression.[2] The proportion of all households with dependent children that are headed by a lone parent has, according to the British General Household Survey, increased some 140 per cent between

Table 14.1 European trends between 1970 and 1988 in (i) divorce and (ii) births outside marriage

	(i) Divorces per 1,000 married population: 1988	Rate increase 1970–88*	(ii) Percentage of all births outside marriage: 1988	Rate increase 1970–88*
Belgium	8.4	2.2	7.9 (1986)	1.8
Denmark	13.1	0.8	44.7	3.1
FR Germany	8.7	0.7	10.0	0.8
France	8.4	1.5	26.3	2.9
Ireland	–	–	11.7	3.3
Italy	2.1	0.6	5.8	1.6
Netherlands	8.1	1.4	10.2	3.9
UK	12.3	1.6	25.1	2.1
EC average	(not available)		16.1	2.3

Source: Eurostat, *Demographic Statistics*, 1990. Divorce data not available for Greece, Portugal and Spain; Luxembourg omitted.
Note: *Rates calculated upon 1970 base figures (1.0) provided by Eurostat.

1971 (8 per cent) and 1990 (19 per cent). Two of the most relevant facets of the complex and interactive changes occurring inside marriage and family form are, first, the increasing propensity for a marriage to end in divorce, and second, the accelerating move away from marital parenthood as the social habit in which to bear and raise children. Yet, conservative attitudes prevail in family matters. Most children are raised in two-parent households and couples still opt to live together in conventional monogamous association rather than in the supposedly broader freedom of radical communes. Traditional family values are also reflected in the British Values study finding that seven out of ten adults (of all ages) disapprove of a woman having a child outside the confines of a stable relationship (Brown *et al.* 1985: 118). The more menial child-rearing duties and household chores continue to fall upon the mother (even when in full-time employment); male hands stay clear of soiled nappies and ironing boards. In a society of declared equal opportunity it remains the woman whose avenues of choice are reduced and who drops existing employment worth through the demands of caring time. Our language has no place for 'househusbands'. Public opinion remains strongly committed to established expectations of sexual fidelity by both spouses. But more permissive attitudes are now displayed towards premarital relationships with less than a third of the same survey informants feeling this behaviour was always or almost always wrong (Jowell and Airey 1984: 137). Individual behaviour is no longer so formally prescribed as it was in 1950. We are witnessing transformation but not revolution in family attitudes and habits.

Individualism and choice

Why has the rate of divorce accelerated upwards over the last two decades? What follows does not attempt to give a definitive answer because there is neither space nor a convincing causal explanation. All that can be done is to outline some of the influences which are associated with the recent family patterns and divorce trends outlined in Part III. Current habits and attitudes, if they continue unchanged in a similar social structure, do suggest future family manners and forms being reset to further challenge the efficacy of our law's intervening powers of adjustment.

Romantic love is seen by the public as the right quality to ensure permanent marital happiness. The law is ill-equipped to assess the intended partnership's suitability, and rightly claims no such specific function. It has always allowed easy entry at low cost and minimal qualification to the commitments and obligations of lifelong marriage. Only in recent times have equally accessible marital exits been provided for those whose attachment and affection has died.

We live in an ambivalent enterprise and free-market culture of individualism in which the licence of choice dominates. The Soviet Union and its allied states have crumbled before the ideology of free democratic self-determination. The provision of choice allows far more citizens to examine and consider what they expect of either the government or their marriage. A higher divorce rate may be indicative of modern couples generally anticipating a superior standard of personal marital satisfaction than was expected by their grandparents (Fletcher 1988). Within a regime of open divorce and against a social ethos of self-fulfilment, every day provides a fresh spousal opportunity to re-examine the barometer of personal marital felicity. The gestational open marriage has reverberated from declining state confidence in its certainty of authority to regulate and uphold the traditional establishment morality.

Informants in a 1971 British study believed the three main determinants of a happy marriage to be (a) 'tolerance, give and take', (b) 'enough money' and (c) 'love, affection'; while almost half (47 per cent) named 'financial troubles' as the most important cause making for an unhappy marriage. This inquiry, and a similar USA survey, both recorded the informants' belief that the quality of marriage and family life were the two most important factors determining personal satisfaction (Abrams 1973: 48).

The family and the home still offer the prime haven from the pressures and problems found in everyday modern living. The workplace functions to provide the means for leisure and private pursuits, and this is especially so for younger (under thirty-five) adults (Abrams *et al.* 1985: 40). Personal fulfilment has become home-centred and marriage is now expected to be the primary provider of satisfaction and pleasure. Into this modernistic conjugal setting the television programmes reinforce the feeling that togetherness is the consummate life style.

The private domain of modernity displays shifting personal values and aspirations. Hedonistic freedom became an acceptable life pattern of the 1980s, encouraged by both the Thatcherite manifesto of unfettered self-seeking interest and the bankers. None the less, continuity of social habit is not assured; witness how the world economic recession of the early 1990s created personal financial uncertainty and caused a half-hearted return to more traditional habits such as thrift and savings deposits. It might be that we are witnessing only a temporary aberration from traditional lifelong marriage form, though this is unlikely. There is not enough supporting evidence to nullify argument for continuing transformations in family patterns.

The difference from past times is that now citizens have a real personal choice, and for women especially such opportunity (though not one of sexual equality) is very much a new phenomena their grandmothers never experienced. In the past the majority of unhappy wives had no means of physical escape or satisfactory legal redress. Improvements in the fields of education, employment, health and fertility, welfare and social security provisions, and a more equalitarian family law are some of the structural features allowing women greater freedom and ability to control their own lives. All this, and the new privatized morality, have encouraged consumer emancipation.

Greater freedom to judge, choose and change their mind has encouraged women to become more confident and assertive about what they expect from a marriage. Evidence from both sides of the Atlantic suggests it is the wife who is the spouse most likely to be dissatisfied within a marriage (Bernard 1976; Thornes and Collard 1979). The institution has better served male interests, but female economic dependency within marriage is being slowly transformed. This latter change, together with the safety net of welfare benefits, has provided the financial support options that allow women to reject their domestic lot if it seems untenable and the viable alternatives appear more attractive. Feminist attitudes and thinking on self-fulfilment have percolated into many areas of women's everyday life and expectation, and encouraged them to question some of the values and assumptions of a male-dominated society. Many now feel they have a right to decide their own life pattern and divorce has become a more readily chosen option for women. In this overall pattern of change it has been wives in the lower-income social classes who have especially utilized the new divorce fields of choice (Haskey 1986: 133). An indicator of the impact of these structural and attitudinal changes upon women are reflected in the increasing proportion of petitions coming from wives: the period 1946–50 recorded 45 per cent, in 1966–70 it was 63 per cent and by 1986–90 the rate had risen to 73 per cent. Within a more open society there is no longer the cold material and moral shadow of the workhouse or the rebuke of community stigma to restrain their decision. There is now a choice.

Divorce as a socio-legal process moulds and reinforces social values. Its institutional availability helps to fashion individual action and choice. The interchange between national trends and personal attitude and practice impacts on both the public and private domain. Contemporary younger couples expect more from their relationships and the associated emotional bonds. If this turns into an icefield of disenchantment the victims know they can more readily judicially extricate themselves from their frozen marital wasteland. The rising resort to divorce occurs within the structure of a more tolerant society in which the publicized rescue pathways have been widened, the risks are less off-putting, social stigmatization of divorcees and their children is becoming morally unacceptable, and participants know that beyond them are others who have safely traversed the same route. The divorced are a social affirmation that the process is a transitional and survivable stage to, they hope, a better life. For many men and women divorce does create a happier future.

Within our pluralistic society it has become increasingly difficult to sustain an identifiable common culture containing generally held values, aspirations and symbols. George Formby and his ukulele had a cultural identity embracing men and women, rich and poor, young and old; the vocal form of Madonna does not offer the same symbolic universality. Public affirmation of transcendental authority has declined to 20 per cent in Britain, with only Hungary reporting lower church attendance (Ashford 1987). A hundred years ago nine in ten marriages were preceded by religious rites, in 1966 it was two-thirds, the proportion has now fallen to half. Secularization has also witnessed the fading of the evangelical bond of rigid morality which intertwined the cultural fabric of conformist social mores and habits and the declared public conscience. This is not to suggest secularization has itself created current family changes, or that history provides a picture of earlier contented and untroubled traditional family life. As previous chapters have indicated neither of these assertions fit the known evidence.

There is no single satisfactory explanation for the transformation in family form. But the power and influence of conscience remains an ingredient worthy of inclusion in the specifiable fare. The prevailing common cultural norms and values provided acknowledgement of what was recognized as 'proper' behaviour at individual, kin and community level. The evangelical conscience did hold respectably together many unhappy couples in a formal and unloving embrace of domesticity. Such marriages will more readily terminate within an increasingly individualistic society promoting the egotism of self-determination for all citizens.

Future patterns and childhood experiences

What are likely to be the observed family patterns at the beginning of the twenty-first century? Such forecasting has to be presented here in broad general-ized strokes. The divorce rate in recent years has been stable. Nevertheless, the ongoing structural and individual changes suggest a slight but steady increase in the rate of divorce, though as the married population aged under fifty-five declines the numbers actually divorcing will drop significantly. Some of these changing features are rising unemployment with its strong association towards divorce; childhood assimilation of, and socialization towards, parental separation as an increasingly standard life event; the ethos of individualism; and growing community acceptance of divorce and single parenting. Those that divorce will do so at an earlier stage and this helps to explain the fewer children per divorcing couple. The majority of parents will marry again, while an increasing proportion will be cohabitors.

The existing broader forms of non-traditional family patterns will continue to grow and incorporate an ever larger segment of children. By the first decade of the new century some 45 per cent of children will, if present trends continue, have experienced some form or other of a non-conjugal household structure by the time they reach sixteen years of age. Movement from one family format to another will occur more often. Recent new findings concerning the impact of parental disruption upon children has come from the impressive longitudinal evidence provided by the National Child Development Study (NCDS) series of interviews with 17,000 children born in early March 1958. Comparison between similarly matched divorcing and non-divorcing households underlines how the long-term damaging consequences of divorce upon children continues over a long period. This evidence of detrimental impact (as recorded by such indicators as leaving school at sixteen, leaving home due to friction, cohabitation by age twenty, parent by age twenty) suggests 'that children who grew up in lone-parent families and particularly step-families are more likely to suffer negative long-term socio-economic and demographic effects compared to contemporaries from families that remain intact' (FPB 1991: 2). Children in step-families are especially vulnerable to unsettling domestic relationships; for example, young women display a threefold greater propensity to leave a step-parent household because of 'friction in the home' than do those brought up within intact families.

Parental breakdown in the new century is likely to be similarly associated with their offspring experiencing social disadvantage. The reduced life chances may be due less to the family situation itself than to the material handicaps experienced by lone-parent households. The NCDS evidence provides a classic confirmation of justifiable public concern: many children suffer from parental separation and divorce. Yet, it is important to also note the same data records that children are affected by unhappy family life and matrimonial conflict whether the parents actually divorce or stay together for the sake of the children. This, and earlier evidence, suggests the distortion of parental relationships is more significant than whether parents actually separate (Rutter 1972: 107–10). In short, the way parents choose to live and raise their offspring has consequences for other, and especially younger, members of the community.

These patterns and projections are relevant to the realm of family law, they raise basic overlapping questions about the law's purpose, efficiency and responsibility. Should legal and social policies and practices be amended as a result of changing habits in and out of wedlock? How effectively does our two-tier judicial system of divorce courts and magistrates courts regulate and process with dignity, justice and humanity the legalized dissolution of a failed marriage? The remainder of this chapter examines some of these issues and presents certain proposals.

ELEMENTS OF FAULT

The legislative philosophy of 1969 accepted that a reformed malleable law did not itself cause breakdown; rather, the reality of marital disharmony induced movement towards divorce. The five designated 'facts' were to be seen as the symptoms and not the cause of irretrievable breakdown, but the new law compromised in readdressing as 'facts' the three previously recognized offence grounds. Twenty years on and the expected decline and withering away of the matrimonial offence has not occurred; instead there has been a steady growth in fault-based 'facts' that are correlated with the intensifying utilization of unreasonable behaviour since 1971. The Matrimonial Causes Procedure Committee under Mrs Justice Booth recorded both the Committee's and the witnesses' dislike of the continuing existence of the fault element (Report 1985: par. 2.10). The Law Commission once again examined the matter, this time with the benefit of two decades of working experience and information to judge the efficaciousness of the substantive law. Evidence from the Bristol study had indicated consumer dissatisfaction with the assiduous momentum of the divorce process (Davis and Murch 1988). The Commission's 1990 report *The Ground for Divorce* believed the most objectional features of the present law and practice were that it: (a) was confusing and misleading, (b) was discriminatory and unjust, (c) distorted the parties' bargaining positions, (d) provided unnecessary hostility and bitterness, (e) did nothing to save the marriage, and (f) could make things worse for the children (Law Commission 1990: 3–9). The Report concluded that the working of the present system offered neither a genuine test of breakdown nor any real brake towards divorce.

Towards a process over time

The Law Commission's radical proposals for a new divorce law for the 1990s scraps the 'facts of breakdown' approach and instead offers a new scheme intending to provide a more conciliatory procedure. The spouses (or spouse, if not both agreed) would register their intent to divorce by notifying the court that their marriage had irretrievably broken down (this remains the sole ground for divorce). Registration is followed by a one-year transitionary period of reflection and adjustment that also allows the possibility of either reconciliation or concilition to be considered. Amicable private resolution is preferred to court-imposed arrangements and orders.

Divorce would normally be automatically obtained after one year from the date of giving notice. The concern of critics is that in many cases there will be a longer waiting period than under the present law. Lower-income wives might well be forced to continue living under the same roof with a violent husband, thereby encouraging the very tension, bitterness and acrimony which the Commission hopes to eradicate.

This one-year period becomes supporting confirmation of the marriage's irreversible collapse. It is a simple no-fault plan intended to minimize spousal hostility and acrimony while providing time to consider, co-operate upon and resolve likely future practical problems resulting from the breakdown. By this approach divorce is transformed from an event to a process of realignment. Arrangements concerning the children, property and finance are to be dealt with as part of the main divorce process rather than at a post-decree stage. The Commission argue their scheme has the advantage of making divorce simpler and more economical while eliminating the problems associated with the use of the fault-based facts.

Such reforms will not make divorce easier nor of themselves are they likely to affect the divorce rate. Parliament will probably accept – after some heart searching – these recommended changes to current divorce law and practice. The proposed procedural framework confirms the desirability of the court's regulatory influence upon the quality of post-divorce arrangements. But there is a danger that the newly formed Child Support Agency's presence seems set to reduce the judiciary's investigatory function and, at the same time, divert potential settlement cases away from the courts. The opportunity for compromise and conciliation may be hindered, thereby reducing the likelihood of a consent order.

Matrimonial hearings and summary courts

Divorce reform has advanced around the institutional belief that shattered spousal relationships should be legally and civilly dissolved. This legislative philosophy has bypassed the matrimonial jurisdication of magistrates which continues as a court of first resort processing marital breakdown within the poorer section of the community. Some eighty years ago the Gorell Commission, after an exhaustive review of this jurisdiction, pungently declared: 'We think there is a serious objection to a court, whose main duties are of a criminal character, entertaining applications which, if granted, may produce the practical although not the legal dissolution of the marriage tie' (Report 1912a: par. 140). The Royal Commission's stringent condemnation is still valid. Nevertheless, a joint Law Commission and Home Office Working Party have justified this jurisdiction's continuing existence on account of its supposedly practical benefits (Law Commission 1973: par. 24). They metaphorically argued the summary courts functioned as a casualty clearing station offering first aid and even resuscitation for those marital war victims who would eventually be reconciled and rehabilitated back to the domestic front. For others, the wounds were 'clearly mortal', or would prove to be so gangrenous that the only antidote was marital amputation by the qualified surgeons of the divorce courts. But the officers' inspections failed to detect and report an important fact: a significant minority of cases never leave the treatment area. Many thousands of conjugal casualties remain shrouded within court-record cabinets as lifeless unions devoid of spousal meaning and marital hope. Such long-preserved separations conduce to a non-conformity of habit that the Gorell Commission had long ago roundly condemned as detrimental to the norms of traditional family life.

This jurisdiction can no longer offer prompt matrimonial relief: as many maintenance orders (21 per cent) are made within one month of application within the County court as by the magistrates courts (Murch 1987: table A9[a]iii). The inadequacy and irrelevance of the analogy of the domestic court functioning as a marital casualty clearing station is underlined by further evidence from a senior magistrates's survey of larger urban courts which indicates up to seventeen weeks are taken for processing patients' claims for maintenance (Gray 1981: 195). Wives and dependent children who are left without sufficient financial assistance require enforceable maintenance orders within a reasonably short period of the complaint.

Though the numbers of newly made orders had fallen sharply, yet a sizeable amount of matrimonial work continues to be undertaken by family proceedings panels. This paradox is explained by the summary matrimonial jurisdiction obtaining a new role in the post-1969 divorce era, this being the enforcement and variation of divorced wives' maintenance orders. Nevertheless, the number of divorce court orders transferred over the last ten years has halved from some 98,000 registrations in 1975–9 down to 47,000 in 1985–9. The latter period records a steady annual decline to some 8,000 registrations in 1989. The Child Support Agency will severely curtail the enforcement role of the magistrates courts, and this will lead to a significant drop in both divorce registrations and summary hearings. Fresh work has come the family proceedings panels' way with the transfer of child-care hearings from the juvenile court to the newly titled Family Proceedings Court, but critics maintain the judicial environment remains unchanged. What then has caused critics to be concerned at matrimonial and family cases still being channelled into the summary courts?

The summary matrimonial legislation began life in 1878 conditional upon and an adjunct to the magistrates' criminal jurisdiction. The Finer Committee could observe in 1974: 'There has been no legislative response to the criticisms which the Gorell Report, more than sixty years ago, made of the summary matrimonial jurisdiction' (Report 1974: 7). Nor has anything changed since 1974; the charge remains that courts designed to process criminal work should not house family matters any more than the Lord Chancellor's Department, the judges and the Bar would entertain the criminal – functioning Crown Courts handling divorce cases.

Lack of government finance to rectify the outdated design of many of the older court buildings together with the few modern purpose-built structures and the overcrowded list of criminal matters set down for hearing means that the criminal and civil arenas can, and do, overlap. In some courts it is not possible, or the magistrates and clerks are unwilling, to separate into different sessions the related criminal assembly of accused, police, lawyers and witnesses from those who are attending domestic hearings. A survey of the domestic jurisdiction at work reports: 'Parties were certainly aware that those charged with criminal offences were waiting close-by. It made them, too, feel like criminals' (Guymer and Bywaters 1984: 20). Little has changed over the two decades from the initial Bedford College, University of London, 1970 findings of spousal dissatisfaction with their experiences in the magistrates courts (McGregor *et al.* 1971: ch. 8). The most recent investigation of family litigation in the summary court similarly reports: 'References to criminal association cropped up in abundance throughout the interviews as our quote material shows' (Murch 1987: 59). One such informant reported: 'The bit I didn't like was, in the Magistrates' Court they're dealing with all petty criminal things as well. And you go into the waiting room and you sit there, and you're amongst all the petty thieves. And you feel a bit of a criminal yourself.' These courts remain to deal with the poorer members of our society.

The magistrates' matrimonial jurisdication operates within a court that handles over 98 per cent of the country's criminal trials. Nor are magistrates always clear about the civil distinction between domestic and criminal matters. A reviewer of a work entitled 'Dictionary of Criminology' could complain 'magistrates might wish for an entry under *Arrears* and more details about *Matrimonial, Maintenance*, and *Domestic* work, none of which was indexed' (*The Magistrate*, November 1983: 185). Until April 1989 the unmarried mother had no choice of venue for her affiliation application, the heritage of the old Poor Law and its criminal pedigree had placed her remedy exclusively in a court setting identified by the *Justice of the Peace* as the 'bedrock of our criminal courts' (31 July 1982). The public see their local magistrates courts in similar vein.The reality of being a 'Police Court' remains chiselled on the stone face of some of the older buildings. A survey of one city's magistrates courts found them to be 'dirty, crowded, have no refreshment facilities and, at best, basic toilets' (*The Times*, 19 February 1990). This is the setting for London, 1990. Two bands of spousal remedy were constructed in past times to adjudicate and regulate the marital needs of two distinct social groups within a court framework partitioned to administer the civil affairs of the middle class and process the petty crime of the working class. The 1990s still finds our system of family law purposefully offering two forms of matrimonial resolution embodied in two separate jurisdictions.

MODERN NEEDS AND NEW INITIATIVES

The most important institution within the social fabric remains the family. The future prosperity of society depends upon the well-being of the family unit. Yet little has been done by either organizations or governmental departments to rectify the mist of ignorance shrouding the intricate interweaving features of family habit, choice and legal structure. Personal behaviour changes and adapts to new expectations and pressures, and minority practices become absorbed and assimilated into accepted everyday life. For instance, the overall indicators of stability in two-parent households can no longer be properly examined without studying the interlinking world of cohabitants and spouses; parental breakdown has numerically broadened beyond marriage, separation and the divorce rate.

Little is known about the life patterns of the 400,000 children inside cohabiting parental households, how stable such relationships are compared with those of married parents, nor why the parents eventually decide to marry or remain outside marriage, or whether legal factors play any part in such decisions.

Today one in seven of all newborn children will have parents living in consensual unions. These movements are changing the accepted boundaries of the traditional family.

A competently organized judicial system needs full information by which to monitor its own efficiency. This is especially true for courts handling family disputes, for without relevant and reliable data any public, political or professional judgement on the effectiveness of the service provided to the law's clients becomes conjecture.

There is special need to rectify the dearth of regularly collated official statistical information on maintenance ordered for wives and children. It is over a decade since the Law Commission's paper on *The Financial Consequences of Divorce* (1981: 3–4) critically observed how 'very little reliable up-to-date information is in fact available about the operation of the existing law. Even the most basic questions about the extent to which the existing private law imposing financial obligations on spouses does, in reality, provide any significant support for their families cannot be answered.' The only statistic provided by the Lord Chancellor's Department *Judicial Statistics* until 1985 was the number of maintenance orders made annually. A more detailed breakdown has been provided since 1985: table 5.10 for 1988, though statistics for 1990 (table 5.5) only report County court orders, these being from 1 April. But interpretation of these published figures remains equivocal, especially regarding probable overlap between 'wife' and 'children' orders. These statistics cannot be used as an indicator of propensity to seek maintenance for they do not directly relate to the current divorcing population. The minimal information necessary to allow a meaningful ongoing legal and social analysis of our maintenance laws and procedures would have to be far more relevant and reliable than the limited figures currently provided. Additionally, there are no satisfactory statistics concerning the resolution of matrimonial property or how such orders may be related to the court's decision on maintenance.

Nor does the paucity of information improve when the magistrates' matrimonial jurisdiction is examined. Reliable and informative data on the utilization of this domestic jurisdiction has never been considered an exercise worthy of serious official effort and expense. Since 1984 the Home Office (1990) has published an annual statistical Bulletin of some fifteen pages upon domestic proceedings. These summary matters are socially and quantitatively a major element in the regulation and processing of marriage breakdown yet the publication remains devoid of any demographic detail; thus nothing is known about such vital matters as ages of spouses, numbers and ages of children, and duration of marriage. This Departmental malaise extends to court level; some case files fail to record such necessary details as the ages of involved children which are essential for the proper administration of justice (Murch 1987: 112).

Parliament has legislated two potentially conflicting modes of assessment; one resides within the courtrooms of the judiciary, the other is set in the high-street offices of public administration. It is proper to ask whether the Child Support Agency offers a workable scheme of distributive economic justice to both the former and the current family dependants of the liable father. Will administrative action be more successful than the judicial process in assessing and collecting maintenance? What will be the impact of effective enforcement upon the divorced husband's new family household? The efficacy of the law in action needs as careful scrutiny and monitoring as other public institutions.

Law's response

Does statute law regulating the conditions for divorce have any impact on the divorce rate? This country's divorce pattern, viewed against long-lasting directional trends, suggests substantive legal changes have made little immediate impression on a generation's chances of divorce. Each successive five-year birth cohort in England and Wales between 1900 and 1944 provides a higher proportion of marriages ending in divorce than the preceding cohort regardless of whether the law was eased or not (Schoen and Baj 1984: 441). Divorce law reform has developed in response to increasing breakdown rather than increasing breakdown being dependent on more liberal laws.

Modern divorce law does not of itself make a noticeable impression on individual conduct. A facet of the law's limited impact is seen when examining the effect of reducing the petitioning time bar after marriage from three years to one year in October 1984 (The Matrimonial and Family Proceedings Act 1984, section 1). The writer's 1972 Oxford divorce data examined those couples who, following marriage, separated within one year and divorced within ten years. The average time between separation and petitioning was three and a half years, there was not a rush to the court at the three-year point. Double the proportion of one-year separation petitioners (33 per cent) recorded mutual agreement (two-year separation by consent) than did those who separated between five and ten years. Two broad conclusions appear. First, the old three-year barrier did not deter early marital disruption but it did prevent early divorce. This explains why the numbers of petitioners in 1986 fell back to the 1984 level once the backlog of previously delayed petitioners had been cleared in 1985 under the revised legislation. Second, spouses do not so much desire to be legally unshackled from the bonds of wedlock as to withdraw from an unhappy relationship. Lord Chancellor Gardiner succinctly described the reality facing legislators of family life: 'I do not believe that people's standards of conduct in their marriages depend upon the state of the divorce law; they spring from social and moral consider-ations which are independent of the law' (*The Times*, 6 May 1967). The law may affect public perception of desirable behaviour but cannot so readily change or regulate private habits.

The truth is the world of the 1990s does not provide divorce law policy makers and legislators with many real intervening options. The authoritarian state could eradicate divorce from its statutes, thereby ensuring a statistically clean face. Effective enforcement of such a draconian new-century legislative policy requires punitive deterrents for the malevolent crimes of desertion (transportation) and adultery (sharia law), curtailment of travel to countries offering easy divorce and remarriage (Ireland), and the outlawry of unmarried cohabitants. The history of divorce shows that neither prohibition nor severe restrictions ensures matrimonial harmony; the law cannot chain unhappy spouses together. Nor does the state have a valid claim to enforce spurious unity upon those who wish to leave a freely entered partnership.

The logic of civil marriage was conceded in 1836. All else follows, and divorce has become the readily dispensed civil prescription for marital unhappiness and disharmony. As George Bernard Shaw facetiously observed in 1908: 'It only re-assorts the couples: a very desirable thing when they are ill-assorted.' This century records the emancipation of divorce, providing access to those previously restricted by income and gender. The state retains *de jure* public control of the process, but now it is couples who *de facto* privately regulate their personal relationships and order their judicial warrant. Before 1937 only adultery sufficed as a wrong of sufficient enormity to justify dissolution of a marriage; today it is the subjective judgement of every unhappy partner. (We have yet to follow Cook County outside Chicago, where uncontested divorces are handled by a sympathetic computer that asks petitioners some 500 questions before it feels confident to judge.) Court adjudication is reserved for the ancillary matters of financial resolution and child welfare disputes. It has been seen how the administrative extension of special procedure transformed the justiciable formality of divorce litigation into a paper exercise. Though spousal agreement is encouraged as the preferred approach to divorce yet fault petitions dominate the desks of district judges. The proposed 'process over time' approach to marriage breakdown offers a realistic and rational improvement over the present system. Access to both nationwide conciliatory services and legal advice and assistance will be a necessary adjunct to effective implementation.

Conciliation: at what cost?

Lord Chancellor Mackay has announced (12 November 1992) the government's intention to severely tighten the financial regulations governing civil legal aid from April 1993. Only those with disposable incomes below income support levels will remain eligible for free legal aid. Others who still qualify for legal aid will be required to make a contribution towards legal costs of one-third of their disposable income that is above the lower limits. At the same time, help under the Green Form Scheme will only be available for those who qualify for assistance without the requirement of a cost contribution. These proposed draconian changes will affect the the lower-income husband or wife seeking advice or representation upon their family troubles. The employed mother involved in an acrimonious parental-contact dispute is especially vulnerable to these financial restrictions upon resort to professional advice and defence of legal rights. The clock has been turned back and access to the courts is narrowed.

At the same time the Lord Chancellor's Department is giving serious thought to two possible options that could be linked to the Law Commission's proposals for a divorce process over a one-year period. The Lord Chancellor believes there should be a wider use of mediation backed up by incentives to reach agreement (*Independent*, 2 November 1992). The first option proposes to cut eligibility for legal aid to those refusing to seek mediation or conciliation. The latter two overlapping terms describe a dispute-resolution approach which holds it best for the couple, their children, and the community if both spouses are encouraged to lessen the intensity of conflict upon troublesome issues and jointly work towards compromise. The mediator's role is directed towards conciliation and a negotiated settlement; the purpose is neither to reunite the spouses (reconciliation) nor to offer therapy on personal issues of marital disharmony. The neutral mediator, operating within an informal setting, helps to steer these voluntarily entered negotiations towards an amicable private resolution as opposed to the judicially imposed order of an adversarial court system of judges and lawyers. Resolution may not always be achieved, but the areas of concord and antagonism are mapped out. Such marital charting reduces the opportunity for full-blown litigation.

The second option the Lord Chancellor's Department are considering is the imposition of mediation as a mandatory scheme for all couples. This official interest suggests mediation procedures could form an intergral part of government plans to reform the divorce process in line with the Law Commission's recommendations; though the latter come out clearly against compulsion (Law Commission 1990: par. 5.35). Similar debate is going on within many countries about the feasibility, effectiveness and desirability of conciliation as an independent and viable consumer service within the process of divorce.

Before conciliation can make any officially approved progress there is need to resolve questions concerning the form, structure, financial support and attachment – if any – of the conciliation process to the court structure. Two models emerge: (a) as a necessary support provision to the adjudicatory procedure, or more radically, as (b) an effective real alternative to the formal legal system. The latter form has especially brought proper warning of the inherent dangers of a loss of legal rights contained within the drift towards de-legalization of the divorce process (see Bottomley 1984: 293–303).

The Report of the Conciliation Project Unit (CPU) of Newcastle University provides an empirical account of family conciliation in England (Ogus *et al.* 1989). In broad terms the Report confirmed that two main types of service exist. The first functions as a court-based conciliation scheme operated by the probation service and is chiefly concerned with disputes involving children. The second form operates as an independent out-of-court scheme. The CPU findings indicate both these existing forms of alternative settlement involve significant financial cost to the divorce process. The 'in-court' based schemes generated, on average, some £150 a case to the net cost of resolving child disputes, while the equivalent figure for the 'out-of-court' scheme was about £250 (Ogus *et al.* 1990). These figures suggest provision of a new multi-purpose national conciliation service will lead to increased expenditure by either citizen or state. The Report accepts an independent service might be effective in providing other consumer gains such as reducing the areas of conflict or creating further psychological well-being. In general the Newcastle researchers conclude there are greater benefits when conciliation is independent of the courts and the probation service though 'whether these resources should be made available is a matter for political, rather than scientific, judgement' (Ogus *et al.* 1990).

The Lord Chancellor's strong feeling towards the benefits of mediation, together with the persuasive views of the Law Commission (1990: 34–5) seem set to propel the conciliation movement into a more widely known and accessible service. This would meet with public approval. Couples interviewed in a 1990 Gallop survey wished to see the process of divorce made more considered, and more protective of children's interests. There was strong backing (87 per cent) for encouraging conciliation before divorce, together with belief that the government should financially support these services (*Daily Telegraph*, 11 June 1990). Even if politicans and civil servants believe conciliation's benefits do compensate for the additional costs (and the Newcastle researchers vacillate on this question), will the government be willing to fund adequately the extra supportive resources?

Family courts

What should be done to see that family disputes are handled in a dignified and proper manner? The preceding 'matrimonial hearings and summary courts' evidence underlines the essential validity of the indictment made against magistrates courts by Sir Jack Jacob, QC, an authority on civil procedure, that 'it is a glaring and palpable anomaly that they should continue to exercise civil jurisdiction' (Jacob 1987: 260). A fundamental transformation of a system designed for the needs of Victorian England is required before the new century arrives. The existing edifice of courts should be replaced by a new purpose-designed unifying family court structure housing and handling all family matters. This would ensure cases were dealt with by a uniform set of legal rules applicable to all citizens. As well as administering family law, the new courts should have supporting services; allowing direct access to provisions such as conciliation, legal help and advice and welfare benefits. But family courts would remain a judicial institution served by judges and magistrates adjudicating family claims and disputes within a format in which legal rules and equitable rights are paramount and therapeutic services remain ancillary. The research of Davis underlines that marital disputants do expect firm responsive adjudicative justice, not delaying ameliorative hoops 'including certain forms of conciliation which they had to jump through in order to achieve (divorce)' (Davis 1988: 207).

Nothing has come of the plan cogently presented in the Report of the Departmental Committee on One-Parent Families (1974: 222). Departmental beliefs, determinations and self-interests which support policy implementation are built up and developed over time. There needs to be departmental conviction that change will produce a distinct improvement in administration. This belief did not exist in 1974 (and it remains absent in 1992). The interests of too many Departments were threatened and the political boundaries of existing Whitehall empires would have been altered. The Home Office resisted the attack on its control of the siting of the magistrates' matrimonial jurisdiction. The Treasury brake to reform emerged once again. The government decided not to proceed with the introduction of family courts because the Treasury's estimated extra expenditure of £32 million was seen as non-essential spending (*The Times*, 17 June 1987). Yet such initial outgoings could be offset by cost savings in other areas. A new integrated structure would more effectively promote pre-court settlement, which in turn causes a reduction in legal aid expenditure. In the one study that purposefully examined the cost factor, Judge Graham Hall and Mr Martin conclude: 'Cost need not be an obstacle or a cause for delaying the setting up of a unified family court' (Graham Hall and Martin 1983: 243).

It is inconceivable that legal architects starting from scratch with instructions to draw up plans for an effective modern consumer-orientated family jurisdiction, would incongruously site a 'family proceedings court' upon the criminal bedrock of the magistrates courts. Reform requires more than just tinkering around by relabelling the court structures. Meaningful change needs ministerial commitment to provide a general one-level tier of family courts offering like remedies in similar buildings, with the Family Division of the High Court continuing its specialized senior role. Governments cannot continue to argue the importance of the family to national life and prosperity and allow matters of domestic misfortune and issues of child welfare, often concerning the least fortunate members of society, to be heard in the setting of a criminal court.

Changes are occurring along the broad front of administrative and legal reform. Paradoxically, it is not Parliamentary concern but the Treasury's commitment to reduce expenditure on lone-parent families that will cause the summary matrimonial jurisdiction to be severely reduced. The Child Support Agency has taken over large amounts of maintenance adjudication and enforcement work from the magistrates courts. Since April 1992 the Lord Chancellor and his Department have responsibility for the magistrates courts as well as the existing courts and tribunals in England and Wales. This must be a major stepping-stone towards establishing a Ministry of Justice, thereby ending the inadequacies of the division of responsibilities between the Lord Chancellor's Department and the Home Office. In time family courts must come. The right time is now.

Notes

3 PARLIAMENTARY DIVORCE

1 The table is based on *Parliamentary Papers*, 1857, Sess. 2 (123): 121; that provides a total of 317 Acts. The Return provides a yearly total of Acts that was initially summarized (Gibson 1972: 38); and reproduced in the Report of the Committee on One-Parent Families (1974, vol. 2: 92). The new table further abridges the 1972 version taking account of more recent evidence. Very similar totals are reached by Anderson, 325 (1984: 230); Phillips, 325 (1988: table 1) and Wolfram, 330 (1987: 98).

2 There was nothing in Standing Orders to stop a husband or wife of English domicile from applying to Parliament for a divorce under circumstances not provided for by the 1857 Act, such as desertion. Standing Orders still allowed private Bills of divorce to be presented from Ireland and other countries of the Empire. Roberts (1906: 33) mentions six Acts to wives upon adultery and cruelty or desertion between 1857 and 1906.

5 CONSTRAINTS OF POVERTY AND GENDER

1 The capital limit was raised from £5 to £25 in 1883. The income limit for a wife could be extended to £2.

2 Translated from Gratian's *Decretum*, published in or around 1140 and quoted in G.G. Coulton *Life in the Middle Ages* (1930, vol. 2: 119). The *Decretum* was the accepted text book of canon law throughout the Middle Ages.

3 *The Englishwoman's Review* (1878: 89) reports a husband being whipped on his fourth conviction of running away and leaving his wife.

4 *Judicial Statistics* for 1894, Pt1 'Criminal Statistics', table XIV. The first year for which such statistics were available was 1893. The Home Office's *Criminal Statistics* was to remain their source until 1968 – a reminder of the jurisdiction's origins.

5 *Hansard*, HC, 1895, vol. 34, col. 62. There is little record of Parliamentary debate covering the passing of the 1895 Act.

6 The newspaper quotations are from Gates (1910: 30 *et seq.*).

7 Table XVA (compiled by Sir John MacDonell: working class being defined by occupations of husbands at date of marriage) (Report, 1912e: 35, appendix 3).

6 BETWEEN THE WARS

1 Section 8(2) of the Guardianship of Infants Act allowed attachment of income or pension as a means of enforcing compliance with the order, thereby preceding the 1958 legislation by some thirty years.

2 Report, (1936: 14–5). Calculated from tables, appendix iii.
3 As quoted by A.P. Herbert when justifying his Bill to the House of Commons (*Hansard* 1937, vol. 317, col. 2082).
4 A.P. Herbert presents a witty account of his Parliamentary success in *The Ayes Have It*, 1937.

9 THE RESORT TO DIVORCE: THE SOCIAL EVIDENCE

1 This conclusion is drawn from the 1986 General Household Survey of Britain (OPCS 1989: tables 4.9 and 10), in which figures from (a) the 1980 and 1981 and (b) 1984 and 1986 surveys are combined to provide data for separating and divorced women who were under thirty at the time of their first marriage in 1970–4. At fifteen years duration 24 per cent of the wives had experienced separation and 22 per cent had divorced. These figures suggest (2/24 = 8 per cent) that only 5 per cent of separated wives eventually will not divorce once allowance is made for wives separated at the time of the interview who will ultimately either become reconciled or divorced.
2 Gregory and Foster (OPCS 1990c: 34, table 3.1) record a much higher unemployment level (14 per cent) for their divorcing sample than for still-married men (8 per cent) aged sixteen to sixty-four. Yet it is unsatisfactory evidence, being nullified when 'economically inactive' is included in the respective totals. Reworking GHS (OPCS 1987: 67) data for 1985 – both 1984 and 1985 report 84 per cent of married men under sixty-four as 'working' – by excluding married men aged fifty-five to sixty-four (because the risk of [a] divorce is small and [b] and 'not working' is high, when compared to younger generations) produces a new pattern for men aged sixteen to fifty-four in which 'unemployment' and 'economically inactive' when totalled together, remain significantly higher for divorcing men (16 per cent) than for married men (9 per cent).
3 The Royal matrimonial troubles of an earlier time occasioned the Act of Supremacy whereby Henry VIII became 'Supreme Head on Earth' of the Church of England (26 Henry VIII, ch. 1). Henry never divorced a wife, he annulled his marriages to Catherine of Aragon, Anne Boleyn and Anne of Cleves.

11 DIVORCE: THE LEGAL EVIDENCE

1 *Counsel* (1987) 2 (3): 13.
2 Law Society *Gazette* (1972) 69: 5.
3 Legal aid statistics report on a major area of social and legal importance affecting a citizen's ability to utilize legal rights and services. The statistics remain a frustrating compendium of tabulations presented on a tax year basis (see Gibson 1980: 610–11) that restricts comparison with other relevant calendar year data. Their presentation continues to attract adverse comment from the Lord Chancellor's Advisory Committee on Legal Aid (LCD 1988: 173). The newly formed Legal Aid Board may choose to present these statistics differently.
4 *R. v. Nottingham County Court, ex parte Byers* [1985] FLR 695.

12 FAMILY BREAKDOWN, PROTECTION AND THE LAW

1 Recent legislation circumvents this block to liability by renaming the divorced mother's 'adult personal allowance' as a 'parent as carer' allowance.
2 Report of the Committee on Statutory Maintenance Limits (1968: 90–135); McGregor and Gibson (1974: 268–9, 290–9); Gibson (1982); Smart (1984); Eekelaar and Maclean (1986); Edwards *et al.* (1990); OPCS (Gregory and Foster) (1990c);

Bradshaw and Millar (1991).
3 Nor can the legal structure defend women who are domestic victims of male violence or mental assault. Generally, see Lorna Smith's concise 'Overview of the Literature' (1989).

13 ACCOUNTING FOR FAMILY SUPPORT

1 Whitehall has never produced an official definition of poverty. Academics disagree as to whether it is a set list of minimum necessities or variable, rising with the improving living standards and expectations of society (the concept of relative poverty).
2 For a brief history of this policy decision see Gibson (1970).
3 The resultant proportions recorded in Table 13.2 would be far higher if the calculation had been undertaken against a base line of only mothers with dependent children.
4 This chapter's discussion of the Child Support Act and the role of the CSA draws on my 1991 article in *Civil Justice Quarterly*: hence this acknowledgement to the journal's publishers.
5 *Annual Report of the Chief Adjudication Officer for 1989/90 on Adjudication Standards* (HMSO 1991: 38, 7).

14 MARRIAGE BREAKDOWN IN THE 1990s

1 See Gallup findings (*Daily Telegraph*, 11 June 1990) of a survey in May 1990 of some 1,000 married or cohabitating men and women. Over four-fifths (81 per cent) of the informants aged eighteen to thirty-four regarded the decline of the traditional family – in which the man supported the family while the wife stayed at home – as positively a good thing. The British Values study of 1981 found disapproval of single parenthood reported by only one-third of a similar age group (of all marital statuses) compared with 65 per cent of those aged fifty-five or more (Brown *et al.* [1985: table 2.7]).
2 The evidence, and some of the conclusions, would alter if an earlier time was chosen as the base line for comparison. For instance, choosing 1900 instead of 1940 would make evident the impact of high mortality rates upon family form and stability.

Bibliography

Abrams, M. (1973), 'Subjective social indicators', *Social Trends* 4: 35–50. HMSO.

Abrams, M., Gerald, D. and Timms, N. (eds) (1985), *Values and Social Change in Britain*. London: Macmillan.

Allan, G. (1985), *Family Life*. Oxford: Blackwell.

Anderson, M. (1983), 'What is new about the modern family: an historical perspective', in OPCS, *The Family*. HMSO.

Anderson, S. (1984), 'Legislative divorce-law for the aristocracy?', in Rubin, G. and Sugarman, D. (eds), *Law, Economy and Society: 1750–1914: Essays in the History of English Law*. Abingdon: Professional Books.

Anntila, K. (1977), 'Finland', in Chester, R. (ed.), *Divorce in Europe*. Leiden: Nijhoff.

Arendell, T. (1986), *Mothers and Divorce: Legal, Economic and Social Dilemmas*. London: University of California Press.

Ashford, S. (1987), 'Family matters', in Jowell, R., Witherspoon, S. and Brook, L. (eds), *British Social Attitudes: Special International Report*. Aldershot: Gower.

Ashton, J. (1886), *The Dawn of the XIXth Century in England*. London: Fisher Unwin.

Barrington Baker, W., Eekelaar, J., Gibson, C. and Raikes, S. (1977), *The Matrimonial Jurisdiction of Registrars*. Oxford: Centre for Socio-Legal Studies, Wolfson College.

A Barrister (1938), *Justice in England*. London: Gollancz.

Bell, F. (1907), *At the Works*. London: Arnold.

Bentham, J. (1789), *An Introduction to the Principles of Morals and Legislation*. London: Payne.

Bernard, J. (1976), *The Future of Marriage*. Harmondsworth: Penguin.

Bhrolcháin, M.N. (1988), 'Changing partners: a longitudinal study of remarriage', *Population Trends* 53: 27–34. London: HMSO.

Blackstone, W. (1783), *Commentaries on the Laws of England*, (9th edn). London: Strahan.

Booth, C. (1902), *Life and Labour of the People in London: Religious Influences* (3rd series, vol. 1). London: Macmillan.

Bottomley, A. (1984), 'Resolving family disputes: a critical view', in Freeman, M. (ed.), *State, Law and the Family*. London: Tavistock.

Bowley, A.L. (1900), *Wages in the United Kingdom in the Nineteenth Century*. Cambridge: Cambridge University Press.

Bradshaw, J. and Millar, J. (1991), *Lone Parent Families in the UK*. HMSO: Department of Social Security Report no. 6.

Brodrick, G.C. (1881), *English Land and English Landlords*. London: Cassel, Petter & Galpin.

Brose, O.J. (1959), *Church and Parliament: The Reshaping of the Church of England 1828–1860*. London: Oxford University Press.

Brown, G. and Harris, T. (1978), *The Social Origins of Depression*. London: Tavistock.

Brown, J., Comber, M., Gibson, K. and Howard, S. (1985), 'Marriage and the family', in Abrams, M., Gerald, D. and Timms, N. (eds), *Values and Social Change in Britain*. London: Macmillan.

Brown, J.C. (1988), *In Search of a Policy*. London: National Council for One-Parent Families.

—— (1989), *Why Don't They Go to Work? Mothers on Benefit*. HMSO, Social Security Advisory Committee Research Paper no. 2.

Bryce, J. (1901), *Studies in History and Jurisprudence*, vol. 2. Oxford: Clarendon Press.

Bumpass, L. and Rindfuss, R. (1979), 'Children's experience of marital disruption', *American Journal of Sociology* 85: 49–65.

Burchinal, L.G. (1964), 'Characteristics of adolescents from unbroken, broken and reconstituted families', *Journal of Marriage and the Family* 26: 44–51.

Burgoyne, J. and Clark, D. (1980), 'Why get married again?', *New Society* 152: 12–14.

—— (1984), *Making a Go of It*. London: Routledge & Kegan Paul.

Burnett, J. (1969), *A History of the Cost of Living*. Harmondsworth: Penguin.

CAB (Citizens Advice Bureaux) (1992), *Not in Labour*. London: National Association of CAB.

CSO (Central Statistical Office) (1988), *Social Trends* 18. HMSO.

—— (1989), *Social Trends* 19. HMSO.

—— (1990), *Social Trends* 20. HMSO.

—— (1992), *Social Trends* 22. HMSO.

CSO:AB (1987), *Annual Abstract of Statistics*. HMSO.

—— (1992), *Annual Abstract of Statistics*. HMSO.

Cairns, J.A.R. (1934), *Drab Street Glory*. London: Hutchinson.

Cannon, J. (1984), *Aristocratic Century: The Peerage of Eighteenth-Century England*. Cambridge, Cambridge University Press.

Canterbury, Archbishop of, Group (1966), *Putting Asunder: A Divorce Law for Contemporary Society*. London: SPCK.

Cecil, D. (1939), *The Young Melbourne*. London: Constable.

Chapman, C. (1925), *The Poor Man's Court of Justice*. London: Hodder & Stoughton.

Cherlin, A. (1978), 'Remarriage as an incomplete institution', *American Journal of Sociology* 84: 634–50.

Chester R. (1971), 'The duration of marriage to divorce', *British Journal of Sociology* 22: 172–82.

—— (1972), 'Is there a relationship between childlessness and marriage breakdown?', *Journal of Biosocial Science* 4: 443–54.

Churchill, W.S. (1909), *The People's Rights* (new [1970] edn). London: Cape.

Clifford, F. (1885), *A History of Private Bill Legislation*, vol. 1. London: Butterworth.

Cobbe, F.P. (1878), 'Wife torture in England', *The Contemporary Review*, April.

Cohen, B. (1988), *Caring for Children*. London: Family Policy Studies Centre.

Cohen, H. (1915), 'The origins of the English Bar, part II', *Law Quarterly Review* 31: 56–74.

Coleman, D.A. (1989), 'The contemporary pattern of remarriage in England and Wales', in Grebenik, E. *et al.* (eds), *Later Phases of the Family Cycle*. Oxford: Clarendon Press.

Coleman, T. (1965), *The Railway Navvies*. Harmondsworth: Penguin.

Coote, H.C. (1847), *The Practice of the Ecclesiastical Courts, with Forms and Tables of Costs*. London: Butterworth.

Cornish, W.F. (1910), *The English Church in the Nineteenth Century*. London.

Coulton, G.G. (1930), *Life in the Middle Ages*. Cambridge: Cambridge University Press.

Crawford, W. and Broadley, H. (1938), *The People's Food*. London: Heinemann.

Cretney, S.M. (1984), *Principles of Family Law*. London: Sweet & Maxwell.

Cretney, S.M. and Masson, J. M. (1990), *Principles of Family Law*. London: Sweet & Maxwell.

Davidoff, L. (1984), 'Statistics of domestic proceedings in magistrates' courts, England

and Wales, 1983', in Marshall, T. (ed.), *Magistrates' Domestic Courts*. HMSO, Home Office Research and Planning Unit, Paper 28.

Davis, G. (1988), *Partisans and Mediators: The Resolution of Divorce Disputes*. Oxford: Clarendon Press.

Davis, G. and Murch, M. (1988), *Grounds for Divorce*. Oxford: Clarendon Press.

Davis, G., MacLeod, A. and Murch, M. (1983a), 'Undefended divorce: should section 41 of the Matrimonial Causes Act 1973 be repealed?', *Modern Law Review* 46.

—— (1983b), 'Divorce: who supports the family', *Family Law* 13: 217–24.

Deech, R. (1977), 'The principles of maintenance', *Family Law* 7: 230–32.

Dewar, J. (1989), *Law and the Family*. London: Butterworths.

Devlin, P. (1965), *The Enforcement of Morals*. Oxford: Oxford University Press.

Dicey, A.V. (1905), *Lectures on the Relation between Law and Public Opinion in England during the Nineteenth Century*. London: Macmillan.

DSS (Department of Social Security) (1992), *Social Security Statistics, 1991*. HMSO.

Duncan, G.I.O. (1971), *The High Court of Delegates*. Cambridge: Cambridge University Press.

Dunnell, K. (1979), *Family Formation 1976*. HMSO.

Edwards, S., Gould, C. and Halpern, A. (1990), 'The continuing saga of maintaining the family after divorce', *Family Law* 20.

Eekelaar, J. (1984), *Family Law and Social Policy*. London: Weidenfeld & Nicolson.

—— (1991), *Regulating Divorce*. Oxford: Clarendon Press.

Eekelaar, J. and Clive, E. (1977), *Custody after Divorce*. Oxford: Centre for Socio-Legal Studies, Wolfson College.

Eekelaar, J. and Maclean, M. (1986), *Maintenance after Divorce*. Oxford: Clarendon Press.

Egerton, R. (1946), *Legal Aid*. London: Kegan Paul, Trench, Trubner.

Elston, E., Fuller, J. and Murch, M. (1975), 'Judicial hearings of undefended divorce petitions', *Modern Law Review* 38: 609–40.

Ermisch, J. (1989), 'Divorce: economic antecedents and aftermath', in Joshi, H. (ed.), *The Changing Population of Britain*. Oxford: Blackwell.

Eurostat Demographic Statistics (1990), Brussels, Statistical Office of the European Communities.

FPB (*Family Policy Bulletin*) (1991).

FPSC (Family Policy Studies Centre) (1990), *One-Parent Families*, Fact Sheet no. 3.

Feinstein, C.H. (1981), 'Capital accumulation and the industrial revolution', in Floud, R. and McCloskey, D. (eds), *The Economic History of Britain since 1700: 1780–1860*. Cambridge: Cambridge University Press.

Fellows, A. (1932), *The Case against the English Divorce Law*. London: Lane.

Finch, J. (1989), *Family Obligations and Social Change*. Cambridge: Polity Press.

Finch, J. and Mason, J. (1990), 'Divorce, remarriage and family obligations', *The Sociological Review* 38: 219–46.

Finer, M. and McGregor, O.R. (1974), 'The history of the obligation to maintain', in *Report of the Committee on One-Parent Families*, vol. 2 (appendices). HMSO (Cmnd 5629–1).

Firth, R., Hubert, J. and Forge, A. (1970), *Families and their Relatives*. London: Routledge & Kegan Paul.

Fletcher, R. (1988), *The Shaking of the Foundations*. London: Routledge.

Freeman, M.D.A. (1978), *The Domestic Proceedings and Magistrates' Courts Act 1978*. London: Sweet & Maxwell.

Furstenberg, F.F. and Spanier, G. (1984), *Recycling the Family: Remarriage after Divorce*. Beverley Hills: Sage.

Gash, N. (1953), *Politics in the Age of Peel*. London: Longmans, Green & Company.

Gates, R.T. (1910), *Divorce or Separation: Which?*. London: Divorce Law Reform Union.

Geeson, C. (1936), *Just Justice? Husbands and Wives in the Police Courts*. London: King.

Genn, H. and Genn, Y. (1989), *The Effectiveness of Representation at Tribunals.* HMSO.

Gibson, C.S. (1970),'The case for state insurance against broken marriages', *Social Work Today* 1: 25–8.

—— (1971a), 'The effect of legal aid on divorce in England and Wales; part 1: before 1950', *Family Law* 1: 90–6.

—— (1971b), 'A note on family breakdown in England and Wales', *British Journal of Sociology* 22: 322–5.

—— (1972), *Matrimonial Breakdown in England and Wales since the Reformation*, unpublished PhD thesis, University of London.

—— (1974), 'The association between divorce and social class in England and Wales', *British Journal of Sociology* 25: 79–93.

—— (1980), 'Childlessness and marital instability: a re-examination of the evidence', *Journal of Biosocial Science* 12: 121–32.

—— (1982), 'Maintenance in the magistrates courts in the 1980s', *Family Law* 12: 138–41.

—— (1987), 'Maintenance in England and Wales: entanglement with reality', *Zeitschrift für Rechtssoziologie* 8: 86–97.

—— (1990), 'Widowhood: patterns, problems and choices', in Bury, M. and Macnicol, J. (eds), *Aspects of Ageing.* Egham: Royal Holloway College.

—— (1991), 'The future of maintenance', *Civil Justice Quarterly* 10: 330–46.

Gillis, J.R. (1985), *For Better, for Worse: British Marriages, 1600 to the Present.* Oxford: Oxford University Press.

Glass, D.V. (1934), 'Divorce in England and Wales, *Sociological Review* 26.

Glass, D.V. and Grebenik, E. (1954), 'The trend and pattern of fertility in Great Britain', in *Papers of the Royal Commission on Population*, vol. vi, pt1. HMSO.

Glick, P.C., and Lin, S.-L. (1986), 'Recent changes in divorce and remarriage, *Journal of Marriage and the Family* 48: 737–47.

Goldthorpe, J.E. (1987), *Family Life in Western Societies: A Historical Sociology of Family Relationships in Britain and North America.* Cambridge, Cambridge University Press.

Goode, W. (1965), *Women in Divorce.* New York: The Free Press.

Graham Hall, J. and Martin, D.F. (1983), 'Towards a unified family court – the cost factor', *Civil Justice Quarterly* 2: 223–43.

Gray, D.E. (1981), 'Domestic proceedings in magistrates courts', *The Magistrate* 37.

Guymer, A. and Bywaters, P. (1984) 'Conciliation and reconciliation in magistrates' domestic courts', in *Magistrates' Domestic Courts: New Perspectives.* HMSO, Home Office Research and Planning Unit paper no. 28.

Hale, W.H. (1847), *Precedents and Proceedings in Criminal Causes from 1475 to 1640. . . Illustrative of the Discipline of the Church of England.* London.

Hardcastle, M.J. (ed.) (1881) *Life of John Lord Campbell.* London: Murray.

Hardy, M. and Crow, G. (eds) (1991), *Lone Parenthood: Coping with Constraints and Making Opportunities.* Hemel Hempstead: Harvester Wheatsheaf.

Hart, N. (1976), *When Marriage Ends: A Study in Status Passage.* London: Tavistock.

Hartley, C. Gasquoine (1913), *The Truth About Women.* London: Eveleigh Nash.

Harvey, C.P. (1953), 'On the state of the divorce market', *The Modern Law Review* 16: 129–39.

Haskey, J. (1983), 'Marital status before marriage and age at marriage: their influence on the chance of divorce', *Population Trends* 32. HMSO

—— (1984), 'Social class and socio-economic differentials in divorce in England and Wales', *Population Studies* 38: 419–38.

—— (1986), 'Grounds for divorce in England and Wales – a social and demographic analysis', *Journal of Biosocial Science* 18: 127–53.

—— (1987a), 'Trends in marriage and divorce in England and Wales: 1837–1987', *Population Trends* 48: 11–19.

—— (1987b), 'Social class differentials in remarriage after divorce: results from a forward linkage study', *Population Trends* 47: 34–42.

—— (1989a), 'Current prospects for the proportion of marriages ending in divorce', *Population Trends* 55: 34–7.

—— (1989b), 'Trends in marriage and divorce, and cohort analyses of the proportions of marriages ending in divorce', *Population Trends* 54: 21–8.

—— (1991), 'Estimated numbers and demographic characteristics of one-parent families in Great Britain', *Population Trends* 65: 35–47.

—— (1992), 'Premarital cohabitation and the probability of subsequent divorce: analyses using new data from the General Household Survey', *Population Trends* 68: 10–19.

Herbert, A.P. (1934), *Holy Deadlock*. London: Methuen.

—— (1937), *The Ayes Have It*. London: Methuen.

Hoggett, B.M. and Pearl, D.S. (eds) (1991), *The Family, Law and Society: Cases and Materials*. London: Butterworth.

Holmans, A.E. (1981), 'Housing careers of recently married couples', *Population Trends* 24, 10–14.

Holmans, A.E., Nandy, S. and Brown, A.C. (1987), 'Housing formation and dissolution and housing tenure: a longitudinal perspective', *Social Trends* 17, 20–8. HMSO.

Holme, A. (1985), *Housing and Young Families in East London*. London: Routledge & Kegan Paul.

Holmes, T. (1900), *Pictures and Problems from London Police Courts*. London: Arnold.

Home Office (1990), *Statistics of Domestic Proceedings in Magistrates' Courts, England and Wales, 1989*: HMSO Statistical Bulletin 21/90.

Horstman, A. (1985), *Victorian Divorce*. London: Croom Helm.

Howard, G.E. (1904), *A History of Matrimonial Institutions*, vol. 2. London: Fisher Unwin.

Jackson, J. (1969), review in *The Law Quarterly Review* 85.

Jacob, J.I. (1987), *The Fabric of English Civil Justice*. London: Stevens.

James, T.E. (1961), 'The Court of Arches during the 18th century: its matrimonial jurisdiction', *The American Journal of Legal History* 5: 55–66.

Johnstone, J. (1851), *A Collection of the Laws and Canons of the Church of England*, vol. 1.

Joshi, H.(1990), 'Obstacles and opportunities for lone parents as breadwinners in Great Britain', in OECD.

Jowell, R. and Airey, C. (1984), *British Social Attitudes*. Aldershot: Gower.

Kahl, J.A. and Davis, J.A. (1955), 'A comparison of indexes of socio-economic status', *American Sociological Review* 20: 317–25.

Kiernan, K. (1983), 'The structure of families today: continuity or change', see OPCS (1983).

—— (1986), 'Teenage marriage and marital breakdown: a longitudinal study', *Population Studies* 40: 35–54.

Kiernan, K. and Eldridge, S.M. (1987), 'Age at marriage: inter and intra cohort variation', *British Journal of Sociology* 28: 44–65.

Kurdek, L. (1991), 'Predictors of increases in marital distress in newlywed couples: a 3-year prospective longitudinal study', *Developmental Psychology* 27: 627–36.

LCD (Lord Chancellor's Department) (1965), *Legal Aid; Annual Reports of the Law Society and the Lord Chancellor's Advisory Committee (1963–64)*. HMSO.

—— (1988), *Annual Reports (1986–7)*. HMSO.

—— (1989), *Judicial Statistics for 1988*. HMSO.

Laslett, P. (1977), *Family Life and Illicit Love in Earlier Generations*. Cambridge: Cambridge University Press.

Law Commission (1966), *Reform of the Grounds of Divorce: The Field of Choice*, Cmnd 3123, HMSO.

—— (1969), *Financial Provision in Matrimonial Proceedings*, Report 25, HMSO.

—— (1973), *Matrimonial Proceedings in Magistrates' Courts*, working paper 53, HMSO.

—— (1981), *The Financial Consequences of Divorce*, Report 112, HMSO.

—— (1988), *Facing the Future: A Discussion Paper on the Ground for Divorce*, Report 170, HMSO.

—— (1990), *The Ground for Divorce*, Report 192, HMSO.

Lecky, W.E.H. (1869), *A History of European Morals*. London: Longman.

Lee, B.H. (1974), *Divorce Law Reform in England*. London: Peter Owen.

Leete, R. and Anthony, S. (1979), 'Divorce and remarriage: a record linkage study', *Population Trends* 16.

Lewis, J.S. (1986), *In the Family Way: Child-bearing in the British Aristocracy 1760–1860*. New Brunswick: Rutgers University Press.

Lewis, R. (1805), *Reflections on the Causes of Unhappy Marriages*. London: Clarke.

Lush, M. (1901), 'Changes in the law affecting the rights, status and liabilities of married women', in Council of Legal Education, *A Century of Law Reform*.

Maclean, M. (1991), *Surviving Divorce: Women's Resources after Separation*. Basingstoke: Macmillan.

McGregor, O.R. (1957), *Divorce in England*. London: Heinemann.

—— (1987), 'Family Courts?', *Civil Justice Quarterly* 6: 44–55.

McGregor, O.R. and Gibson, C. (1974), 'Matrimonial Orders', in *Report* of the Committee on One-Parent Families, Cmnd. 5629–1, HMSO.

McGregor, O.R., Blom-Cooper, L. and Gibson, C. (1970), *Separated Spouses*. London: Duckworth.

MacQueen, J.F. (1842), *A Practical Treatise on the Appellate Jurisdiction of the House of Lords and Privy Council*. London: Maxwell.

—— (1858), *Divorce and Matrimonial Jurisdiction*. London.

Madan, M. (1780), *Thelphothora, or, A Treatise on Female Ruin*, vol. 2. London.

Maddox, B. (1975), *The Half-Parent: Living with Other People's Children*. London: André Deutsch.

Maidment, S. (1984), *Child Custody and Divorce*. London: Croom Helm.

Marchant, R.A. (1969), *The Church under the Law: Justice, Administration and Discipline in the Diocese of York, 1560–1640*. Cambridge: Cambridge University Press.

Marsden, D. (1969), *Mothers Alone; Poverty and the Fatherless Family*. London: Allen Lane.

Martin, J. and Roberts, C. (1984), *Women and Employment: A Lifetime Perspective*. HMSO.

Massie, J. (1758), *A Plan for the Establishment of Charity-Houses for Exposed or Deserted Women and Girls*. London.

Masters, B. (1981), *Georgiana*. London: Hamish Hamilton.

Mathieson, W.L. (1923), *English Church Reform 1815–1840*. London

Menefee, S.P. (1981), *Wives for Sale*. Oxford: Blackwell.

Merrivale (Lord) (1936), *Marriage and Divorce*. London: Allen & Unwin.

Mill, J. (1821), *Essay on Government*. Encyclopaedia Britannica.

Mill, J.S. (1869), *The Subjection of Women*. London: Dent (Everyman edn).

Millar, J. (1989), *Poverty and the Lone-Parent Family: The Challenge to Social Policy*. Aldershot: Avebury.

Mitchell, A. (1985), *Children in the Middle: Living through Divorce*. London: Tavistock.

Monahan, T. (1958), 'The changing nature and instability of remarriages', *Eugenics Quarterly* 5: 73–85.

Money, L.C. (1911), *Riches and Poverty*. London: Meuthen.

Morgan, H.D. (1826), *The Doctrine and Law of Marriage, Adultery and Divorce*, vol. 2. Oxford.

Morris, C. (1963), 'A consistory court in the Middle Ages', *Journal of Ecclesiastical History* 14: 150–7.

Mueller, G. (1957), 'Inquiry into the state of a divorceless society', *University of Pittsburg Law Review* 18: 545–78.

Mullins, C. (1935), *Wife v. Husbands in the Courts*. London: Allen & Unwin.

Murch, M. (1987), *The Overlapping Family Jurisdiction of Magistrates' Courts and County Courts*. Bristol, Bristol University.

Murphy, M.J. (1984), 'Fertility, birth timing and marital breakdown: a reinterpretation of the evidence', *Journal Biosocial Science* 16: 487–500.

—— (1985), 'Demographic and socio-economic influences on recent British marital breakdown patterns', *Population Studies* 9: 441–60.

NAB (1954), *Report of the National Assistance Board for 1953* (cmd. 9210). HMSO.

NCH (National Children's Home) (1992).

Newman, W.L. (1867), 'Questions for a reformed Parliament', in Pollock (1883).

Noble, T. (1970), 'Family breakdown and social networks', *British Journal of Sociology* 21: 135–150.

Ogus, A., Walker, J. and Jones-Lee, M. (1989), *Report to the Lord Chancellor on the Costs and Effectiveness of Conciliation in England and Wales*. Newcastle: University of Newcastle-upon-Tyne.

Ogus, A., Jones-Lee, M., Cole, W. and McCarthy, P. (1990), 'Evaluating alternative dispute resolution: measuring the impact of family conciliation on costs', *The Modern Law Review* 53: 57.

OPCS (Office of Population, Censuses and Surveys), HMSO.

—— (1974), *Marriage and Divorce* (series FM2), no. 1.

—— (1979), Dunnell, K. *Family Formation 1976*.

—— (1983), *The Family*, (occasional paper 31).

—— (1987), *General Household Survey* (GHS), no. 15.

—— (1989), *GHS* 16.

—— (1990a), *FM2*, no. 15.

—— (1990b), *FM2*, no. 16.

—— (1990c), Gregory, J. and Foster, K., *The Consequences of Divorce*.

—— (1990d), *Population Trends* 61.

—— (1990e), *GHS* 18.

—— (1991a), *GHS* 19.

—— (1991b), *FM2*, no. 17.

—— (1992a), *GHS* 21.

—— (1992b), *FM2*, no. 18.

O'Donovan, K. (1978), 'The principles of maintenance: an alternative view', *Family Law* 8, 180–4.

OECD (Organisation for Economic Co-operation and Development) (1990), Duskin, E. (ed.), *Lone-Parent Families: The Economic Challenge*. Paris and London: HMSO.

O'Gorman, F. (1989), *Voters, Patrons and Parties: The Unreformed Electorate of Hanoverian England, 1734–1832*. Oxford: Oxford University Press.

Parker, S. (1990), *Informal Marriage, Cohabitation and the Law, 1750–1989*. London: Macmillan.

—— (1991), 'Child support in Australia: children's rights or public interests', *International Journal of Law and the Family* 5: 24–57.

Parry, E. (1914), *The Law and the Poor*.

Phillips, R. (1988), *Putting Asunder: A History of Divorce in Western Society*. Cambridge: Cambridge University Press.

Pinchbeck, I. (1930), *Women Workers and the Industrial Revolution 1750–1850*. London: Routledge.

Pollock, F. (1883), *The Land Laws*. London: Macmillan.

Pollock, F. and Maitland, F.W. (1968), *The History of English Law (Before the time of Edward I)*, vols 1 and 2. Cambridge: Cambridge University Press.

Poynter, T. (1824), *Doctrine and Practice of the Ecclesiastical Courts in Doctors'*

Commons . . . relative to . . . Marriage and Divorce. London.

Prater, H. (1834), *Law Relating to Husband and Wife*. London.

Price, F.D. (1942), 'The abuses of excommunication and the decline of ecclesiastical discipline under Queen Elizabeth', *English Historical Review* LVII.

Quinlan, M. (1941), *Prelude: A History of Manners 1700–1830*. New York: Columbia University Press.

Rathbone, E. (1924), *The Disinherited Family*. London: Arnold.

Registrar General (1965), *Statistical Review of England and Wales* for 1965, Pt III, HMSO.

Reid, I. (1981), *Social Class Differences in Britain*. London: McIntyre.

Report(s), HMSO (Chairman's name in brackets).

—— (1832), *. . . Commissioners on the Practice and Jurisdiction of the Ecclesiastical Courts of England and Wales* (199).

—— (1844), *Return of Matrimonial Suits in each Metropolitan and Diocesan Court in England and Ireland, 1840 to 1843* (354).

—— (1853), *Royal Commission on the Law of Divorce* (1604). (Campbell).

—— (1871), *Royal Commission upon the Administration and Operation of the Contagious Diseases Acts*.

—— (1912a), *Royal Commission on Divorce and Matrimonial Causes*. (Cd. 6478). (Gorell).

—— (1912b), *Minutes of Evidence*, vol. 1 (Cd. 6479).

—— (1912c), *Minutes of Evidence*, vol. 2 (Cd. 6480).

—— (1912d), *Minutes of Evidence*, vol. 3 (Cd. 6481).

—— (1912e), *Appendices to the Evidence* (Cd. 6482).

—— (1919), *Committee to Enquire into Poor Persons' Rules* (Cmd. 430). (Lawrence).

—— (1925), *Poor Persons' Rules Committee* (Cmd. 2358).

—— (1934), *Committee on Imprisonment by Courts of Summary Jurisdiction in Default of Payments of Fines and Other Sums of Money* (Cmd. 4649). (Fischer Williams).

—— (1936), *Committee on the Social Services in Courts of Summary Jurisdiction* (Cmd. 5122). (Harris).

—— (1946), *Second Interim Report of the Committee on Procedure in Matrimonial Causes* (Cd. 6945). (Denning).

—— (1956), *Royal Commission on Marriage and Divorce* (Cmd. 9678). (Morton).

—— (1967), *Committee on the Age of Majority* (Cmnd. 3342). (Latey).

—— (1968), *Committee on Statutory Maintenance Limits* (Cmnd. 3587). (Graham Hall).

—— (1974), *Committee on One-Parent Families* (Cmnd. 5629), appendices, vol. 2 (Cmnd. 5629–1). (Finer).

—— (1985), *Matrimonial Causes Procedure Committee*. (Booth).

—— (1988), *Report of the Inquiry into Child Abuse in Cleveland* (Cm. 412). (Butler-Sloss).

—— (1990) (White Paper), *Children Come First* (Cm.1264), vol. 1 (the proposals), vol. 2 (the background).

Roberts, J. (1906), *Divorce Bills of the Imperial Parliament*. Dublin.

Routh, G. (1965), *Occupation and Pay in Great Britain, 1906–60*. Cambridge: Cambridge University Press.

Rowntree, G. and Carrier, N. (1958), 'The resort to divorce in England and Wales, 1857–1957', *Population Studies* 11: 186–233.

Rowntree, S. (1901), *Poverty: A Study of Town Life*. London: Macmillan.

Rutter, M. (1972), *Maternal Deprivation Reassessed*. Harmondsworth: Penguin.

Sanctuary, G. and Whitehead, C. (1972), *Divorce and After*. Harmondsworth: Penguin.

Schoen, R. and Baj, J. (1984), 'Twentieth-century cohort marriage and divorce in England and Wales', *Population Studies* 38: 439–49.

Shaw, C. Sir (1843), *Manufacturing Districts*. London.

Shrapnel, N. (1969), 'The cathedral in the Strand', in Macy, C. (ed.), *Marriage and Divorce*. London: Pemberton.

Slatter, M.D. (1953), 'The records of the Court of Arches', *Journal of Ecclesiastical History* 4: 139–53.

Soames, M. (1987), *The Profligate Duke*. London: Collins.

Smart, C. (1984), *The Ties that Bind: Law, Marriage and the Reproduction of Patriarchial Relations*. London: Routledge & Kegan Paul.

Smith, L. (1989), *Domestic Violence: An Overview of the Literature*, (Home Office Research Study 107). HMSO.

Stone, L. (1977), *The Family, Sex and Marriage in England, 1500–1800*. London: Weidenfeld & Nicolson.

—— (1990), *Road to Divorce: England 1530–1987*. Oxford: Oxford University Press.

Stone, L. and Stone, J.C. (1984), *An Open Elite? England 1540–1880*. Oxford: Clarendon.

Tate, W.E. (1969), *The Parish Chest*. Cambridge: Cambridge University Press.

Thornes, B. and Collard, J. (1979), *Who Divorces?* London: Routledge & Kegan Paul.

Thornton, A. (1985), 'Changing attitudes towards separation and divorce: causes and consequences', *American Journal of Sociology* 90: 856–72.

Tozer, B. (1909), 'Divorce versus compulsory celibacy', *The Nineteenth Century* 65.

Trumbach, R. (1978), *The Rise of the Egalitarian Family: Aristocratic Kinship and Domestic Relations*. New York: Academic Press.

United Nations (1976), *Demographic Yearbook for 1974*. New York.

—— (1984), *Demographic Yearbook for 1982*. New York.

Virgin, P. (1989), *The Church in an Age of Negligence: Ecclesiastical Structure and Problems of Church Reform 1700–1840*. Cambridge: James Clarke.

Wallerstein, J. and Kelly, J. (1980), *Surviving the Breakup*. London: Grant-MacIntyre.

Walsh, J. (1953), *Not Like This*. London: Lawrence & Wishart.

Warne, A. (1969), *Church and Society in Eighteenth Century Devon*. Newton Abbot: David & Charles.

Weitzman, L.J. (1985), *The Divorce Revolution*. New York: Free Press.

Werner, B. (1985), 'Fertility trends in different social classes: 1970 to 1983', *Population Trends* 41.

Whetham, W.C.D. and C.D. (1909), *The Family and the Nation: A study in National Inheritance and Social Responsibility*. London: Longman.

Wilson, W.J. (1987), *The Truly Disadvantaged: The Inner City, the Underclass and Public Policy*. Chicago: University of Chicago Press.

Wolfram, S. (1984), 'Divorce in England 1700–1857', *Oxford Journal of Legal Studies* 5: 155–86.

—— (1987), *In Laws and Outlaws*. London: Croom Helm.

Woodcock, B.L. (1952), *Medieval Ecclesiastical Courts in the Diocese of Canterbury*. London: Oxford University Press.

Woolf, H. (1990), *Protection of the Public: A New Challenge*. London: Stevens.

Worsley-Boden, J.F. (1932), *Mischiefs of the Marriage Law*. London: Williams & Norgate.

Wybrow, R.J. (1989), *Britain Speaks Out, 1937–87: A Social History as Seen through the Gallup Data*. Basingstoke: Macmillan.

Young, E. (1876), 'The Anglo-Saxon family law', in Adams, H. *et al*. (eds), *Essays in Anglo-Saxon Law*.

Name index

Subject index